IMPORTANT

⟨ **W9-AOQ-215**

Here is your registration code to access *Connect Personal Health* to accompany *Personal Health: A Concise Guide.* This registration code is only valid if you have purchased a new book.

You need this code to gain access to *Connect Personal Health.*

To gain access to *Connect Personal Health:*

1. Your instructor will provide you with a web address (URL) to *Connect Personal Health.* Click on that link.

2. At the Connect registration site, click the "Register Now" button.

3. When prompted, enter your email address, and then click the "Submit" button.

4. Enter the personal access code that is found on this card.

5. Follow the instructions to setup your personal UserID and Password

6. Write your UserID and Password down for future reference. Keep it in a safe place.

If you forget your password and would like to reset it, please visit the Support website at www.mhhe.com/support for help. Support hours and telephone numbers can be found at this site.

Thank you. Welcome to *Connect Personal Health!*

BN 978-0-07-731531-3
HID 0-07-731531-6
A SPARLING. PERSONAL HEALTH: A CONCISE GUIDE 2009 EARLY RELEASE

DY8F–EDNU–PDH4–AQ3E–6M

REGISTRATION CODE

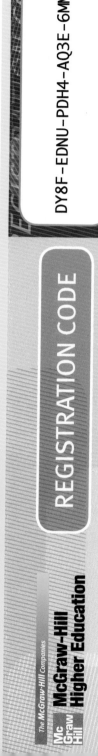

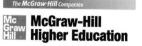

The McGraw-Hill Companies

McGraw-Hill Higher Education

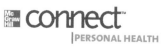

connect™

| PERSONAL HEALTH

The McGraw-Hill Companies

McGraw-Hill Higher Education

PERSONAL HEALTH: A CONCISE GUIDE

PERSONAL HEALTH: A CONCISE GUIDE

Phillip B. Sparling

Georgia Institute of Technology

Kerry J. Redican

Virginia Polytechnic Institute and State University

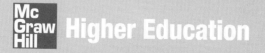

Boston   Burr Ridge, IL   Dubuque, IA   Madison, WI   New York
San Francisco   St. Louis   Bangkok   Bogotá   Caracas   Kuala Lumpur
Lisbon   London   Madrid   Mexico City   Milan   Montreal   New Delhi
Santiago   Seoul   Singapore   Sydney   Taipei   Toronto

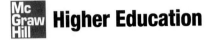 **Higher Education**

Published by McGraw-Hill, an imprint of The McGraw-Hill Companies, Inc., 1221 Avenue of
the Americas, New York, NY 10020. Copyright © 2009. All rights reserved. No part of this
publication may be reproduced or distributed in any form or by any means, or stored in a
database or retrieval system, without the prior written consent of The McGraw-Hill
Companies, Inc., including, but not limited to, in any network or other electronic storage or
transmission, or broadcast for distance learning.

1 2 3 4 5 6 7 8 9 0 DOC/DOC 0 9 8

ISBN: 978-0-07338086-5
MHID: 0-07-338086-5

Editor-in-Chief: *Michael Ryan*
Editorial Director: *William Glass*
Executive Editor: *Christopher Johnson*
Director of Development: *Kathleen Engelberg*
Development Editor: *Erin Strathmann*
Editorial Coordinator: *Sarah Hill*
Marketing Manager: *William Minick*
Media Project Manager: *Ron Nelms*
Production Editor: *Anne Fuzellier*
Art Director: *Preston Thomas*
Art Manager: *Robin Mouat*

Art Editor: *Sonia Brown*
Cover Designer: *Cassandra Chu*
Interior Designer: *Ellen Pettengel*
Photo Manager: *Brian J. Pecko*
Photo Researchers: *Nora Agbayani and
Sonia Brown*
Production Supervisor: *Randy Hurst*
Composition: *9/11 Palatino by Aptara-York*
Printing: *45# New Era Matte Plus by R. R.
Donnelley, Crawfordsville*

Cover image: istock/copyright Skip O'Donnell

Credits: *The credits section for this book begins on page 467 and is considered an extension of the
copyright page.*

Library of Congress Cataloging-in-Publication Data

Sparling, Phillip B. (Phillip Belton), 1949-
    Personal health : a concise guide / Phillip Sparling; Kerry Redican.—1st ed.
        p. cm.
    Includes index.
    "2009 Early Release Version."
    ISBN-13: 978-0-07-338086-5 (alk. paper)
    ISBN-10: 0-07-338086-5 (alk. paper)
    1. Health—Textbooks. I. Redican, Kerry J. II. Title.
    RA776.S696 2009
    613--dc22

                                        2008038256

The Internet addresses listed in the text were accurate at the time of publication. The inclu-
sion of a Web site does not indicate an endorsement by the authors or McGraw-Hill, and
McGraw-Hill does not guarantee the accuracy of the information presented at these sites.

www.mhhe.com

To our students and colleagues, who inspire us to be better teachers, and to our wives, Phyllis and Barbara, for their support and understanding.

BRIEF CONTENTS

CONTENTS

Part III

MEDICAL CONDITIONS

Part IV

NAVIGATING THE HEALTH CARE SYSTEM

PERSONAL HEALTH: A CONCISE GUIDE is a new kind of health textbook, created in response to the needs of today's students *and* today's instructors: a brief, dynamic text accompanied by an innovative and engaging Online homework manager called *Connect Personal Health.*

In large-scale surveys and ethnographic studies recently undertaken by McGraw-Hill, students told us they want a textbook that is:

- light and easy to carry
- engaging and relevant to their own lives
- inexpensive
- supported by digital activities that help them learn and succeed in their course

Instructors told us they want a textbook that addresses their two greatest challenges:

- covering a large number of topics in a limited amount of time
- keeping students engaged in learning

In response to students' needs, the text is designed to highlight **visual appeal, brevity, portability,** and **function.** In response to instructors needs, the text focuses on the **essential topics in health** that are most fundamental to students' overall wellness. The text covers the core principles and common language of personal health and distills content down into small, manageable portions. The focus on core content gives instructors more time for exploring special topics or issues during class sessions, supported by *Connect Personal Health.* Together, the text and reader give instructors ample **opportunities to elicit and promote greater student engagement.**

➤ Essential Topics in Personal Health

Part I contains a single chapter, "Foundations of Personal Health." We set the stage for the rest of the book by discussing the concept of health and introducing four cross-cutting themes—health literacy, health risk, health advances, and lifestyle modification. Part II focuses on health behaviors and includes chapters on diet, fitness, drugs, sexuality, and stress. Part III addresses medical conditions, with chapters on mental disorders, heart disease and stroke, cancers, diabetes, and infections. And lastly, Part IV covers the health care system, with chapters on health care fundamentals and health care decision making.

➤ *Connect Personal Health:* Engaging, Flexible, Innovative

An online companion to the printed text, *Connect Personal Health* is designed to address a number of core teaching issues and to provide instructors with a vehicle for truly contextualizing health issues. While the *Concise Guide* teaches essential health concepts, *Connect Personal Health* expands on these topics in original and thought-provoking ways. Two important instructional benefits of *Connect Personal Health* are

- **Emphasis and Customization:** The *Connect Personal Health* allows instructors to focus on and integrate those special topics and themes that are important to them personally, whether the environment, diversity, genetics, globalization, or an other current concern.
- **Content in Context:** The *Connect Personal Health* provides the context that gives students a broader perspective about health topics. Articles are chosen for their relevance to students' lives and their ability to engage students and promote behavior change.

Connect Personal Health will present three to four thought-provoking and often controversial readings for each chapter of *Personal Health: A Concise Guide*. Each reading will be selected to align with a given chapter content (primary theme) as well as to address issues such as diversity, consumerism, genetics, mind/body, technology, globalization, culture, and the environment (secondary themes). The readings will include a range of formats—news reports, essays, op/ed, interviews, and visual essays. The readings will be drawn primarily from the mainstream media (newspapers, magazines, and related Internet sites) and scientific journals and will be authored by prominent journalists and scientists.

The key features of *Connect Personal Health* include

- **Germane Introductions and Article Abstracts:** Engaging introductions will capture students' attention and tie *Connect Personal Health* to the printed textbook both philosophically and pedagogically. Abstracts will summarize articles and orient students to their main points.
- **Thoughtful and Relevant Articles:** Readings will put health concepts in a real-world, contemporary context.
- **Key Terms:** Lists of key terms and definitions, cross-referenced to the textbook, will help students build health literacy.
- **Critical Thought Questions:** Critical Thought questions accompanying each article will help students develop their cognitive strategies and motivate behavior change.

- **Content Questions:** Additional practice activities will help students test their knowledge of key concepts discussed in the textbook.
- **Video Discussion Board Activities:** Students can watch discussions by college students on health topics that are relevant to them. After watching the videos, students can then post their own opinions to an online discussion board.
- **Online Health Assessments:** Students will be able to assess their own health and submit their findings to their instructor online.

Faculty Reviewers

The quality of this book is a testament to the skills and abilities of so many people, and we are tremendously grateful to the following individuals whose insightful contributions during the book's development and production have improved it immeasurably.

EDITORIAL BOARD MEMBERS

Eric	Buhi	University of South Florida Tampa
Gail	Dial	University of Florida
Steve	Dion	Salem State College
Whitfield B.	East	United States Military Academy
Dan	Gerber	University of Massachusetts Amherst
James E.	Graves	University of Utah
Jimmy H.	Ishee	Texas Woman's University
Beverly	Mahoney	Liberty University
Eric	Nehl	Emory University
Beverly	Zeakes	Radford University

PERSONAL HEALTH SYMPOSIUM PARTICIPANTS

Daniel Adame	Emory University
Vikki Armstrong	Fayetteville State University
Donna Bacon	Nassau Community College
Brian Barthel	Utah Valley State College
Deborah Blair	Sacramento City College
Jodi Brookins Fisher	Central Michigan University
Charlene Brown	Western Michigan University
Larry Bryant	Georgia Southern University
Karen Camarata	Eastern Kentucky University
Steve Chandler	Florida Agricultural and Mechanical University
Kim Clark	California State University, San Bernardino

Steve Dion — Salem State College
Shae Donham-Foutch — Northeastern State University
Eva Doyle — Baylor University
Kathi Fuller — Western Michigan University
Kim Hyatt — Weber State University
Allen Jackson — Chadron State College
David Jolly — North Carolina Central University
Emina Ibragic-Burak — The University of Vermont
Mark Kittleson — Southern Illinois University Carbondale
John Kowalczyk — University of Minnesota Duluth
Grover Pippin — Baylor University
Elaine Popp — Humber Institute of Technology and Advanced Learning
Linda Rankin — Idaho State University
Thurman Robins — Texas Southern University
Linda Shaffer — Mira Costa College
Shawna Shane — Emporia State University
Carol Smith — Elon University
John C. Smith — Springfield College
Jiri Stelzer — Valdosta State University
Debra Sutton — James Madison University
Michele Sweeney — Salem State College
Laura Sweet — Eastern Michigan University
Steve Trujillo — University of Western Ontario
Holly Turner Moses — University of Florida Gainesville
Karen Vail-Smith — East Carolina University
Resa Walch — Elon University
Cecilia Watkins — Western Kentucky University
Wayne Wylie — Texas A&M University

FOCUS GROUP PARTICIPANTS

Eric Buhi — University of South Florida
Harry Davakos — The Citadel
Paul Finnicum — Arkansas State University
Guoyuan Huang — University of Southern Indiana
Mark Kittleson — Southern Illinois University
Jo Anne Jackson — Middle Georgia College
Beverley Mahoney — Liberty University
Holly Turner Moses — University of Florida
Eric J. Nehl — Emory University
Steve Owens — Tallahassee Community College
Jennifer Petit — University of Akron
Monica Webb — University of South Florida
Chris Wirth — University of Florida
Beverly S Zeakes — Radford University

A.J.	Baca	North Harris Montgomery Community College District
Debbie	Blair	Sacramento City College
Curtis	Baird	Riverside Community College-Moreno Valley Campus
Christine	Bouffard	Waubonsee Community College
Elizabeth	Constandy	University of North Carolina Wilmington
Dick	Dalton	Lincoln University
Cathy	Dooly	Lander University
Max	Faquir	Palm Beach Community College-Boca Raton
Lisa	Fender-Scarr	University of Akron
Jennifer	Han	University of Oklahoma
Jody	Hart	John A. Logan College
Dina	Hayduk	Kutztown University of Pennsylvania
Allen	Jackson	Chadron State College
Mark	Kittleson	Southern Illinois University Carbondale
Garry	Ladd	Southwestern Illinois College
Grace	Lartey	Western Kentucky University
Barbara	Long	Bridgewater College
Susan	Lyman	University of Louisiana Lafayette
Calvin	Maginel	Southeast Missouri State University
Patty	Marcum	University of Southern Indiana
Catherine	Mckay	Bridgewater College
Bridget	Melton	Georgia Southern University
Tomas	Mendez	College of Charleston
Julie	Merten	University of North Florida
Juli	Miller	Ohio University
Peggy	Oberstaller	Lane Community College
Ramani	Rangavajhula	San Jose State University
Raymond	Reinertsen	University of Wisconsin-Superior
Karen	Vail-Smith	East Carolina University
Scott	Wolf	Southwestern Illinois College
Ottley	Wright	Chadron State College
Connie	Zuercher	Sacramento City College

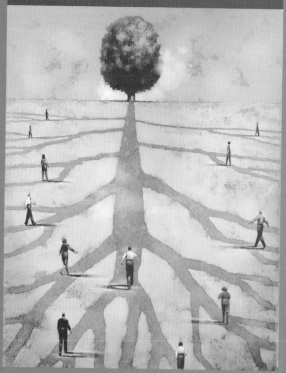

Learning is like rowing
upstream. Not to
advance is to fall
backward.

— CHINESE PROVERB

Chapter 1

FOUNDATIONS OF PERSONAL HEALTH

In Chapter 1, we provide a framework for understanding
fundamental health topics from health behaviors and medical
conditions to health care considerations. This orientation can
guide you in optimizing your health. We review the modern
concept of health followed by the crosscutting themes of health
literacy, health risk, impact of health advances, and health
behavior change.

LIFE EXPECTANCY rose dramatically in the United States during the 20th century. Life expectancy for Americans born in 1900 was 47 years, whereas for those born in 2000, life expectancy is 77 years. Thirty years is a phenomenal gain in average lifespan. Yet, researchers who study the biology of human aging believe that most of us are still dying prematurely. They contend that with prudent lifestyles, young people in America today can expect to live to an average age of 90 years.

The trends are evident. In the year 2000, over 9 million Americans were 80 years or older, and about 75,000 were centenarians—100 years or older. Lizzie Brown of Fayetteville, Georgia, took everything in stride and lived to 111. At 110 she was still tending her garden at the house in which she had lived for the past 62 years. Among long-lived celebrities, Bob Hope reached 100 and was still performing in his mid-90s. Yet, we all also know of older folks in assisted care homes or convalescent centers who are only in their 70s. Many of them will reside in these facilities for many years or even decades. This thought gives us pause.

Undeniably, a full life is what we long for, and it is much more than merely being alive. How does this relate to being healthy? How do we go about making smart decisions and establishing healthy behaviors? If we invest the time and effort to truly improve our health status, are there immediate paybacks, or are the benefits only to be gained in the years and decades ahead? How much control do we actually have in living a long and full life? Our aim in writing the *Concise Guide* is to address these fundamental questions.

➤ Modern Concept of Health

Health is a universal term used widely in everyday language. We all have a general sense about what the term means but are unsure about specific definitions. Has the definition of *health* changed over time? How should the term *health* be used today? Let's take a closer look. We'll begin by defining health and then discuss its dimensions and how the meaning of health is influenced by social and cultural factors.

DEFINITION OF HEALTH

For over 50 years, the World Health Organization (WHO) has defined health as a state of complete physical, mental, and social well-being and not merely the absence of disease or infirmity. Yet, for most of us, the importance of health becomes clear only when we are sick or injured. Consequently, our

Health is a dynamic human condition with multiple but intertwined dimensions—physical, emotional, social, intellectual, and spiritual. Health can be viewed as a continuum with positive and negative poles. Positive health is associated with a capacity to enjoy life and to withstand challenges. Negative health is associated with illness and disease and, in the extreme, with premature death.

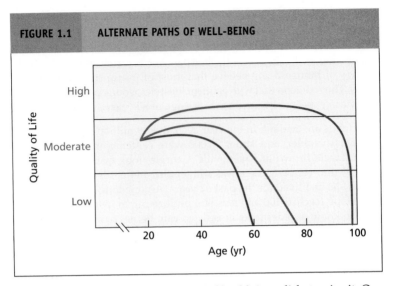

FIGURE 1.1   ALTERNATE PATHS OF WELL-BEING

reflexive perspective on the meaning of health is to dichotomize it. One is either healthy or unhealthy, with a continuum existing only on the unhealthy side depending on the severity of the illness. This lopsided and mistaken view has a serious unintended consequence—it limits human development and potential. This narrow view overlooks the existence of the broad continuum on the positive side of health. With little conscious intention, most young adults simply drift along on the positive side of the continuum. The good news is that by becoming more aware of what it means to be healthy, we can take steps to improve our own health.

Quality of life is an important related concept. Most succinctly, the phrase *quality of life* refers to our overall sense of well-being. **Quality of life** is a subjective rating of the difference between our hopes and expectations and our present experience. Health professionals sometimes have patients rate their quality of life to measure the effects of disorders and disabilities as well as medical treatments. These ratings can then be used to help guide medical decisions. Some treatments can seriously impair a person's ability to enjoy normal life activities without providing appreciable benefit, while others can greatly enhance quality of life. For most young adults, quality of life is synonymous with overall enjoyment of life and highly dependent on their current and expected health.

The relationship between quality of life and longevity is illustrated in Figure 1.1. From adolescence into young adulthood, we have increasing

Quality of life is one's overall sense of well-being or enjoyment of life. It's a subjective rating of the difference between a person's hopes and expectations and his or her present experience, and it is sometimes used in medical settings to help assess the effects of disease, disability, and treatments.

control over lifestyle choices and set the trajectory for our quality of life. The lower curve and the upper curve represent two hypothetical boundaries within which individual lifespan curves can be drawn. The upper curve reflects an individual who maximizes lifestyle choices and healthy behaviors. This leads to *both* a full life and a long life, reaching the 90-year potential and perhaps beyond. Ideally, the end of life is preceded by a sharp decline of short duration, with only a few weeks or months of deteriorating function and loss of independence, as in the case of Lizzie Brown.

In contrast, the lower curve represents a person who is unaware of or uninterested in a healthy life and adopts unhealthy behaviors. This compromises quality of life and substantially shortens a normal biological lifespan. Death at 60 rather than 90 is life truly cut short, yet sadly we all have first-hand knowledge of premature deaths and incomplete lives. Moreover, in this scenario, many years of low quality of life may precede the person's early death.

The middle curve depicts the path of many Americans who are aware of key health issues but unsuccessful in effectively translating their knowledge into healthier lifestyle behaviors. Note that the area between the lower and upper curves is large—it is high (along the Quality of Life axis) and wide (along the Age, or longevity, axis). Within these broad bounds, we can have enormous control on setting our own course. This is the potential area for growth available to us.

As in the WHO definition, health is often referred to as a state of optimal functioning, which implies the highest achievable level physically, mentally, and socially. In contrast, a contemporary perspective views health not as a state of being but as a goal that people continually work toward throughout their life. In Figure 1.2, health is depicted as a continuum extending from critical illness to optimal health. The traditional "treatment model" focuses on the left side of the continuum, and its emphasis is on freedom from sickness and disease. The proactive "wellness model" focuses more on the right side of the continuum and the challenge of maximizing potential and quality of life.

Humans are goal-oriented creatures. We like to set goals and then work to achieve them. The goal of better health is no exception. To craft a plan, we need to know what factors influence movement along the health continuum, especially those we can control or modify. As it turns out, the most important factors are those associated with lifestyle—for example, factors related to eating, exercising, sleeping, drug use (including alcohol and tobacco), and stress. To a great extent, we are in charge on these matters. By choosing which behaviors to develop and which to avoid, each of us sets the course for moving forward (or falling back) along the health continuum.

Uncontrollable (or nonmodifiable) factors can also influence our health. These include heredity, age, gender, and race. Occasionally unfavorable

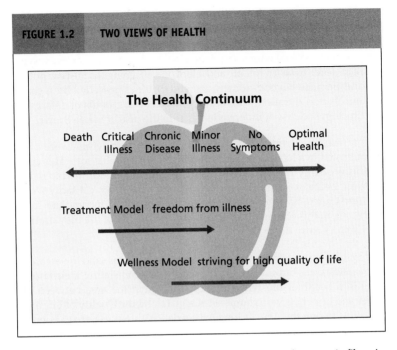

FIGURE 1.2   TWO VIEWS OF HEALTH

The Health Continuum

Death   Critical   Chronic   Minor   No   Optimal
Illness   Disease   Illness   Symptoms   Health

Treatment Model   freedom from illness

Wellness Model   striving for high quality of life

genetic combinations result in hereditary diseases such as cystic fibrosis, sickle cell anemia, and type 1 (juvenile) diabetes. Fortunately, today most inherited diseases can be effectively treated or managed. The uncontrollable factors of age, gender, and race—in addition to being essential parts of who we are—are useful categories for researchers studying diseases in populations. Yet, for us as individuals, our gender and race have no inherent positive or negative qualities that limit our movement along the health continuum across the broad span of our adult years (except for the very old).

Throughout the *Concise Guide* an emphasis is placed on understanding modifiable factors and how to maximize lifestyle behaviors for a full and long life. Admittedly, there are no guarantees, because life is unpredictable. Every day, unexpected accidents and deaths occur that are beyond people's control. This serves to remind us that good health is about having the best quality of life possible for whatever conditions we face or however many years we may have. In short though, a healthy lifestyle dramatically improves the odds for a full life, both today and in the future. Men and women of all races can be proactive about their health and reap the benefits today as well as tomorrow.

DIMENSIONS OF HEALTH

The modern view of health holds that health is multidimensional. Scholars point out that the characteristic of multidimensionality is of fundamental importance to truly understanding health. This view counters the popular notion that health is simply physical well-being. Expanding upon the three dimensions (physical, mental, social) cited in the WHO definition, the contemporary view typically encompasses five dimensions of health: physical, emotional, social, intellectual, and spiritual (some authors also include occupational and environmental). A brief description of each dimension follows.

Physical Dimension of Health

The physical dimension of health encompasses the functional operation and soundness of the body. How well are you able to perform activities of daily living such as dressing, cooking, walking, and driving? Can you perform routine tasks efficiently without becoming overly fatigued? Do you get regular medical checkups? Do you follow preventive health practices known to optimize physical health—namely, eating prudently, exercising regularly, avoiding substance abuse, wearing seat belts, minimizing sun exposure, and getting immunizations? For centuries, health was equated only with physical health. Today, physical health, although the predominant dimension at times, is recognized as only one of five dimensions that underlie our health.

Emotional Dimension of Health

The emotional dimension is associated with the ability to deal with personal feelings in a positive and constructive manner, to cope with stress, and to live independently. How is your outlook on life? Could your outlook be improved? Positive approaches to our emotions characterized by flexibility, balance, and resiliency help us deal effectively with feelings such as anger, happiness, fear, guilt, and love. A strong emotional dimension is a key to greater life satisfaction.

Social Dimension of Health

Closely tied to emotional health, the social dimension is the ability to interact effectively with other people, to develop satisfying interpersonal relationships, and to fulfill social roles. Do you have friends in whom you can confide? Do you have friends who feel comfortable confiding in you? Do you get along well with others and show respect regardless of your differences? Hallmarks of social health are the capacity for intimacy, meaningful relationships with family and friends, and participation in community activities. Young adulthood is a particularly important time for developing and broadening social skills.

Intellectual Dimension of Health

The intellectual dimension is reflected in our ability to question and evaluate information, to think and learn from a variety of experiences, and to be open to new ideas. Do you enjoy solving problems, learning new skills, and exploring new ideas? The academic challenges of college emphasize the development of intellectual health. Make the most of these opportunities. Critical thinking and problem solving are fundamental lifelong pursuits that enable us to continue learning new material and master new skills.

Spiritual Dimension of Health

Being spiritual doesn't mean belonging to a formal religion, although religion is part of this dimension for many people. The essential component of spiritual health is a commitment to a set of values or principles that guide our actions. This commitment is usually but not always based on a belief in a greater force. This greater force may be a god or simply an acknowledgement of a higher power or order in the universe. Atheists can have sacred sets of values to live by just as Christians, Muslims, and Jews have divine beliefs to guide them. Spiritual health often involves a dedication to nurture all living beings out of respect for the interrelatedness of all life. The basis for leading a moral and ethical life is rooted in spiritual health.

The dimensions of health do not exist as separate elements. Rather, each dimension relates to all others. As one dimension is affected, so too are the others. Just as individual threads are braided together to form a single cord, so too are the dimensions of health. Each thread or dimension contributes to the overall balance, quality, and strength of the whole.

DIVERSITY AND HEALTH

Over the past decade, the issue of diversity has come to the forefront. The changing demographics of the United States are illustrated with the following examples from the U.S. Census of 2000:

- The nonwhite population is growing three times faster than the white population.
- The Hispanic population is increasing at a rate five times faster than the rate for the entire U.S. population (Hispanics were 12.5 percent of the population in 2000).
- Family structures have changed significantly, with a 50 percent chance that married partners will reach their 25th anniversary.
- Thirty-three percent of all children (and 66 percent of Black children) live part of their lives in one-parent households.
- Fifty-five percent of college students are women, and over 60 percent of adult women are in the workforce.
- Immigration to the United States continues to be high: over 600,000 people every year since 1980 and in some years over 1 million.

We see diversity in ordinary encounters with individuals and groups who may differ widely in attitudes, values, and beliefs—cumulatively referred to as *culture*. Diversity is sometimes criticized as a form of political correctness, but that is an unfortunate and shortsighted view. The following quote from Sara Corbett's *New York Times* article "The Long

Road from Sudan to America" introduces us to three young refugees from Sudan:

> One evening in late January, Peter Dut, 21, leads his two teenage brothers through the brightly lit corridors of the Minneapolis airport, trying to mask his confusion. Two days earlier, the brothers, refugees from Africa, had encountered their first light switch and their first set of stairs. An aid worker in Nairobi had demonstrated the flush toilet to them—also the seat belt, the shoelace, the fork. And now they find themselves alone in Minneapolis, three bone-thin African boys confronted by a swirling river of white faces and rolling suitcases.

This description sets a sharp contrast between the lives of these African refugees and those of the Americans who walked by them in the airport. What is ordinary and routine for many may indeed be novel and wondrous for others. Most of us can hardly imagine the environment and circumstances from which these three brothers escaped. Should it be surprising that cultural background and life experiences invariably shape how we perceive each other and the world in which we live?

Of all the places in America, colleges and universities are among the most diverse. A large lecture class may have students who are urban and rural, wealthy and poor, and religious and nonreligious. Students may include devout Christians, Jews, and Muslims alongside agnostics and atheists. Students representing many nationalities from both developed and developing countries and various ethnic groups may be present. Many may speak English as a second language. Students may differ in sexual orientation, and some may be part of a nontraditional family structure. With this medley in mind, it's easier to understand why perceptions and knowledge of health concepts and issues vary so widely.

Discussing diversity is important because many health topics such as stress, mental health, nutrition, drug use, chronic diseases, and infectious diseases are strongly related to culture. Examples include social stressors (prejudice, economic oppression), mental health disorders (depression, suicidal behavior), food choices (ethnic diets), and drug use patterns (tobacco, alcohol, other drugs). Gaining insight into how the concept of health varies among different religious, ethnic, and cultural groups helps each of us better define the meaning of health in our own lives. This theme will be followed throughout the *Concise Guide* and highlighted in selected readings.

The diversity of the American population is a great asset. It is also one of our nation's greatest challenges because profound health disparities exist between the mainstream population and various subpopulations such as African Americans, Hispanics, American Indians, and residents of Appalachia. Health disparities are a reality faced daily by employers, educators, and health professionals. A primary goal of public health is to reduce health disparities through research, education, and improved access to heath care. In the wealthiest and most technologically-advanced country in the world, affordable and equitable health care should be available to everyone.

✓ **NEED TO KNOW**

The concept of health is much more than simply not being sick. Health is multidimensional, dynamic, and influenced by social and cultural norms. Our overall health status and the associated quality of life are largely determined by our lifestyle choices and behaviors.

➤ Health Literacy

Health literacy can be defined as the degree to which individuals have the capacity to obtain, process, and understand basic health information and services needed to make appropriate health decisions. Health literacy programs are traditionally targeted to the poor, the elderly, and those with little education. Yet, health literacy is not solely a matter of formal education or access to health information. The Institute of Medicine estimates that nearly half of all American adults have difficulty understanding and using health information. The challenge of becoming health literate becomes clearer when considered within the context of our consumer-driven society. More than ever before, consumption defines who we are and what we do.

We are immersed in advertising throughout our waking hours. American children and adolescents watch an average of three to four hours of television a day. Young children recall Ronald McDonald, Tony the Tiger, and the Budweiser Frogs as easily as Santa Claus, Mickey Mouse, and Bugs Bunny. Beyond the screen, advertising in other forms from signage to apparel is increasingly found throughout schools. The American Academy of Pediatrics is one of many professional groups to point out that excessive or uncontrolled exposure to television, movies, music, video games and the Internet is associated with increased risk for an array of health problems from obesity and eating disorders to substance abuse, promiscuity, and aggressive behaviors.

Advertisers shape our consumer desires and create values in products by portraying them as having the power to change us into "more desirable" people. Commercials feature adults who are attractive, happy, energetic, and often hip or sensuous too. The underlying message is we can be like them if we use those products. Mega shopping malls have become a cultural primer for telling us how we should dress, furnish our homes, and spend leisure time. Luxuries have become necessities and lifestyles can be purchased. As an interesting side note, Barry Schwartz, Ph.D., a professor of psychology at Swarthmore College, suggests that our nearly unlimited choices have resulted in additional stress for the modern consumer—the paradox of choice.

Health literacy is the ability to obtain, process, and understand basic health information and services needed to make appropriate health decisions.

Health & the Media Public Service Announcements

Advertising, a major industry in itself, is adept at creating messages to sell products. In the 1940s, the nonprofit Ad Council created a new type of advertising known as public service announcements (PSAs) to bring about positive social change, including better health. The Ad Council remains active today but its resources are limited **(www.adcouncil.org).**

Another approach to communicating healthy messages is to dispel the illusion of advertising with spoof ads. Cigarette and alcohol ads are especially ripe targets. Adbusters, a Canadian advocacy advertising agency and publisher of *Adbusters* magazine, has produced several memorable ones. Their "Absolute on Ice" parody ad evokes a stark contrast to the original ad and makes one think twice about the downsides of excessive drinking. (The product being parodied is Absolut, a vodka.) See other spoof ads such as Joe Chemo, a takeoff on Joe Camel, at **http://adbusters.org/spoofads.**

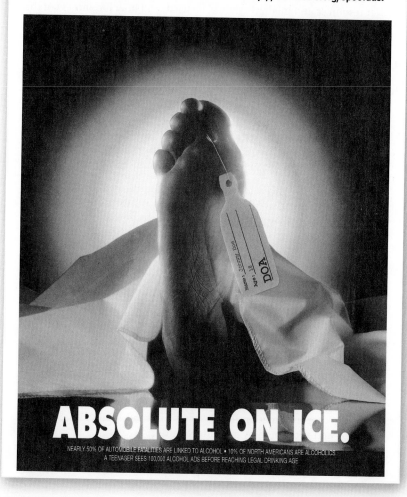

In the health marketplace, frauds and hoaxes remain commonplace. For any ailment or disease, there exist literally hundreds of products, most of which are bogus. Regardless of the source—the Internet, newspapers, magazines, radio, television, neighbors, colleagues—the best advice remains "buyer beware." It is tempting to assume that being college educated ensures the ability to sort out the confounding influences and misleading claims from science-based information. But this is true only if we remain health literate. Health literacy is dependent upon self-directed learning, effective communication, and critical thinking.

SELF-DIRECTED LEARNING

Self-directed learning is a process in which the individual controls both the learning objectives and the means of learning, with or without the help of others. You are in charge—you determine what should be learned, what resources and methods should be used, and how the success of the effort should be measured. This is in contrast to most college courses and workplace training classes, in which the learning objectives, methods, and evaluation are set by the teacher or employer.

To a large degree, most adult learning is self-directed. A person's objective may be to improve family life, enjoy the arts, participate in a hobby, or to research a medical question. For many people, however, the extent of self-direct learning is quite limited. They may not engage in self-directed learning because they lack the confidence, resources, independence, or some combination of the three. Thankfully, these barriers can be overcome with motivation and guidance.

First and foremost, the Internet is a rich resource for the self-directed learner. To become a savvy health consumer, it's essential to learn the basic skills of using the Internet. This will allow you to expand on and update material presented in the *Concise Guide*. The first step is to recognize that you need to carefully and critically evaluate information on the Internet because anyone can post information. For instance, you and your friends may have your own Web sites. Unlike reference books and refereed journal articles, a rigorous review and evaluation by experts prior to posting or "publishing" on the Internet is not required.

As an initial screening procedure, note that certain Web addresses (or URLs)—namely, those with the ".org" (nonprofit organization), ".gov" (federal government), and ".edu" (college/university) extensions—are more likely than the ".com" (commercial business) Web sites to lead to authoritative information. As health decision makers, our primary aim is to find credible and reliable information—not to buy a product! We should look for information that is factual, current, written in everyday language, and sponsored by a reputable group.

The following four Web sites are excellent general resources for health information and are listed in the Top Ten Most Useful Web sites by the

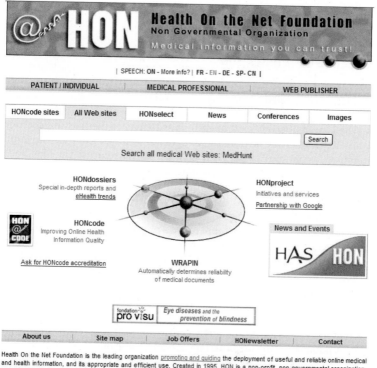

Medical Library Association. All four abide by the Health on the Net (HON) Foundation Code of Conduct which comprises a set of ethical principles for justifiability, attribution, and transparency of health and medical information (www.hon.ch). Look for the HON icon (upper left) as a sign of credibility and trustworthiness. Even among reputable Web sites though, it's a good practice to search several to cross-check information.

MedlinePlus **http://medlineplus.gov** Sponsored by the National Library of Medicine and the National Institutes of Health (NIH)

Healthfinder.gov **www.healthfinder.gov** Sponsored by the Office of Disease Prevention and Health Promotion, U.S. Department of Health & Human Services (HHS)

Centers for Disease Control and Prevention (CDC) **www.cdc.gov** Leading federal agency for preventing and controlling disease, injury, and disability

Mayo Clinic **www.mayoclinic.com** Sponsored by the renowned Mayo Clinic, the world's first and largest not-for-profit medical practice

A few carefully selected Web sites will be presented in each chapter. Since Web addresses sometimes change, occasionally there may be a link that no longer works. If that happens, refer to the *Concise Guide*'s Web page for updates.

EFFECTIVE COMMUNICATION

The importance of developing written and oral communication skills cannot be overstated. Every day we communicate with different people in a variety of settings. Yet, good communication skills are not routinely learned in school so it's left to each of us to master them as self-directed learners. Let there be no doubt that regular investments of time and effort to improve communication skills will yield great returns. The likelihood for miscommunication when dealing with medical or health issues is enormous. Let's consider three different scenarios.

Scenario One

You are waiting in the exam room to see a physician. You have been told to take off your clothes and put on an exam gown. You have an odd illness you have never experienced before. Or you may have a hunch about what's going on but hope it's not true. You know your time with the doctor will be short, perhaps 5 to 10 minutes. And on top of that, you are feeling really lousy—that's why you've come to the doctor in the first place! This situation is predictably stressful and not conducive to good communication. Common barriers are intimidation, embarrassment, and fear. Many people are intimidated by the medical setting, being half-clothed, and the status of the doctor. They may be embarrassed due to the personal nature of the condition they need to reveal. Some are fearful they may have a serious condition. It's no wonder we often cannot recall exactly what the doctor said or we forget to ask a question. How to prepare for a doctor's appointment and how to get your questions answered are discussed in Chapter 13, "Health Care Decision Making."

Scenario Two

Your elderly neighbor has asked you to drive her to her doctor's appointment. As you take her home, she tells you that she has diabetes. But she is confused. She relates, "I think some of the words . . . [during the office visit and in brochures], they ought to explain in simple English. Everybody hasn't graduated from high school or college. They should just speak or put them down in plain English." Like millions of Americans, she is struggling with "medspeak," the specialized language of health professionals. The overuse of medical jargon has created a communication barrier for the public. As health professionals work to minimize their use of medspeak with patients, we as health consumers should increase our understanding of basic health and medical terms.

Scenario Three

You are in the pharmacy line at the drugstore and hear a disjointed conversation between the pharmacist and a Hispanic man in front of you. Although he has a heavy accent, his English is understandable.

But it is unclear if he completely comprehends the pharmacist's instructions about how the medication should be taken. Communication problems are not limited to obvious language differences between patients and health care providers. They may also exist between people who come from different regions of the country or who have different values or expectations about health care. It is important to remember that one's customs and beliefs should be considered when communicating health messages.

CRITICAL THINKING

The term *critical thinking* is widely used but not well understood. Most would say it has something to do with logic or analysis, but these terms provide only a partial description. Essentially, critical thinking is careful and deliberate determination of whether to accept, reject, or suspend judgment. These are often the *why* questions. Critical thinking has two components: first, a set of skills to process and generate information and beliefs, and second, the habit—based on intellectual commitment—of using those skills to guide behavior. This is in contrast to the mere acquisition of information, the simple possession of skills, or the use of those skills as an exercise without giving any thought to their results.

Critical thinking is driven by asking the *right* questions. Critical thinking is *not* involved when teachers feed students endless facts for simple recall or when students sit in silence except for superficial or ill-informed questions. Both examples are dead ends. In contrast, good teaching and good questions lead to more questions and eventually to true learning. Overcome lifeless classrooms by asking thought-provoking questions. Learn the skills and establish the habit of critical thinking. From time to time, we are all subject to undisciplined and irrational thought. But is it the norm or the exception? The practice of critical thinking can be developed and refined during the college years but doesn't stop upon graduation. Critical thinking can serve us well in all endeavors and should be a lifelong pursuit.

Breaking It Down Does Listening to Classical Music Make You Smarter?

A few years ago the "Mozart effect"—an alleged increase in brain development in children when they listen to the music of Mozart—received wide coverage in the popular print and broadcast media. Since that time, the Mozart effect has taken on a life of its own. It's featured in parenting, education, and music oriented publications. Governors of several states started programs that give a Mozart CD to every newborn. Dozens of toys suddenly appeared proclaiming themselves "educational" because they played snippets of Mozart's "Rondo Alla

Turca" rather than "Mary Had a Little Lamb." The Mozart effect has also been used to sell music lessons and music products. Moreover, claims have expanded: classical music can not only increase a child's intelligence but also aid an adult's healing process. What caused this Mozart love fest?

The Mozart effect is an example of how science and the media can mix in our world. First, a scientific paper is published in a prestigious journal that reports a new and potentially important finding. The scientific study receives attention from the media, as it should. But next comes the over-simplification of the science. Sometimes reporters innocently misstate facts because of lack of scientific understanding. Other times, businesses may intentionally exaggerate a study's findings in order to publicize products and boost their sales. Regardless of the cause, once these mis-statements are embraced by the general public, what started as a trickle of misinformation can become a raging river of exaggeration that affects all in its flow—scientists and the general public alike.

In this case, Frances Rauscher and two colleagues (1993) from the Center for Neurobiology of Learning and Memory at the University of California–Irvine reported in *Nature* that listening to a composition of Mozart briefly increased scores among college students on a paper-folding task that measures spatial abilities. The increase in scores lasted only about ten minutes. Nonspatial tasks measured on the same IQ test were unaffected by listening to the music. The boost in scores was widely reported, but the short-lived effect and narrow nature of the improvement received a lot less attention. The accuracy of the original findings was lost over the years as the Mozart effect morphed into the popular notion that "Mozart makes you smarter." This notion is, of course, a gross oversimplification. Does it really make sense to talk about being "smarter" if it only lasts ten minutes?

Accuracy is needed in science *and* in the media. Too often, important re-search is trivialized and misrepresented in the popular media. The case of the Mozart effect can teach us several lessons. First, we should be careful not to abandon common sense when we read health-related news. If a claim seems a bit extreme or too good to be true, then this ought to be a warning flag that the news might be incomplete or distorted. Second, we should allow the data to speak for themselves. When findings are contro-versial, explore reputable Web sites for summaries, read the original re-port and the opinions of experts, and reach your own conclusions. Apply those critical thinking skills!

Consider critical thinking as a process that stresses an attitude of suspended judgment, incorporates logical inquiry and problem solving, and leads to an evaluative decision or action. In today's information age, critical think-ing is more important than ever before. In addition to being an essential part of our intellectual health, critical thinking allows us to filter and analyze the maze of facts, claims, and hoaxes that surround health and medical issues. Critical thinking is what we must rely on if we are to successfully separate science from marketing and find solutions to complex questions.

✓ **NEED TO KNOW**

Health literacy is the knowledge and skills that enable us to successfully access, analyze, and interpret relevant information, to answer personal health questions, to provide guidance in dealing with a health condition, and to change a health behavior. Key aspects of health literacy include self-directed learning, effective communication, and critical thinking. These characteristics require related skills that must be developed. Health literacy also assumes a mindfulness and inquisitiveness that motivates continual learning.

➤ Concept of Risk

To fully appreciate the impact of our behaviors on our health, it's essential to understand what a health risk is and how to interpret it. Simply stated, a **health risk** is the probability that an adverse event (an outcome) will occur if one engages in a certain behavior (exposure). For example, those who do not buckle up when riding in a car are at greater risk for a serious injury should an accident occur than those who do buckle up. The negative behavior (exposure) is not using a seat belt, and serious injury is the likely outcome if an accident occurs. The risk factors (behaviors and other factors) that are associated with specific diseases or injuries are established primarily by epidemiological studies.

Epidemiology is the study of the causes, distribution, and control of diseases in populations. Many medical findings reported in the popular media are based on epidemiological studies in which large numbers of people (hundreds or thousands) have been evaluated repeatedly over

A **health risk** or **risk factor** is any factor which increases susceptibility or has a strong association with the occurrence, onset, or progression of a disease or injury.

Epidemiology is the scientific discipline studying the occurrence, distribution, control, and prevention of disease, infection, injury, and other health-related events in a defined human population. It includes the study of factors affecting the progress of an illness and, in the case of many chronic diseases, their natural history.

many years or decades. The goal of these studies is to investigate the links (associations) between the characteristics (including health behaviors) of the participants and the occurrence of specific outcomes across time (e.g., onset of diseases or death). Epidemiological studies help scientists sort through many, many factors and eventually identify those that are most highly related to a given disease.

Statistical correlations in population studies are based on observational data. That is, changes over time are observed and measured but no experimental treatment or intervention is being tested. As such, epidemiological findings by themselves cannot prove cause and effect. Just because variable A is highly related to variable B does not prove that A causes B. Does smoking cause cirrhosis of the liver? Probably not. Excessive consumption of alcohol is the likely cause. Yet, since heavy drinkers tend to be heavy smokers, the statistical association is there. More often than not, evidence from experimental research, such as controlled laboratory studies or clinical trials, is used in conjunction with epidemiological findings to support or refute potential causal relationships.

RISK PERCEPTION

David Ropeik and George Gray, researchers at the Center for Risk Analysis at the Harvard School of Public Health, have shown that risk perception is not a straightforward, logical process based on the best science. How we decide what to be afraid of and to what degree to be afraid is heavily influenced by psychological factors. Here are three examples of how we decide what's safe and what's risky:

1. People tend to be less afraid of risks that are natural than those that are man-made. There is greater fear of radiation from cell phones or power lines than from the sun, which presents a much greater risk.
2. People are less afraid of a risk they choose to take than one imposed on them. Smokers are less fearful of smoking than they are of asbestos or other indoor air pollutants in the workplace, over which they may have little control.
3. Most of us are less afraid of a risk that comes from people or organizations that we trust and more afraid if the risk comes from a source that we don't trust. We are more likely to accept the risk assessment of a drug's safety from a trusted physician than from the pharmaceutical company that makes it.

In their book *Risk: A Practical Guide for Deciding What's Really Safe and What's Really Dangerous in the World Around You* (2002), Ropeik and Gray provide evidence-based information to help put the risks in life in perspective. These researchers have found that Americans tend to overestimate small risks and underestimate large risks, regardless of age, race, or socioeconomic status. When you are making decisions about health risks, be aware that perceptions can be shaped by emotions and feelings. Consider taking a step back and relying on careful objective analysis when a major health risk must be evaluated.

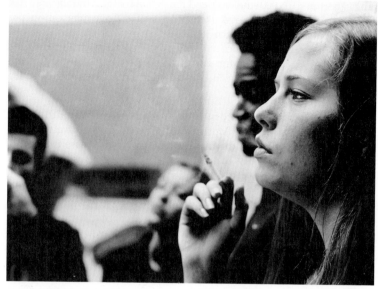

Smokers have both a greater relative risk and absolute risk of developing certain cancers than nonsmokers.

RELATIVE RISK

Health risks are generally discussed in the language of medical statistics. **Relative risk** is a common way to quantify and report a health risk. Although statistics can be complex, relative risk is a straightforward concept and one we should know as medical consumers. Relative risk is the "times-greater chance" a person has of acquiring a specific negative health effect (e.g., a disease) based on the extent to which a certain variable (e.g., a characteristic or behavior) is present. Relative risk is the ratio of the rate of disease among those exposed to a variable compared to those not exposed or having limited exposure.

To illustrate, the American Cancer Society reports that the annual death rate from lung cancer among people who smoke is approximately 50 deaths per 100,000 people per year while the death rate of people who don't smoke is only 2.5 deaths per 100,000 people per year. In this case, the relative risk—the ratio of the lung cancer death rates of those exposed (smokers) to those not exposed (non-smokers)—is 20 (50 divided by 2.5). Put another way, relative risk is the ratio of two absolute risks: the numerator is the absolute risk among those with the risk factor (50 deaths from

Relative risk is a measure of comparative risk of a health-related event such as disease or death between two groups. It is the chance that a person receiving an exposure will develop a condition compared to the chance that a non-exposed person will develop the same condition.

lung cancer per 100,000 smokers), and the denominator is the absolute risk among those without the risk factor (2.5 deaths from lung cancer per 100,000 non-smokers). A relative risk of 20 means that those who smoke have a 20-times-greater chance of dying from lung cancer than those who don't smoke. (Relative risk for smoking versus not smoking and death from lung cancer varies between 10 and 20 depending primarily upon the amount of smoking.)

Often a relative risk is reported by itself. A relative risk of 10 to 20 (as with smoking) is extremely high. Most relative risks are in the range of 1.5 to 3.0. Let's assume the absolute risk for developing a disease is 4 in 100 among people who exercise regularly, and the risk is increased 50 percent in those who do not exercise. The 50 percent relates to the absolute risk number, 4, so the increase in the risk is 50 percent of 4, or 2. Consequently, non-exercisers' absolute risk of developing the disease is 6 out of 100, and the relative risk is 1.5 for the non-exercisers compared to the exercisers (6 divided by 4). On the one hand, a 50 percent increase sounds alarming, but on the other, because the absolute risk is small, a 50 percent increase is not that significant overall—the risk only increased from 4 out of 100 to 6 out of 100. Consequently, when possible, find out both relative and absolute risks, and do your own calculation to determine the overall risk.

We believe that "knowing the numbers" is important. The trend in public health, however, is to not report any numbers when communicating risk, but simply to rate the risk of a behavior as low, moderate, or high. This may be fine for some risks but not for others. You must be the judge. When in doubt, continue to ask or research your questions until you completely understand the risks associated with a specific behavior, intervention, or treatment. From the examples presented, the value of using the concepts of absolute and relative risk should be evident. Interpreting results from epidemiological and clinical studies and applying them to individual situations will enable you to make more informed decisions.

✓ **NEED TO KNOW**

Health risk is the concept that relates specific health-compromising factors (exposures) to increased likelihood of developing diseases or higher death rates (outcomes). Conversely, from a proactive viewpoint, adopting health-enhancing or health-protective behaviors can reduce the probability of unwanted outcomes. Epidemiologists study the disease process in populations and quantify health risk in terms of absolute risk and relative risk.

➤ Advances in Public Health

The health concerns and health care services available when Lizzie Brown, the centenarian mentioned at the beginning of the chapter, was born in 1892 are vastly different from those that exist for a baby born today. A century ago, America was in the midst of the Industrial Revolution. Large numbers of people were migrating to the cities for jobs in factories. City housing was crowded, dirty, unheated, and unventilated. Clean water and proper sanitation (waste disposal) were limited, and food supplies were unreliable and often contaminated. These conditions allowed **infectious diseases** such as influenza, pneumonia, and tuberculosis to thrive.

Death rates fluctuated widely from year to year depending on disease (epidemics), severe weather (snowstorms, floods, hurricanes), and the harvest (varying from poor to bountiful). Infant mortality was high. In some cities, up to 30 percent of babies did not live to their first birthday. Many women died during childbirth. In short, life was hard. Under these conditions, it's understandable that good health would be thought of as being simply one step beyond the necessities for survival—that is, having adequate food and shelter and not being ill. The life expectancy for an American born in 1900 was less than 50. A century later, life expectancy was over 75.

ADVANCES OVER THE PAST CENTURY

Several major public health advances contributed to the 50 percent increase in life expectancy over the past 100 years. Leading the way was the provision of clean water, improved sanitation (the building of sewer systems), and the development of vaccines and antibiotics—collectively these markedly improved the control of most infectious diseases. Other notable public health achievements were safer and healthier foods, greater access to health care, and technologic improvements in health care. For example, since 1900, infant mortality has decreased 90 percent and maternal mortality has decreased 99 percent. Substantial reductions in disability (morbidity) and death (mortality) have also resulted from improvements in workplace safety (e.g., regulations in mining, manufacturing, and construction) and motor vehicle safety (e.g., better-engineered vehicles and highways and seat belt use). Most of these public health advances have been translated into public policy, such as school immunization policies and seat belt laws. Americans today can hardly imagine the difficulties their ancestors faced only four or five generations ago.

As infectious diseases were controlled with public health advances, the leading causes of death and disability in America shifted. In 1900 the three leading causes of death were pneumonia, tuberculosis, and diarrheal diseases. In 2000 the three leading causes of death were not infectious diseases

---

An **infectious disease** is a medical condition typically resulting from a disease-causing organism—usually a bacterium, virus, or parasitic worm—known as a pathogen. Most infectious diseases are short-term or highly treatable illnesses, such as the common cold and strep throat. Other infectious diseases such as AIDS are long-term diseases for which no medical cure has yet been developed.

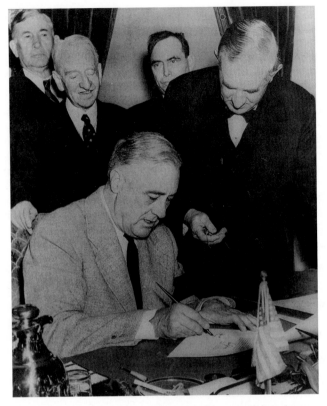

President Franklin Delano Roosevelt contracted polio as an adult and was paralyzed from the waist down for the rest of his life. Polio epidemics are now practically unheard of in the developed world thanks to the invention of immunizations.

but chronic diseases—heart disease, cancer, and stroke. **Chronic diseases** are medical conditions that are prolonged, do not resolve spontaneously, and are rarely cured completely. And, just as with infectious diseases, chronic diseases impose huge human and economic costs.

As we once faced the scourge of infectious diseases, we now face a different challenge to our health, one that won't be solved solely by breakthroughs in medical technology or new drugs. Over the years, we've learned that the rise of chronic diseases, particularly over the second half of the 20th century, was due primarily to our lifestyle habits. Hence, chronic diseases are often referred to as "lifestyle diseases." As seen in

A **chronic disease** is a medical condition that is permanent, leaves a residual disability, is caused by a nonreversible pathological condition, and requires special training of the patient for rehabilitation or is expected to require a long period of supervision or care. Coronary heart disease and cancer are two common examples.

TABLE 1.1	LEADING CAUSES OF DEATH IN THE U.S. IN 2000
CAUSE	**NUMBER OF DEATHS**
Heart disease	710,760
Cancer	553,091
Stroke	167,661
Chronic lower respiratory disease	122,009
Unintentional injuries	97,900
Diabetes	69,301
Influenza and pneumonia	65,313
Alzheimer disease	49,558
Kidney disease	37,251
Septicemia	31,224

Source: Mokdad AH, Marks JS, Stroup DF, et al. Actual causes of death in the United States, 2000. *JAMA* 291 (10): 1238–1245, 2004.

TABLE 1.2	ACTUAL CAUSES OF DEATH IN THE U.S. IN 2000
ACTUAL CAUSE	**ESTIMATED NUMBER OF DEATHS**
Tobacco	435,000
Poor diet/activity patterns	400,000
Alcohol consumption	85,000
Microbial agents	75,000
Toxic agents	55,000
Motor vehicles	43,000
Firearms	29,000
Sexual behavior	20,000
Illicit use of drugs	17,000

Source: Mokdad AH, Marks JS, Stroup DF, et al. Actual causes of death in the United States, 2000. *JAMA* 291 (10): 1238–1245, 2004.

Table 1.1, the first four causes of death, and six of the top ten, are chronic diseases attributed largely to daily habits associated with eating, physical activity, and tobacco use. National estimates indicate that about 50 percent of disease and premature deaths (i.e., death before age 65) are due to unhealthy lifestyles. Heart disease, cancer, stroke, and diabetes will be discussed in Part 3. As Pogo proclaimed in the 1970s, "We have met the enemy and he is us." (Walt Kelly's *Pogo*, a long-running comic strip [1948–75] provided social satire and laughs for both kids and adults.)

When considering lifestyle diseases, another approach is to consider deaths by actual causes as opposed to medical conditions. In Table 1.2, tobacco use is shown to be the number one cause of mortality, responsible for an estimated 435,000 deaths per year. These tobacco-attributed deaths would cut across several of the chronic diseases, including about 90 percent of deaths from lung cancer and pulmonary disease (chronic lower respiratory disease) and lower percentages of deaths from heart disease, stroke, and other cancers. Deaths due to poor diet and physical inactivity (400,000) combined with alcohol abuse (85,000) account for another 485,000 annual deaths. Clearly, our habits regarding eating, physical activity/exercise, and use of tobacco and alcohol have a major impact on our individual health as well as on population health.

Because most of you are young adults, let's also consider the leading causes of death for your age groups (CDC Table 10, 2005). For the age group 15–24, the leading cause of death is unintentional injury (over 15,750 deaths/year), with the majority being motor vehicle accidents. The second and third leading causes of death among this age group are homicide and suicide (combined, over 9,600 deaths/year). For the 25–44 age group, accidental death remains number one. However, cardiovascular diseases and cancers are the second and third leading causes of deaths in this age group. These statistics highlight the importance of using seat belts, being alert to thoughts of suicide, screening for cardiovascular diseases and cancers, and behaving responsibly regarding alcohol, drugs, and firearms. Even if you are alert to these risks, consider the positive influence you might have with your peers. A few words of concern and caution from a friend can make a difference.

What Is Your Risk? Campus Binge Drinking

Alcohol abuse is a problem on nearly all college campuses. But how big a problem is it, and what is the risk? Let's use binge drinking—consuming five or more drinks on a single occasion—as an indicator of alcohol abuse. The table below summarizes recent findings on drinking behavior from the ongoing National College Health Assessment (American College Health Association, 2000–2007).

DRINKING BEHAVIOR OF COLLEGE MEN AND WOMEN

Over the last two weeks, how many times, if any, have you had five or more alcoholic drinks at a sitting?

	NONE	1-2 TIMES	3 OR MORE TIMES
Men	53%	24%	23%
Women	68%	21%	11%

Based on statics from the five most recent years, the proportion of college students who report binge drinking is consistently in the range of 45 to

50 percent for men and 30 to 35 percent for women. Clearly, these results indicate that alcohol abuse among college students—both men and women—is widespread. But how dangerous is it?

To assess the degree of risk associated with binge drinking, let's correlate the prevalence of binge drinking with the leading causes of death among this age group. Unintentional injuries—motor vehicle accidents, falls, and drowning—followed by homicides and suicides are the major causes of death among people ages 18–24. In the United States, these amount to over 25,000 deaths per year (0.8 deaths per 1,000 persons), with 75 percent of these young adult deaths occurring among men rather than women.

The vast majority of these deaths are linked to alcohol and other drug abuse. Many of the deaths are casualties of those who are drunk—the friends in the car or the people in the other car or those folks trying to assist or merely standing nearby during a violent encounter. Although the absolute risk of dying due to binge drinking is low, remember that for every death that occurs, there are many more individuals who survive an alcohol-related incident but are seriously injured or disabled. We all know of someone who has been affected either directly or indirectly.

Certainly, the problem of binge drinking varies greatly among colleges and among groups on a single campus. In general though, alcohol abuse among young adults is a behavior that is widespread and dangerous. The risk of death among young adults in America is low, yet most of those deaths are linked to alcohol and drug abuse. Stepping in to counter poor judgment or simply taking the time to consider the possible dire consequences goes a long way in preventing dangerous situations. As my grandmother use to say, "Have fun but be careful."

HEALTHY PEOPLE 2010

Grounded on the best scientific and medical evidence, *Healthy People 2010* is a comprehensive document that outlines our national health objectives. It identifies the most significant preventable threats to public health and sets specific goals to reduce these threats. Two overarching goals, 10 leading health indicators and 28 focus areas are presented (see Table 1.3). Both overarching goals should sound familiar. The first is to help individuals of all ages increase life expectancy and improve their quality of life. The second, based on an obvious need, is to eliminate health disparities among different segments of the population.

The nation's health experts have identified our 10 most pressing public health issues and present them as leading health indicators. They are intended to help Americans understand how healthy we are as a nation and which are the most important changes we can make to improve our health and the health of our families and communities. The health indicators are in turn expanded into 28 focus areas, each of which are detailed in *Healthy People 2010*. Both the health indicators and focus areas emphasize *our* role in

TABLE 1.3	*HEALTHY PEOPLE 2010:* GOALS, HEALTH INDICATORS, AND FOCUS AREAS

OVERARCHING GOALS

1. Increase quality and years of healthy life
2. Eliminate health disparities

LEADING HEALTH INDICATORS

1. Physical activity
2. Overweight and obesity
3. Tobacco use
4. Substance abuse
5. Responsible sexual behavior
6. Mental health
7. Injury and violence
8. Environmental quality
9. Immunization
10. Access to health care

FOCUS AREAS

1. Access to quality health services
2. Arthritis, osteoporosis, back conditions
3. Cancer
4. Chronic kidney disease
5. Diabetes
6. Disability and secondary conditions
7. Educational and community-based programs
8. Environmental health
9. Family planning
10. Food safety
11. Health communication
12. Heart disease and stroke
13. HIV
14. Immunization and infectious diseases
15. Injury and violence prevention
16. Maternal, infant, and child health
17. Medical product safety
18. Mental health and disorders
19. Nutrition and overweight
20. Occupational safety and health
21. Oral health
22. Physical activity and fitness
23. Public health infrastructure
24. Respiratory diseases
25. Sexually transmitted diseases
26. Substance abuse
27. Tobacco use
28. Vision and hearing

Source: *Healthy People 2010* **www.healthypeople.gov**

making healthy choices—better choices for ourselves and those close to us about doctors, health insurance, health information, and a healthy lifestyle.

You will find chapters (or chapter sections) on eight of the 10 leading health indicators in the *Concise Guide.* Although we do not treat injury and violence (indicator 7) and environmental quality (indicator 8) as distinct topics, we do recognize their importance as leading health indicators. Both are intertwined with related main topics and discussed within that context. They are also briefly discussed in the following paragraphs.

The public health goal reflected by indicator 7 is to reduce injuries, disabilities, and deaths due to unintentional injuries and violence. Most people sustain a significant injury at some time during their lives. Many mistakenly believe that most injuries happen by chance and are the result of unpreventable accidents. In fact, many injuries are predictable and preventable. As noted previously, the leading cause of death among young adults is injury. Injuries—both unintentional and intentional—are due to a variety of causes, such as motor vehicle crashes, firearms, poisoning, suffocation, falls, fires, and drowning. The majority are related to alcohol or drugs. Many accidents could be prevented or minimized by taking standard precautions such as using seat belts and wearing helmets and safety glasses. Violence is sometimes a factor in an injury as well. Date rape, spousal abuse, gang violence, and the mass murders at Virginia Tech in 2007 are all examples, from the more common to the rare. None are acceptable. Violence can be reduced by identifying potential and actual perpetuators and intervening with community-based counseling and enforcement as appropriate. Consider injury and violence issues as you study the chapters on drugs, sexuality, stress, mental disorders, and personal health care.

For public health indicator 8, the goal is to promote health for all through a healthy environment. Environmental quality encompasses all aspects of health, disease, and injury that are determined or influenced by the environment. Examples include preventing or managing exposures to hazardous agents (biological, chemical, physical) in the air, water, soil, and food, as well as minimizing the unhealthy effects of the broader physical and social environment (housing, land use, transportation, industry, agriculture). As noted earlier, protecting the environment in which we live has long been a mainstay of public health practice. Ensuring clean air and safe supplies of food and water along with preventing and controlling hazardous waste continue to be important priorities.

Global environmental health issues also need to be faced. For instance, the effects of pathogens (disease-causing microbes) on food supplies and health are an increasing concern as world markets and international travel continue to expand. This concern includes bioterrorism. A second concern is the impact of overpopulation and related environmental change on health. Can planetary overload and environmental degradation be averted by controlling population growth and managing environmental resources? Is multinational cooperation possible? Although it may be difficult to think of ourselves as members of a global community, it is, in fact, becoming more of a reality every day and warrants our attention and action. Consider issues of environmental health as you read the chapters on diet, cancers, infections, and health care.

PROSPECTS FOR THE 21ST CENTURY

Descriptions of today's achievements in science, technology, and medicine read like the science fiction of your grandparents' generation. What medical advances are on the horizon over the next decade? And, importantly, what are the implications for such progress? Selected health trends associated with key scientific concepts provide examples of what the future holds:

- Based on human genome research, the ability to screen for genetically based diseases and to tailor interventions will be greatly expanded.

Issues associated with genetic counseling, patient privacy, and insurability will continue to be debated.

- Major advances will continue to be made in noninvasive medical imaging designed to screen for and diagnose cancers, heart disease, and neurological disorders such as depression and Alzheimer's disease. These sophisticated scanners will be faster, more accurate, and less burdensome on patients.
- The concept of racial blending will begin to replace the traditional racial-categories paradigm. Reducing health disparities among groups will no longer be based on race per se, but rather on economic, educational, and cultural factors.
- A grand melding of molecular biology, genetic engineering, and nanotechnology will strengthen the drug discovery and delivery process. At huge expense, pharmacological research will develop drugs to treat every major disease.
- Advances in biomedical engineering will yield a new generation of tissue and organ replacements and improve the transplantation process. Growing and harvesting tissues in the laboratory will become a reality.

The examples listed above give a sense of the wondrous medical advances that are being made. Yet, such scientific and technological developments must be seriously considered and debated in light of ethical, social, and economic implications and the development of public policy.

Our health will continue to be influenced by a wide array of scientific advances, public health goals, changing societal expectations, and new and revised governmental policies. Yet, at the level of the individual and the family, it's ironic that the greatest potential benefit for the future health of Americans is not biomedical research. Rather, as prominent scientific and medical experts increasingly agree, the greatest promise for improved health lies with preventive medicine and a focus on understanding health as a consequence of human behavior.

✓ **NEED TO KNOW**

Over the past century, tremendous gains have been made in the average lifespan and quality of life for Americans due largely to major advances in public health, drug discovery, and medical technology. Today the major causes of death are chronic diseases, not infectious diseases. Chronic diseases—such as heart disease, cancer, and diabetes (type 2)—are strongly tied to how we chose to live, to our routine daily habits. The nation's high-priority health issues are summarized in the 10 leading health indicators of *Healthy People 2010*. We need to remain mindful that technology, advertising, and the built environment have both positive and negative influences on our health.

Personal health texts focus primarily on knowledge and secondarily on contextual factors that influence our views and behaviors. However, a reminder is apropos—*knowledge by itself does not assure positive decision making*. If it did, we would not see doctors and nurses who smoke or nutritionists who are overweight. Attitudes, beliefs, and values as well as knowledge underlie our decisions about health. This combination of influences makes it unlikely that a single factor is the basis of any given health decision. How can knowledge be separated from attitudes? Or attitudes from values? Decision making is clearly dependent on multiple factors.

The presentation of content is never done in a vacuum. Attitudes, beliefs, and values are shaped by our environment. The influence of family, friends, school, workplace, the media, and societal customs should be recognized. Both formal and informal learning occur within these social and societal contexts. No individual among us makes decisions that are truly independent of all others and the society in which we live. The process by which we learn a new behavior or modify a current one is multifaceted. An appreciation of this from the onset will serve you well.

Many of us have good intentions about changing an unhealthy habit (e.g., stopping smoking) or adopting a healthier behavior (e.g., eating more fruits and vegetables). The challenge is *how* to do it. As pointed out, our behaviors are complex, and from personal experience we know habits are not changed easily. So if we wish to change a behavior, we need a well-grounded plan. But before we can make a plan, we must first have an understanding of how people change.

To better understand health habits, psychologists have developed **health behavior theories** to explain individual behavior change. Briefly reviewing a few selected theories can be instructive because each theory takes a different approach to explaining the why and how about a particular behavior change. Seeing the components of a behavior and the logic that connects them can provide insights to our own behaviors. Three of the most practical theories are social cognitive theory, the health belief model, and the stages of change model. A brief overview of each theory is presented; more complete explanations are available in the National Cancer Institute's online booklet *Theory at a Glance* (for the URL, see "Web Site Resources" at the end of this chapter). These behavior-change theories will be referred to from time to time throughout the *Concise Guide* to illustrate their use in formulating plans for translating good intentions into action.

A **health behavior theory** is a conceptual framework of key factors or variables hypothesized to influence health behavior. An established theory is logical, supported by evidence, and underpins behavior change plans and strategies.

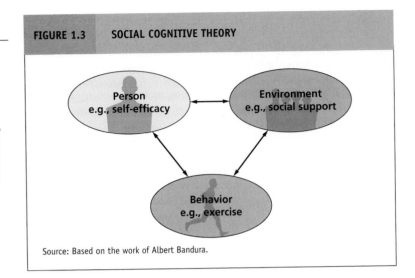

FIGURE 1.3   SOCIAL COGNITIVE THEORY

Source: Based on the work of Albert Bandura.

SOCIAL COGNITIVE THEORY

Albert Bandura's social cognitive theory is based on the principle that behavior is dynamic, depending on individual and environmental factors, all of which influence each other simultaneously. As illustrated in Figure 1.3, there is an ongoing interaction among a person's characteristics (biological, psychological, experiential), the environment within which the behavior is performed (social influences, physical environment, societal norms), and the specific behavior's characteristics.

A change in one component of the model will affect the others. To see how this works, let's use exercise as a behavior we wish to increase (target behavior). A personal characteristic such as confidence in being able to exercise for 30 minutes on a treadmill (an example of self-efficacy) will influence whether the person does, in fact, perform that behavior. Characteristics of the environment include available facilities (e.g., fitness center or exercise equipment) and associated factors such as affordability, convenience, and safety. The environment also includes the social environment (e.g., the degree to which family and friends encourage and support the person's new exercise routine). Finally, the positive and negative characteristics of the behavior itself must be considered (e.g., whether the exercise was invigorating, challenging, and completed with a sense of accomplishment or exhausting, boring, and frustrating).

Social cognitive theory holds that the interactions among the individual, the environment, and the specific behavior are subtle and complex, but it provides a framework for understanding them. This ecological approach attempts to encompass all possible determinants of health behavior for individuals in their everyday lives. A key point is that success in changing a health behavior is just not a matter of self-determination. In addition to intention and commitment, an awareness of other potential intervening factors is necessary.

HEALTH BELIEF MODEL

Irwin Rosenstock's health belief model, one of the first theories of health behavior, was developed to understand why so few people participated in health screening programs such as chest X-rays to screen for tuberculosis (in the 1950s) or mammograms for breast cancer. The hypothesis was that many people hold mistaken beliefs about the disease or the screening process and that this keeps them from taking advantage of beneficial medical screening. Researchers wanted to understand what factors were encouraging or discouraging people from participating in screening programs.

In the current version of the health belief model, five factors appear to be central in influencing people's decisions about whether to take action to prevent, screen for, or manage a medical condition (see Figure 1.4). The model predicts that individuals will take action if they perceive themselves to be susceptible (first factor) and if they believe that the condition will have potentially serious consequences (second factor)—these two beliefs become the perceived threat. In addition, they believe a successful course of action to reduce susceptibility or minimize consequences is available (third factor) and that the benefits of taking action outweigh the barriers (fourth factor)—this translates into a belief in a positive outcome. Other variables that can influence the perceived threat and outcome expectation

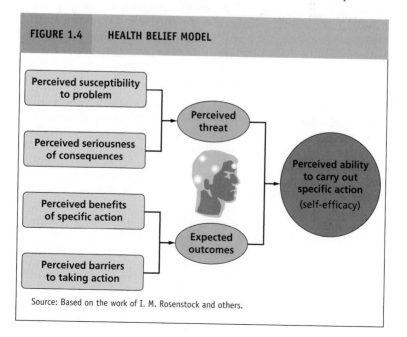

FIGURE 1.4   HEALTH BELIEF MODEL

- Perceived susceptibility to problem
- Perceived seriousness of consequences
- Perceived benefits of specific action
- Perceived barriers to taking action

Perceived threat

Expected outcomes

Perceived ability to carry out specific action (self-efficacy)

Source: Based on the work of I. M. Rosenstock and others.

include cues to action (media campaigns, symptoms of the condition), personal characteristics (personality, age, gender, ethnicity), and social circumstances (education, income). The fifth key factor is one's confidence in his or her ability to take appropriate action and to follow through. This is the self-efficacy concept borrowed from Bandura.

The health belief model has been applied to prevent the spread of HIV/AIDS. For this disease, the model predicts with some success that individuals would be more likely to practice safe sex if they believe that they are at risk of HIV infection, that the consequences of the infection are serious, that safe sex practices (e.g., condom use) are effective in reducing the risk of infection, that the benefits of safe sex practices outweigh the potential costs and barriers, and that they are confident in their ability to actually follow safe sex practices. This model provides a framework for individuals, health care workers, and educators to use in understanding and intervening in the spread of the disease.

STAGES OF CHANGE MODEL

James Prochaska and Carlo DiClemente's stages of change model—technically known as the transtheoretical model—is often integrated with other theories (hence *trans-*, or across, theories). The central premise is that behavior change is a process, not an event, and that individuals have varying levels of motivation or readiness to change. For most health behaviors, there appear to be five stages of change: 1) pre-contemplation—not thinking about change, 2) contemplation—thinking about change, 3) preparation—making small changes toward the desired behavior, 4) action—actually engaging in the desired behavior, and 5) maintenance—sustaining the new behavior over a prolonged period (refer to Figure 1.5). The model predicts that individuals progress through these stages, but it also recognizes that setbacks occur. People can and do relapse to previous stages. This is accepted as a normal part of the change process.

The stages of change model was initially developed as a framework to understand smoking cessation programs. Over the years, the model has been adapted and used with a number of other health behaviors including eating and physical activity. The conceptual appeal of the stages of change model is that specific behavior-change strategies can be matched to specific stages. The type of information, counseling, incentives, or reinforcement can be tailored to an individual's level of readiness or motivation (stage of change). Time frames may be associated with specific stages; for example, the "action stage" typically refers to the first six months of change, and the "maintenance stage" refers to continuing the behavior beyond six months. After several years, the target behavior becomes an established habit and part of one's lifestyle.

Across many different behavior-change theories, four factors appear to be necessary for successful change to occur: a knowledge or awareness of the benefit of the change, the motivation to take action, the opportunity in

FIGURE 1.5   STAGES OF CHANGE MODEL

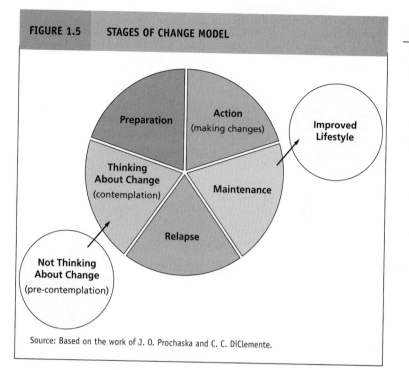

Source: Based on the work of J. O. Prochaska and C. C. DiClemente.

terms of resources and time, and the necessary behavioral skills. Your personal health course and the *Concise Guide* are primarily oriented toward increasing knowledge. Yet, we are also committed to assisting you in developing the requisite skill set (planning, organizational, and behavior-specific skills) to modify or adopt a target behavior. Increased motivation may be a byproduct of the class experience as well. When thinking about changing a health behavior, use the behavior-change models and keep the four common factors in mind: knowledge, motivation, opportunity, and skills.

✓ NEED TO KNOW

Behavior change is a complex process and often difficult to sustain. Developing healthy behaviors sometimes means competing against ingrained social and environmental practices. Information by itself is typically not enough. The benefits of behavior change must be compelling and outweigh the barriers. Three widely-used health behavior models are social cognitive theory, the health belief model, and the stages of change model. Across models, four factors appear to be necessary for successful behavior change: knowledge, motivation, opportunity, and skills. Use conceptual frameworks and these four factors to guide you in making healthful lifestyle changes.

Web Site Resources

Ad Council
www.adcouncil.org
Adbusters
http://adbusters.org
Centers for Disease Control and Prevention (CDC)
www.cdc.gov/
Health Literacy (National Library of Medicine, NIH)
http://nnlm.gov/outreach/consumer/hlthlit.html
Healthfinder.gov
www.healthfinder.gov
Healthy People 2010
www.healthypeople.gov
How Stuff Works: Health
http://health.howstuffworks.com/
Issues in Science and Technology
www.issues.org/issues/about.html
Media Literacy
www1.medialiteracy.com
MedlinePlus
http://medlineplus.gov
Mayo Clinic
www.mayoclinic.com
Office of Minority Health (U.S. Department of Health and
Human Services)
www.omhrc.gov
Resources for Health Consumers (Medical Library Association)
www.mlanet.org/resources/consumr_index.html
Theory at a Glance (National Cancer Institute, NIH)
www.nci.nih.gov/PDF/481f5d53-63df-41bc-bfaf-5aa48ee1da4d/
TAAG3.pdf
U.S. Census Bureau
www.census.gov

Knowing the Language

chronic disease
epidemiology
health
health behavior theory
health literacy

health risk
infectious disease
quality of life
relative risk

1. Contrast the treatment model and the wellness model of health.
2. What is meant by *health literacy*? What are the underlying factors that contribute to a person's health literacy?
3. What is epidemiology? Contrast the terms *absolute risk* and *relative risk*. As a young adult, what are your greatest risks for injury/illness and death?
4. Contrast the terms *infectious disease* and *chronic disease*. What is meant by the term *lifestyle disease*? What are the leading *actual* causes of disease in the United States?
5. Describe two behavior change theories and how they could be used to help a person improve a health behavior.

Exploring Ideas

1. Why should health be thought of as having different dimensions? How can this be helpful in improving our health or achieving personal goals?
2. To what degree do you have control over your current quality of life? Is it determined by your conscious decision making or by factors beyond your control?
3. How should one go about gathering information on a health topic? Select a health question, investigate it, and report on the process and your findings.

Selected References

American Academy of Pediatrics, Committee on Public Education. Children, adolescents, and television. *Pediatrics* 107: 423–426, 2001.

American Cancer Society. Cancer Facts & Figures 2007
www.cancer.org

American College Health Association. ACHA–National College Health Assessment (NCHA) Data: Publications and Reports, 2000–2007.
www.acha-ncha.org/pubs_rpts.html

Atlanta Journal Constitution. Lizzie Brown, 111, calm, kind, centenarian. Obituary section, January 6, 2003.

Bandura A. Self-efficacy: Toward a unifying theory of behavior change. *Psychological Reviews* 84: 191–215, 1977.

Bandura A. *Self-efficacy: The Exercise of Control.* New York: W. H. Freeman, 1997.

Centers for Disease Control and Prevention (CDC). *Health, United States, 2007.*
www.cdc.gov/nchs/hus.htm

CDC. Table 10: Number of deaths from 113 selected causes by age, 2005. **www.disastercenter.com/cdc/Age%20of%20Deaths%20113%20 Causes%202005.html**

Corbett S. The long road from Sudan to America. *The New York Times*, April 1, 2001.

Glanz K, Rimer BK, Lewis FM. *Health Behavior and Health Education: Theory, Research, and Practice* (3rd ed.). San Francisco: Jossey-Bass, 2002.

Health Promotion Advocates. Definition of health promotion. **http://healthpromotionadvocates.org/resources/definitions.htm/**

Institute of Medicine (IOM). *Health Literacy: A Prescription to End Confusion.* Washington, DC: National Academies Press, 2004. **www.iom.edu/report.asp?id=19723**

McMichael AJ. *Planetary Overload: Global Environmental Change and the Health of the Human Species.* New York: Cambridge University Press, 1993.

Medical Library Association. "Top Ten" Most Useful Consumer Health Websites. **www.mlanet.org/resources/userguide.html#5**

Morbidity & Mortality Weekly Report (MMWR). Ten great public health achievements—United States, 1900–1999. *MMWR:* 48 (12): 241–243, 1999.

MMWR. Achievements in public health, 1900–1999: Healthier mothers and babies. *MMWR:* 48 (38): 849–858, 1999.

Mokdad AH, Marks JS, Stroup DF et al. Actual causes of death in the United States, 2000. *JAMA* 291 (10): 1238–1245, 2004.

National Institutes of Health (NIH). Understanding risk. *Word on Health.* April 2004. **www.nih.gov/news/WordonHealth/apr2004/risk.htm#ask**

Prochaska JO, DiClemente CC. Stages and processes of self-change of smoking: toward an integrated model of change. *Journal of Consulting and Clinical Psychology* 51: 390–395, 1983.

Prochaska JO, DiClemente CC, Norcross JC. In search of how people change: Applications to addictive behaviors. *American Psychologist* 47 (9): 1102–1114, 1992.

Rauscher FH, Shaw GL, Ky KN. Music and spatial task performance. *Nature* 365: 611, 1993.

Rimer BK, Glanz K. *Theory at a Glance: A Guide for Health Promotion Practice* (2nd ed.). National Cancer Institute, National Institutes of Health, U.S. Department of Health & Human Services. Washington, DC: NIH, 2005.

Ropeik D, Gray G. *Risk.* Boston: Houghton Mifflin, 2002.

Rosenstock IM. Historical origins of the health belief model. *Health Education Monographs* 2: 328–335, 1974.

Rosenstock IM, Strecher VJ, Becker MH. Social learning theory and the health belief model. *Health Education Quarterly* 15 (2):175–183, 1988.

Schwartz B. *The Paradox of Choice: Why More Is Less.* New York: HarperCollins, 2004.

U.S. Census Bureau. **www.census.gov**

World Health Organization (WHO). Definition of health. **www.who.int/suggestions/faq/en/index.html**

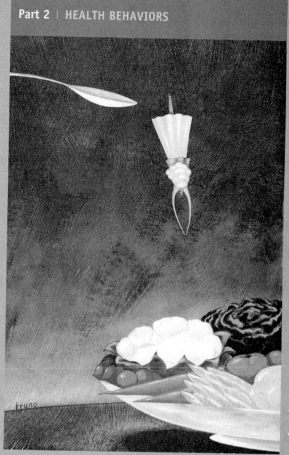

It's difficult to think
anything but pleasant
thoughts while eating
a homegrown tomato.

— LEWIS GRIZZARD

Chapter 2

CHOOSE A HEALTHY DIET

In Chapter 2 we discuss food, a subject near and dear to all.
We present the basic vocabulary of nutrition and current recommendations for a healthy diet, and we discuss steps and strategies to improve our eating habits. We give special attention to
the topic of weight control because it is of particular interest
and relevance. Our aim is to separate the science from the
advertising and show you how to navigate the gray areas.

A CENTURY AGO, the majority of Americans still lived on farms and raised their own food. Nearly every family had a vegetable garden and kept chickens for eggs. Working the garden and canning (and later freezing) the "produce" (vegetables and fruits) was standard practice. It was essential to stock the pantry to provide for food throughout the winter and into the spring. Many homesteads had a milk cow. Some also raised hogs or cattle for meat. Sausage and hams or beef cuts were bartered with neighbors in exchange for other goods. Grains were taken to a central stone mill to be ground into flour. The food supply was direct and simple; food was minimally processed. Agribusiness and the food industry were in their infancy.

Life was physically demanding, whether working on the farm or in a mill, mine, or factory. And the way people ate reflected the physical demands of how they lived. Breakfast, a hearty hot meal, included meat and eggs, not cereal out of a box. Dinner—the midday meal—was the largest meal of the day, with meats, vegetables, and bread or biscuits that were made from scratch every day. Lunch was a meal that evolved in the cities. The evening meal, known as supper, was a lighter meal, often simply leftovers from dinner.

Unlike today, an ample food supply was not a given. There were good years and lean years, depending on the weather, crop infestations, natural disasters, and human and animal epidemics. A plentiful harvest was celebrated, and hard times were endured. Think of the changes that your great-grandparents lived through and how those changes affected their eating patterns. Examples include transitioning from rural to city life, the development of refrigeration and modern appliances, new job opportunities not dependent on manual labor, and the ever-expanding grocery store.

Over the past century, dramatic changes have occurred in nearly every aspect of American life, including how and what we eat. Moreover, thanks to the scientific research of the past 30 to 40 years, we have an excellent understanding of the connections between nutrition and health. Without question, our food resources and nutrition knowledge are far more extensive than they were only a few generations ago. By considering the historical perspective, you can better appreciate our current food environment and understand the origins of the diet-related health challenges we now face. Your generation can share in the bounty of food choices available today but must also face pressing contemporary issues such as obesity, eating disorders, and dietary supplements. Keep this in mind as you study the material presented in this chapter and learn how to choose a healthy diet.

➤ Nutrition Basics

Nutrition is the science of food and how the body uses it in health and disease. A nutrient is simply a substance found in food that is used by the body to support normal growth, maintenance, and repair. The six nutrient classes are carbohydrates, fats, protein, vitamins, minerals, and water. Nutrients can be broadly categorized based on the quantity that should be consumed. The **macronutrients**—carbohydrates, fats, protein, and water—are the main constituents of our food and form the bulk of what we eat every day. In contrast, the **micronutrients**—vitamins and minerals—are needed only in small quantities, and many are not required daily. Micronutrients occur naturally in many of our unprocessed foods such as fruits, vegetables, and whole grains. Nutrients are also categorized based on whether they are energy sources. Carbohydrates, fats, and protein are the energy nutrients. Vitamins, minerals, and water do not yield energy, but their presence in the body is necessary to aid in the proper use of the energy nutrients. Consequently, vitamins, minerals, and water are known as regulatory nutrients.

From a biological perspective, good nutrition is about providing both the right blend of nutrients and adequate fuel (energy) for the body's many needs. Balancing energy intake with energy expenditure is fundamental to maintaining a healthy weight. Weight control is a hotly debated and controversial topic that we address later in this chapter. In terms of basic nutrition, energy density and recommended energy intake by macronutrient are summarized in Table 2.1. At 9 Cal (Calories or kilocalories) per gram, fats have more than twice the energy (per weight) of carbohydrates and protein, which yield 4 Cal per gram. As we discuss carbohydrates, fats, and protein in turn, refer back to Table 2.1 to see what the recommended relative contributions should be.

For the sake of clarity, a comment about energy units is warranted. The common energy unit in the United States is the **Calorie (Cal),** or **kilocalorie (kcal).** (For the curious, the rest of the world uses the kilojoule, abbreviated kj.) Technically, 1 Cal, or kcal, is the amount of heat needed to raise 1 kg of water 1° Celsius. Yes, a Calorie (with a capital "C") is the same as a kilocalorie. Both terms are widely used: food labels typically report Calories, while energy expenditure is often expressed in kilocalories. For example, a 12-oz. can of Coca-Cola contains 140 Cal, which is equivalent to the 140 kcal expended in walking 1.5 mi. To remove any confusion, our convention in the *Concise Guide* is to use only Calories (Cal) when reporting energy intake or expenditure values. Lastly, a point on documentation in this chapter: unless specifically cited otherwise, all recommendations that contain specific nutritional values or dietary intakes are based on two federal documents, either *Dietary Guidelines for Americans* (2005) or *Dietary Reference Intakes* (2006), both of which are available online.

Macronutrients are the nutrients required in the greatest amounts, namely carbohydrates, fats, protein, and water. **Micronutrients** are nutrients that are required only in small amounts, the vitamins and minerals.

Calorie (Cal), or alternately the **kilocalorie (kcal),** is the standard unit of energy used in the United States to define and describe human energy intake and energy expenditure.

TABLE 2.1 RECOMMENDED ENERGY INTAKE BY MACRONUTRIENT

		PERCENTAGE OF TOTAL DAILY CALORIES	
		TARGET*	RANGE
Carbohydrates	4 Cal per gram	55%	45–65%
	Emphasize complex carbohydrates		
	Minimize added sugars	[≤25%]	
Fats	9 Cal per gram	30%	20–35%
	Emphasize unsaturated fats		
	Minimize saturated fats	[≤10%]	
Protein	4 Cal per gram	15%	10–35%
		100%	

Based on the *Dietary Guidelines* and the *Dietary Reference Intakes.*

*Although percentages can vary within the given ranges, it is useful to have specific percentages to use as guidelines.

CARBOHYDRATES AND FIBER

The main function of **carbohydrates** is to provide energy. They are your body's main energy source, the primary fuel for your cells. Each gram of carbohydrate yields approximately 4 Cal, the same as a gram of protein. Carbohydrates should compose the largest percentage of daily caloric intake, at about 55 percent (within a range of 45–65 percent). Carbohydrates include both starches and sugars. Starches, or complex carbohydrates, are found in bread, rice, pasta, cereals, and vegetables. Sugars, or simple carbohydrates, are found in fruits, milk, and many processed foods and drinks that have added sugar, such as candy, pastries, desserts, and soft drinks.

In addition to supplying energy, complex carbohydrates and sugars from fruits and milk supply fiber, vitamins, minerals, and water. Consequently, they should be emphasized over sugars from candy, other sweets, and soft drinks. In addition, your body absorbs complex carbohydrates more slowly than it absorbs simple sugars, providing more energy for a longer period. Remember that snacks and desserts with added sugar, such as candies, cakes, cookies, doughnuts, fruit drinks, and ice cream, provide many calories but offer negligible amounts of other nutrients. That is why typical junk foods are often referred to as having "empty calories," or as having low nutrient density. In the United States, soft drinks are the top source of added sugars.

Carbohydrates are organic compounds (i.e., they contain carbon, oxygen, hydrogen) divided into two types—simple and complex; they are generally known as sugars and starches.

Fiber—also referred to as roughage—is the indigestible part of plant-based foods. Nutritionists divide fiber into two types: soluble and insoluble. Soluble fiber may improve your cholesterol and blood sugar (glucose) levels. It's found in oats, dried beans, and some fruits. Insoluble fiber adds bulk to your stool and helps prevent constipation. It also reduces your risk of colorectal cancer. It's found mainly in vegetables, whole grains, and wheat bran. The average American consumes only 10 to 15 g (grams) of total fiber per day. Federal guidelines recommend 25 g per day for women and 38 g per day for men.

What's the best way to increase fiber? Eat a variety of whole grains, vegetables, legumes (peas, beans, lentils), and fruits. When buying bread, look for the word *whole* next to the name of the grain in the list of ingredients (e.g., whole wheat). Select bread with at least 3 g of fiber per slice and cereals with 3 g or more of fiber per serving. Try whole-wheat pasta—it typically has three times the amount of fiber as regular pasta.

To help encourage Americans to eat a variety of fruits and vegetables every day, the Centers for Disease Control and Prevention (CDC) and the Produce for Better Health Foundation administer an online public health initiative called Fruits & Veggies—More Matters (**www.fruitsandveggiesmatter .gov**). This Web page calculates how many fruits and vegetables you need and provides tips for adding more servings into your daily routine. As a general guide, most Americans should have five or more servings of fruits and vegetables every day.

FATS AND CHOLESTEROL

Fats, or lipids, in the diet serve several purposes. They are the most concentrated energy source, yielding about 9 Cal per gram, more than twice that of carbohydrate or protein. Fats should constitute about 30 percent or less of total calories consumed each day (range: 20–35 percent). Fats satisfy hunger because of their slow absorption rate from the digestive system. Fats also play a role in many other functions, such as the maintenance and function of cell membranes and the absorption of the four fat-soluble vitamins (A, D, E, and K).

It is extremely important to understand the different kinds of dietary fats. Saturated fats are generally from animal sources such as meat, poultry, eggs, and dairy products (butter, cream, whole milk, cheese). Yet palm and coconut oils, which come from plants, are also saturated fats. Saturated fats are solid at room temperature. Diets high in saturated fats elevate blood cholesterol levels and risk of cardiovascular disease. *Trans* fats, which are vegetable oils chemically converted to a solid form, also raise blood cholesterol and should be minimized (refer to "Breaking It

Fats, or lipids, are organic compounds that provide the most concentrated source of calories in a diet. Saturated fats are found primarily in animal products, and unsaturated fats come from plants.

Down" for the full story). No more than 10 percent of total calories should come from saturated fats and *trans* fats.

Remember though, all fats do not get the thumbs down. Unsaturated fats are actually good for us. These fats are mainly plant-based and are liquid at room temperature. Polyunsaturated fats like corn, safflower, and sunflower oils are healthy choices. And monounsaturated fats like olive, peanut, and canola oils are even better, being the most healthful of the unsaturated fats. Also, substantial evidence indicates that omega-3 fatty acids—found in certain types of fish, such as salmon—bestow a variety of benefits, particularly to the maintenance of heart and tissue health.

Breaking It Down *Trans Fats— From Healthy to Harmful*

The unusual story of *trans* fats deserves mention in any discussion of dietary fats. *Trans* fats are produced when unsaturated oils are partially hydrogenated (through the addition of hydrogen), a process that converts vegetable oils to more solid forms. This conversion increases shelf life and flavor stability. In 1911 Procter & Gamble introduced Crisco, a product of hydrogenation. It was the first solidified shortening product made entirely of vegetable oil. Crisco provided an economical alternative to lard (animal fat) and butter. In the 1940s stick margarines were introduced, followed by tub margarines and vegetable oil spreads in the 1960s. With a growing awareness of the health risks of saturated fats, the scientific community promoted the use of margarine—an unsaturated fat—as the healthy alternative to butter. The resulting increase in the use of *trans* fats occurred not only in our kitchens but also in restaurants and the fast-food and baking industries as hydrogenated vegetable oils replaced lard.

At that time, there was no way to know that the process of hydrogenation chemically altered vegetable oil in a detrimental way. Yet, by the 1990s, substantial evidence had come to light showing that *trans* fats are actually as harmful (or even more harmful) in increasing blood cholesterol levels as the saturated fats they were meant to replace. In recent years, the challenge has been to update the American consumer. In 2003, after further study and careful review, the Food and Drug Administration (FDA) mandated that by 2006 all food labels must report the amount of *trans* fats as well as saturated and unsaturated fats. Many food companies have already reduced or eliminated *trans* fats in their products. The bottom line: check the food labels and eat as few *trans* fats as possible.

So we have come full circle. Vegetable shortening and margarine (*trans* fats from hydrogenation) were initially hailed as the healthy option to lard and butter and widely accepted by the public. In the ensuing years, the effects of eating the new *trans* fats were studied, and they were found to be as dangerous as or worse than animal-based fats. What's the lesson? Creating new food products can have both upsides and downsides, and sometimes only time will reveal them.

Cholesterol is a fatlike substance found throughout cells of the body. It is an essential substance that the body can obtain through diet or by production in the liver. Dietary intake should be less than 300 mg per day. All animal fats contain cholesterol, whereas fats from plant sources do not. Concentrated sources include eggs yolks (about 200 mg per yolk) and meats (60–100 mg per 3-oz. serving). Limit cholesterol; however, don't overemphasize its importance. Focus on reducing animal fats, and in turn, you will also be minimizing dietary cholesterol. Remember that the primary dietary determinant of high blood cholesterol has been shown to be saturated fats and *trans* fats, not cholesterol.

PROTEIN

Protein, which is contained in every cell in your body, is necessary for tissue growth and maintenance. Protein is found in foods from animal and plant sources. Each gram of protein yields about 4 Cal, the same as carbohydrate. However, its role as an energy source is secondary to that of carbohydrate and fat. Poultry, seafood, meat, dairy products, legumes (beans, peas, peanuts, soy products), nuts, and seeds are the richest sources of proteins. About 15 percent of total daily calories should come from protein (range, 10–35 percent). There is some evidence that a higher protein intake (20–35 percent of total calories) may be beneficial for certain individuals. As more studies are published regarding this issue, dietary advice will evolve.

The basic components of proteins are amino acids. Of the 22 amino acids used in the body, only 9 are necessary in the diet and thus are known as the essential amino acids. The body has the ability to manufacture the remaining 13. Animal protein is complete, containing all 9 essential amino acids in sufficient amounts. In contrast, plant proteins are incomplete, lacking one or more of the essential amino acids. However, different plant foods can be eaten together to supply a complete protein, such as beans with rice or peanut butter on whole-grain bread. These complementary plant-protein relationships are especially important to vegetarians.

The amount of protein your body needs depends primarily on your body size. Recommended protein intake is 0.8 g per kg of body weight per day. For example, if you weigh 154 lb. (70 kg), then you should be consuming 56 g of protein per day. Most Americans typically consume far more protein than they need. What happens to those excess calories? If your body does not need the protein, it converts and stores those extra calories as fat. A final tip: remember to choose your sources of proteins wisely. Many of the high-protein animal-based foods are also high in saturated fat and cholesterol. Emphasize meats that are lean, skinless, and nonfried, and consider obtaining some of your protein from plant sources.

Proteins are complex organic compounds made up of amino acids that perform a wide variety of functions that include serving as enzymes or structural components and signaling molecules.

Vitamins and **minerals** are found in only small quantities in our food, yet these micronutrients have multiple and diverse roles in regulating and maintaining our bodies' normal functions. Although a review of the many vitamin and mineral micronutrients is beyond the scope of the *Concise Guide*, we offer a brief overview that can set the stage for further self-directed study. Micronutrients play special roles in the prevention and treatment of common chronic diseases. For example, certain minerals are linked to particular medical conditions: among these, sodium is linked to hypertension, calcium to osteoporosis, and iron to anemia. The potential benefits of vitamins E, C, and A (beta-carotene) as antioxidants are of high interest; antioxidants counter the harmful oxidative effects of free radicals and in so doing may protect body cells from damage. Federal standards for good nutrition (technically known as Dietary Reference Intakes) are available for 13 vitamins and 15 minerals. These standards are organized by age, gender, and special conditions such as pregnancy. Comprehensive and detailed information on the micronutrients, including the federal standards, as well as recommendations on the macronutrients are pro-vided by the Food and Nutrition Board of the Institute of Medicine **(www .iom.edu/CMS/3788.aspx).**

WATER

Water is the most essential nutrient. For many Americans though, water could just as well be called the forgotten nutrient as sweetened beverages dominate everyday fluid consumption patterns. People can ingest too few (or none) of the other nutrients for days or weeks before problems arise—not so with water. Insufficient water intake can result in symp-toms ranging from lethargy to disorientation to death, depending on the degree of dehydration. Loss of water occurs primarily through urination, perspiration, and respiration (water vapor in the air we breathe out).

Women who appear to be adequately hydrated consume an average of about 90 oz. (2.7 liters)—from all beverages and foods—each day, while men average about 125 oz. (3.7 liters) daily. About 80 percent of people's total water intake comes from drinking water and beverages—including caffeinated drinks—and the other 20 percent comes from food. Based on these estimates, women should be drinking about nine 8-ounce glasses of water and beverages per day (72 oz.), and men about 12–13 glasses (100 oz.). Due attention should be given to *what* we are drinking, however. The

---

Vitamins are a class of diverse organic substances that occur in many foods in small amounts and are necessary in trace amounts for the normal metabolic functioning of the body. **Minerals** are a group of inorganic elements that are es-sential to the life processes and are obtained through the foods and beverages we consume.

Beverage Guidance Panel reports that about 50 percent of Americans' excess calories come from sweetened (nondiet) beverages (Popkin et al., 2006). The panel recommends that water be the drink of choice and consumption of sweetened beverages be reduced.

Individual water needs may vary widely with body size, environmental conditions, and exercise patterns. A more reliable measure for checking hydratation is to weigh every morning to insure that fluids consumed in the hours following prolonged heat exposure or exercise have restored (water) weight. Individuals can easily lose 1–3 percent of their body weight after several hours of exertion in the heat. Under these conditions, thirst alone may not be a good indicator of dehydration. Other measures for monitoring hydration are recommended: for example, checking body weight on a daily basis to insure (water) weight is regained by drinking plenty of fluids in the hours following prolonged heat exposure or exercise. For more information, see "Dietary water and sodium requirements for active adults" (Kenney, 2004).

✔ **NEED TO KNOW**

Nutrition is about understanding what types and how much food a person needs. To appreciate and apply nutrition principles, we must know that nutrients are composed of macronutrients (carbohydrates, fats, proteins, water) and micronutrients (vitamins, minerals), and we must learn the basics about each type of nutrient. This fundamental knowledge serves as the foundation for making wise decisions about what we eat.

➤ Recommendations for Healthy Eating

The American public is under siege from an information blitz about nutrition and food. And much of the news is bleak. Obesity has become a major public health problem. As a society we eat too much and exercise too little. Many of the foods we eat are high in saturated fat, low in fiber, and stripped of naturally occurring vitamins and minerals. We live in a fast-paced, affluent society where convenience rules. Established restaurants regularly revamp menus, and new restaurants launch every day. Supermarkets are open round-the-clock. New food products are released on a regular basis. Today's large supermarkets carry over 200 fruits and vegetables in their fresh produce sections and stock over 20,000 items on their shelves. In our food and nutrition landscape, the choices are plentiful, affordable, and ever changing.

The challenge is to make smart choices and establish healthful habits. Doing so requires sorting the marketing from the science, but it can be difficult because the two are blended together. Should we be surprised that the average consumer is confused about nutrition issues? Yet, since the connection between what we eat and how we feel and function is indisputable, it's clearly worth the effort to be informed and to stay informed.

As part of public health policy, the federal government disseminates science-based dietary guidelines to aid the American consumer. Let's apply the basic nutrition terms and concepts reviewed in the previous section to the current guidelines. And let's look below the surface. The dietary guidelines deserve more than a superficial glance. These are not simply a list of "rules" to eat by. As self-directed learners, our aim is to develop a working knowledge of the recommendations—not only the *what* but also the *why* and the *how*.

Primarily through the U.S. Department of Agriculture (USDA), the government has provided nutrition information and advice to Americans for over a century. In 1994 the USDA bolstered its role in this regard by creating the Center for Nutrition Policy and Promotion. The formal establishment of the center came at a time when the American public was becoming increasingly aware of the importance of diet yet was receiving conflicting nutrition messages. Thus, a major role of the center is to serve as a trusted source to assure the public that nutrition information disseminated by USDA is based on sound research and analysis. At its Web site—**www.cnpp.usda.gov/**—links are provided to the most recent *Dietary Guidelines for Americans* (Department of Health and Human Services, 2005) and the consumer-oriented MyPyramid food guidance system (USDA, 2005). Become familiar with both.

2005 DIETARY GUIDELINES FOR AMERICANS

The *Dietary Guidelines for Americans* are the cornerstone of federal nutrition policy and nutrition education activities. They are jointly issued by the U.S. Department of Health and Human Services (HHS) and the USDA. They were first released in 1980 and are updated every five years. The following questions and answers provide an overview of the *Dietary Guidelines* and insight on how they were developed. Key recommendations are then highlighted.

What Are the Dietary Guidelines?

The *Dietary Guidelines* are based on what experts have determined to be the best scientific knowledge about diet, physical activity, and other issues related to what we should eat and how much physical activity we need. The *Dietary Guidelines* are designed to help Americans choose diets that meet nutrient requirements, promote health, support active lives, and reduce risks of chronic disease.

Why Are the Dietary Guidelines Important?

The *Dietary Guidelines* allow government agencies to speak with one voice when presenting advice about proper dietary habits for healthy Americans. All federal dietary guidance for the public must be consistent with the *Dietary Guidelines*. They also influence the direction of government nutrition programs, including research, labeling, and promotion.

Health & the Media The Milk Mustache Ad Campaign

Launched in 1996, the national "Got milk?" campaign, portraying celebrities wearing milk mustaches, has been one of the most enjoyed and recognized of any food product ad campaign. The print ads have featured dozens of celebrities over the years, each with a catchy story line linking his or her persona with the health benefits of drinking milk. Tiger Woods, Spike Lee, Sheryl Crow, Jackie Chan, and Kermit the Frog are a few of the notables who have posed with a contented look, sporting the "milk mustache." This one features *Jeopardy* game show host Alex Trebek. This ad campaign, which blends celebrity, creativity, and flair, has become a part of American pop culture. Funded by America's milk processors and dairy farmers, the milk mustache ads continue today. Who has been the latest athlete or entertainer urging us to drink our milk?

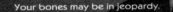

Your bones may be in jeopardy.

One in five osteoporosis victims is male. Luckily, fat free milk has the calcium bones need to help beat it. Beating your Harvard Ph.D. opponents? Well, that's another story.

got milk?

The *Dietary Guidelines* were prepared in a three-stage process. In the first, an independent advisory committee of eminent scientists compiled a report based on the best available evidence. In the second, government scientists and officials reviewed the advisory committee's report and, based on the report and agency and public comments, developed the *Dietary Guidelines*. In the third stage, health communication specialists translated the *Dietary Guidelines* into meaningful messages for the public and educators. This resulted in the MyPyramid Guide, which is presented in the next section.

What Are the Key Recommendations of the 2005 Dietary Guidelines?

The *Dietary Guidelines* make recommendations to the public in nine different areas. Five of these involve the specific selection of some foods and the moderation or avoidance of others.

Recommendations regarding **fats:**

- Consume less than 10 percent of calories from saturated fats and less than 300 mg/day of cholesterol, and keep consumption of *trans* fats as low as possible.
- Keep total fat intake between 20 and 35 percent of calories, with most fats coming from sources of polyunsaturated and monounsaturated fats, such as fish, nuts, seeds, and vegetable oils.
- When selecting and preparing meat, poultry, dry beans, and milk or milk products, make choices that are lean, low-fat, or fat-free.
- Limit intake of fats and oils high in saturated and/or *trans* fats, and choose products low in such fats and oils.

Recommendations regarding **carbohydrates:**

- Choose fiber-rich fruits, vegetables, and whole grains often.
- Choose and prepare foods and beverages with little added sugar or other caloric sweetener.
- Reduce the incidence of dental cavities (caries) by practicing good oral hygiene and consuming sugar- and starch-containing foods and beverages less frequently.

Recommendations regarding **sodium** and **potassium:**

- Consume less than 2,300 mg (approximately 1 tsp of salt) of sodium per day.
- Choose and prepare foods with little salt. At the same time, consume potassium-rich foods, such as fruits and vegetables.

Recommendations regarding **alcohol:**

- Those who choose to drink alcoholic beverages should do so sensibly and in moderation—defined as the consumption of up to one drink per day for women and up to two drinks per day for men.
- Alcoholic beverages should not be consumed by some individuals, including those who cannot restrict their alcohol intake, women of

childbearing age who may become pregnant, pregnant and lactating women, children and adolescents, individuals taking medications that can interact with alcohol, and those with specific medical conditions.

- Alcoholic beverages should be avoided by individuals engaging in activities that require attention, skill, or coordination, such as driving or operating machinery.

Recommendations regarding **food groups to encourage:**

- Consume a sufficient amount of fruits and vegetables while staying within energy needs. Two cups of fruit and 2½ cups of vegetables per day are recommended for a reference 2,000-Calorie intake, with higher or lower amounts depending on energy expenditure.
- Choose a variety of fruits and vegetables each day. In particular, select from all five vegetable subgroups (dark green, orange, legumes, starchy vegetables, and other vegetables) several times a week.
- Consume three or more ounce-equivalents of whole-grain products per day, with the rest of the recommended grains coming from enriched or whole-grain products. In general, at least half the grains should come from whole grains.
- Consume three cups per day of fat-free or low-fat milk or equivalent milk products.

The key recommendations here are also available in interactive and visual versions via the MyPyramid guide. Other key recommendations in the *Dietary Guidelines* concern the areas of food safety, weight management, physical activity, and general nutrition. These are woven into subsequent sections in this chapter.

USDA MyPYRAMID GUIDE

The federal initiative to make the *Dietary Guidelines* consumer-friendly (the third stage of the process) resulted in a new food guidance system known as MyPyramid. Does MyPyramid replace the original Food Pyramid Guide? Yes, it does. Unveiled in 1992, the original Food Pyramid was developed with the same aim—to help Americans select healthier diets. The Food Pyramid had limitations though; for example, information about the number of servings was confusing, and the Pyramid didn't distinguish between good choices and poor choices within food groups. Although consumers became familiar with the Food Pyramid, only a small percentage of Americans actually used it in planning meals or making food choices. Overall, the impact of the Food Pyramid among the public was disappointing and spurred communication specialists to entirely rethink ways to better translate nutrition information for Americans. This led to the development of the new food guidance system, MyPyramid, which was launched in 2005.

The primary goal for developing a different approach was to better enable dietary and physical activity behavior change among consumers. MyPyramid includes a new symbol and slogan—Steps to a Healthier

FIGURE 2.1   USDA FOOD PYRAMID

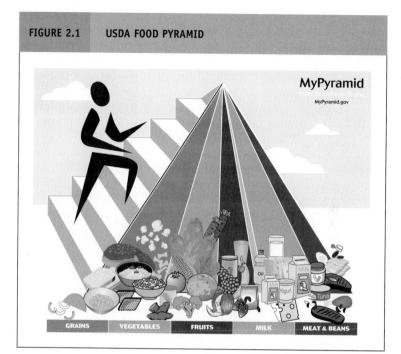

You—with explanatory messages and interactive Web-based tools. My-Pyramid highlights six points (refer to Figure 2.1 and Figure 2.2).

Activity—be physically active every day; illustrated by the person climbing the steps.

Moderation—choose foods that limit intake of saturated or *trans* fats, added sugars, cholesterol, salt, and alcohol; represented by the narrowing of each food group band from bottom to top.

Personalization—tailor a plan to your own situation; reinforced with the MyPyramid Internet address and developed using the MyPyramid Plan Web tool.

Proportionality—eat more of some foods and less of others; shown by the different widths of the food group bands.

Variety—eat foods from all food groups and subgroups; represented by the six-color band.

Gradual Improvement—aim for small, reachable goals; incremental improvement as captured in the "steps to a healthier you" slogan.

The MyPyramid symbol was designed to be simple and remind consumers to make healthy food and physical activity choices every day. Overall, it symbolizes an individualized approach to healthy eating and physical activity as captured in "one size doesn't fit all."

FIGURE 2.2   USDA FOOD PYRAMID

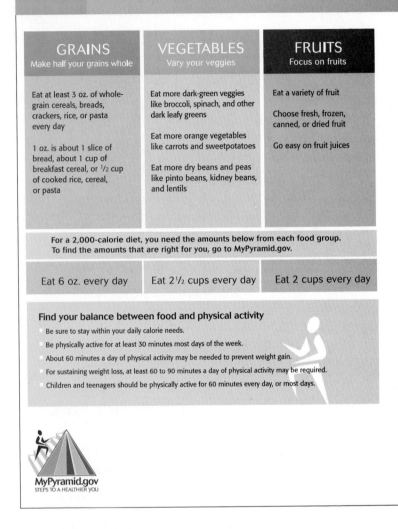

GRAINS
Make half your grains whole

VEGETABLES
Vary your veggies

FRUITS
Focus on fruits

Eat at least 3 oz. of whole-grain cereals, breads, crackers, rice, or pasta every day

1 oz. is about 1 slice of bread, about 1 cup of breakfast cereal, or ½ cup of cooked rice, cereal, or pasta

Eat more dark-green veggies like broccoli, spinach, and other dark leafy greens

Eat more orange vegetables like carrots and sweetpotatoes

Eat more dry beans and peas like pinto beans, kidney beans, and lentils

Eat a variety of fruit

Choose fresh, frozen, canned, or dried fruit

Go easy on fruit juices

For a 2,000-calorie diet, you need the amounts below from each food group. To find the amounts that are right for you, go to MyPyramid.gov.

Eat 6 oz. every day   Eat 2½ cups every day   Eat 2 cups every day

Find your balance between food and physical activity
- Be sure to stay within your daily calorie needs.
- Be physically active for at least 30 minutes most days of the week.
- About 60 minutes a day of physical activity may be needed to prevent weight gain.
- For sustaining weight loss, at least 60 to 90 minutes a day of physical activity may be required.
- Children and teenagers should be physically active for 60 minutes every day, or most days.

MyPyramid.gov
STEPS TO A HEALTHIER YOU

Two excellent resources are available to help pull everything together and answer specific questions. Inside the Pyramid is an easy-to-use, engaging Web tool that provides in-depth information on each food group (including portion sizes) in addition to many practical tips (**www.mypyramid.gov/pyramid/index.html**).

The second resource is the Food Guidance System Education Framework, which presents the primary concepts by topic—such as calories, physical activity, grains, vegetables, and so forth. This material is organized in

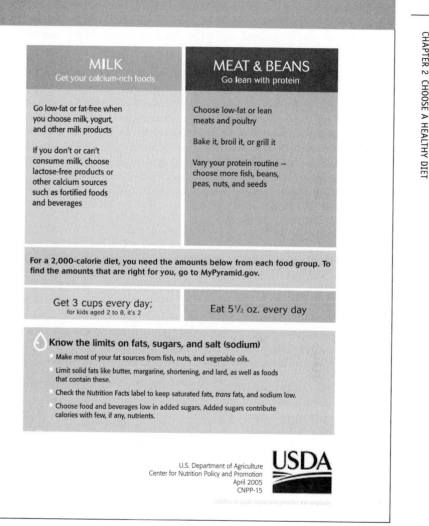

MILK
Get your calcium-rich foods

Go low-fat or fat-free when you choose milk, yogurt, and other milk products

If you don't or can't consume milk, choose lactose-free products or other calcium sources such as fortified foods and beverages

MEAT & BEANS
Go lean with protein

Choose low-fat or lean meats and poultry

Bake it, broil it, or grill it

Vary your protein routine — choose more fish, beans, peas, nuts, and seeds

For a 2,000-calorie diet, you need the amounts below from each food group. To find the amounts that are right for you, go to MyPyramid.gov.

Get 3 cups every day; for kids aged 2 to 8, it's 2

Eat 5½ oz. every day

Know the limits on fats, sugars, and salt (sodium)

- Make most of your fat sources from fish, nuts, and vegetable oils.
- Limit solid fats like butter, margarine, shortening, and lard, as well as foods that contain these.
- Check the Nutrition Facts label to keep saturated fats, *trans* fats, and sodium low.
- Choose food and beverages low in added sugars. Added sugars contribute calories with few, if any, nutrients.

U.S. Department of Agriculture
Center for Nutrition Policy and Promotion
April 2005
CNPP-15

USDA

USDA is an equal opportunity provider and employer

tables that highlight the *what, how,* and *why* for each concept **(www.mypyramid.gov/professionals/pdf_framework.html).**

Due to the enormous variability in both food preferences and food choices, learning to eat healthier—let alone maintaining the good habits we already have—can be quite a challenge. To assist us in implementing healthy changes, the MyPyramid Tracker is an online dietary assessment tool that provides a detailed analysis of one's eating behavior **(www.mypyramidtracker.gov).** After entering at least one day's worth of dietary information, you will receive a diet rating. Your rating is determined by the types and amounts of food you ate as compared to those recommended by the *Dietary Guidelines*. It calculates how many total calories you consumed and provides an analysis of the macro- and micronutrients in your diet.

To get a representative picture of your eating habits, an analysis based on at least three days (two weekdays and one weekend day) is recommended. Remember, just as with any computerized analysis, the output is only as good as the input. If you want an accurate report, become familiar with the MyPyramid Tracker features, keep detailed written records of everything you eat and drink, and enter your information carefully. This will take time and effort, but getting an objective and comprehensive report of your diet is worth the effort. Try it and see how you score. A history function allows you to track progress over time, up to one year.

Some of you may want a food plan to get you started on the path to healthier eating. The MyPyramid Plan, the final tool in the MyPyramid toolbox, contains many excellent resources that will meet this need. MyPyramid Plan provides food guidelines for 12 different calorie levels. It creates a customized food plan based on one's age, gender, and physical activity level. After you enter your information, a food plan is generated at the appropriate calorie level and will specify daily amounts from each food group and a limit for discretionary calories (fats, added sugars, alcohol). Such a plan can provide a template or guide to set short-term goals and also allow for a general comparison with current eating patterns. To generate a customized plan, go to **www.mypyramid.gov/mypyramid/index.aspx.**

In closing this section, we should point out that the recommendations from the *Dietary Guidelines* reviewed in this section are for the general adult population. Be aware that the *Dietary Guidelines* also contain recommendations for more specific populations such as infants and young children, pregnant and breastfeeding women, and older adults. (The full document—*Dietary Guidelines for Americans*—is available at **www .healthierus.gov/dietaryguidelines.**)

FOOD LABELS

Reading food labels is an important step in making sound nutritional choices. By law the "Nutrition Facts" panel on food labels is standardized to give consumers easy access to key information. A sample food label is shown in Figure 2.3. A few of the key facts should be highlighted. Note that "a serving" is defined by the manufacturer—usually by size (e.g., one cup) or pieces (e.g., three cookies). While some manufacturers use the definition of a serving as given by the *Dietary Guidelines*, many do not. What constitutes a single serving can vary, sometimes widely, from one product line to another. Consider how many servings are in the food package, then ask yourself, "How many servings am I consuming?" Is it half a serving, one serving, or more? Note that serving size is always

FIGURE 2.3   UNDERSTANDING A FOOD LABEL

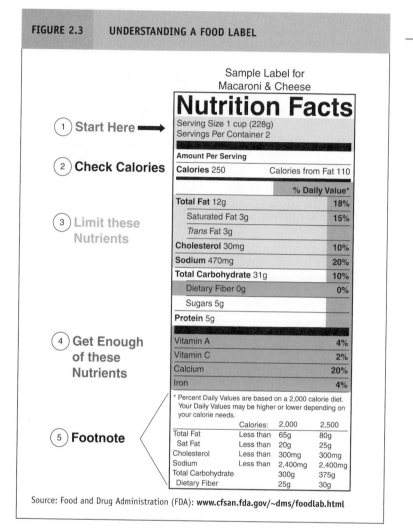

Sample Label for
Macaroni & Cheese

Nutrition Facts

(1) **Start Here** ➡

Serving Size 1 cup (228g)
Servings Per Container 2

Amount Per Serving

(2) **Check Calories**

Calories 250   Calories from Fat 110

	% Daily Value*
Total Fat 12g	**18%**
Saturated Fat 3g	**15%**
Trans Fat 3g	
Cholesterol 30mg	**10%**
Sodium 470mg	**20%**
Total Carbohydrate 31g	**10%**
Dietary Fiber 0g	**0%**
Sugars 5g	
Protein 5g	

(3) **Limit these Nutrients**

Vitamin A	**4%**
Vitamin C	**2%**
Calcium	**20%**
Iron	**4%**

(4) **Get Enough of these Nutrients**

* Percent Daily Values are based on a 2,000 calorie diet.
Your Daily Values may be higher or lower depending on
your calorie needs.

	Calories:	2,000	2,500
Total Fat	Less than	65g	80g
Sat Fat	Less than	20g	25g
Cholesterol	Less than	300mg	300mg
Sodium	Less than	2,400mg	2,400mg
Total Carbohydrate		300g	375g
Dietary Fiber		25g	30g

(5) **Footnote**

Source: Food and Drug Administration (FDA): **www.cfsan.fda.gov/~dms/foodlab.html**

listed first, followed by the calories. In the calorie line (point 2), the fat percentage of the product can be calculated by simply dividing the calories from fat by the total calories. In this macaroni and cheese product, 44 percent (110/250) of the calories are from fat!

Grams for each of the energy nutrients are reported next, with additional information on the types of fat and carbohydrate. Under "Total Fat," a breakdown is given for saturated fat and *trans* fat. Under "Total Carbohydrate," a breakdown is given for dietary fiber and sugars. Saturated fat, *trans* fat, cholesterol, and sodium are nutrients that Americans generally need to limit, whereas dietary fiber, vitamins A and C, calcium, and iron are nutrients that most of us should aim to increase. With practice, using information from the

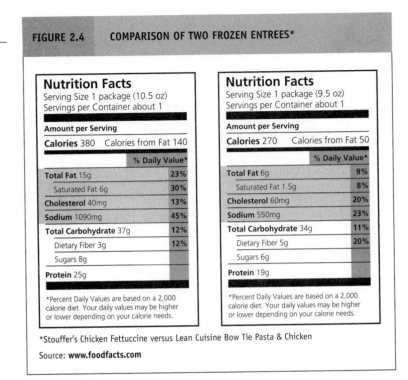

FIGURE 2.4   COMPARISON OF TWO FROZEN ENTREES*

Nutrition Facts
Serving Size 1 package (10.5 oz)
Servings per Container about 1

Amount per Serving

Calories 380   Calories from Fat 140

	% Daily Value*
Total Fat 15g	23%
Saturated Fat 6g	30%
Cholesterol 40mg	13%
Sodium 1090mg	45%
Total Carbohydrate 37g	12%
Dietary Fiber 3g	12%
Sugars 8g	
Protein 25g	

*Percent Daily Values are based on a 2,000 calorie diet. Your daily values may be higher or lower depending on your calorie needs.

Nutrition Facts
Serving Size 1 package (9.5 oz)
Servings per Container about 1

Amount per Serving

Calories 270   Calories from Fat 50

	% Daily Value*
Total Fat 6g	9%
Saturated Fat 1.5g	8%
Cholesterol 60mg	20%
Sodium 550mg	23%
Total Carbohydrate 34g	11%
Dietary Fiber 5g	20%
Sugars 6g	
Protein 19g	

*Percent Daily Values are based on a 2,000 calorie diet. Your daily values may be higher or lower depending on your calorie needs.

*Stouffer's Chicken Fettuccine versus Lean Cuisine Bow Tie Pasta & Chicken

Source: **www.foodfacts.com**

"Nutrition Facts" label along with the list of ingredients will allow you to quickly determine the nutritional characteristics of the food. How healthy would you rate this macaroni and cheese product (Figure 2.3)?

In Figure 2.4, nutrition labels from two brand-name packages of one-serving chicken-pasta-broccoli frozen entrees are presented. Although both are essentially the same size (total weight: 10.5 vs. 9.5 oz.), the meal on the left has 41 percent more calories than the meal on the right (380 vs. 270 Cal). The difference in total energy is due almost entirely to higher fat intake: 15 versus 6 grams, more than twice as much. The saturated fat comparison is 6 g versus only 1.5 g—four times as much. Finally, the meal on the left has significantly more sodium, less fiber, and more sugar than the one on the right. It's easy to make the healthy choice between these two meals, especially since the costs are similar and the low-fat, low-calorie entree tastes just as good. In recent years, food scientists have developed many flavorful low-fat food products. Be ready to be surprised.

Use food labels to apply your nutrition knowledge and make informed choices. Review and compare the nutrition facts, critically analyze, and make your own judgments. For additional information on the nutrition facts panel as well as links to related nutrition labeling issues, go to the Food and Drug Administration (FDA) Web site Food Labeling and Nutrition (**www.cfsan.fda.gov/label.html**).

Foodborne illness or disease—routinely called "food poisoning"—is caused by consuming contaminated foods or beverages. Many different disease-causing microbes (pathogens) can contaminate foods as can poisonous chemicals. Most foodborne diseases are infections, caused by a variety of bacteria, viruses, and parasites. For example, *Salmonella* in chicken and eggs and *E. coli* (strain 0157:H7) in ground meat are bacterial pathogens that received media attention in recent years when they were identified as the "bugs" (microbes) responsible for outbreaks of foodborne illness. In nearly all cases, infections were preventable and resulted from inattention to safe food-handling practices. Unintended poisonings caused by harmful toxins or chemicals—accidentally eating poisonous mushrooms, for example—are less common.

Restaurants are inspected routinely (or should be) by local health departments to make sure they are clean, have adequate kitchen facilities, and follow established food safety practices. Look at the score from the most recent inspection report (usually posted), and use that score to help guide your choice in where you eat. Some restaurants have specifically trained their staff in principles of food safety. Simple observation of the kitchen staff and servers in their handling of the food and cleaning of tables can reveal whether hygienic practices are being followed.

Whether the "food handler" is the cook at a restaurant or you at home, a few simple precautions can greatly reduce the risk of microbial foodborne diseases. Key recommendations regarding food safety from the *Dietary Guidelines* include

- *Clean hands, food contact surfaces, and fruits and vegetables.* Wash your hands with soap and water before and after preparing food. Don't be a source of foodborne illness yourself.
- *Separate raw, cooked, and ready-to-eat foods while shopping, preparing, or storing foods.* Avoid cross-contaminating by washing hands, utensils, and cutting boards after they have been in contact with raw meat or poultry and before they touch another food.
- *Cook foods to a safe temperature to kill microorganisms.* For example, cook ground beef to an internal temperature of 160° Fahrenheit. Eggs should be cooked until the yolk is firm.
- *Chill (refrigerate) perishable food promptly and defrost foods properly.* Bacteria can grow quickly at room temperature, so refrigerate leftovers within 4 hours.
- *Avoid raw (unpasteurized) milk or any products made from unpasteurized milk, raw or partially cooked eggs or foods containing raw eggs, raw or undercooked meat and poultry, unpasteurized juices, and raw sprouts.*

Foodborne illness, or "food poisoning," is an acute gastrointestinal disorder caused by the consumption of food contaminated with harmful microorganisms and, less often, toxic chemicals; it is marked by nausea, vomiting, and diarrhea.

A comprehensive explanation of foodborne illness and food safety for the consumer is provided by the nonprofit Partnership for Food Safety Education: **www.fightbac.org.**

What Is Your Risk? Sick as a Dog

"I was sick as a dog last night." This phrase conjures up images of a dog vomiting, its entire body convulsing with the effort, generally a result of a dietary indiscretion (eating garbage or worse). Or the saying might prompt a personal memory of a long, sleepless night in the bathroom combating nausea and dealing with gastrointestinal distress while hunched over the toilet. Thankfully, for most of us, these "bad food" experiences—although often intense, with symptoms of nausea, stomach cramps, diarrhea, vomiting, and fever—are generally short lived.

But the fact remains that we are more likely to experience foodborne illness than nearly any other health risk. About one in four, or roughly 75 million Americans, suffer a bout of food poisoning every year. The consequence for the vast majority of those afflicted is a day or two of distress. However, foodborne illness also kills about 5,000 Americans a year. With prevention in mind, let's consider the primary risk factors and identify those people who are most vulnerable.

Dozens of different "bugs," or pathogens, are responsible for foodborne illnesses—more than 200 have been identified. Yet no matter which of the various agents spread these diseases, there are several common characteristics. They are carried by food that isn't handled carefully, washed adequately, cooked thoroughly, or stored properly. This simple knowledge and the associated food safety practices can go a long way in reducing exposure. In addition, Americans now eat away from home between 30 and 50 percent of the time. This requires additional vigilance and precautions as you make choices about where and what you eat. For example, be observant and select carefully at salad bars, buffets, and those prolonged group picnics or summer reunions.

Because it is the immune system that protects the body against pathogens, the most severe effects of foodborne diseases occur in the very young, the very old, or anyone with a compromised immune system. In newborns and infants, the immune system is not fully developed. Similarly, pregnant women and their fetuses are at higher risk. In the elderly the immune system is less robust due to age. And literally millions of other individuals are immunocompromised because they are undergoing chemotherapy, taking steroidal or antimicrobial medication, or have an immune deficiency disease (whether genetically based or acquired, such as AIDS). Foodborne diseases in these vulnerable groups can cause serious complications and even death.

To lower the risk of foodborne illnesses, follow safe food practices when handling, preparing, and storing food. Moreover, it's important to watch over those who are most vulnerable (e.g., infants and young children, residents in nursing homes or chronic care facilities, and cancer patients) as they must depend on others to insure that their food is wholesome and safe. In short, for most Americans the overall risk of food poisoning is high—about one out of four per year—but the consequences are relatively low—acute gastrointestinal distress for 6–48 hours—except for those in vulnerable groups. Yet even the healthiest among us should be smart about prevention. No one wants to be sick as a dog, not even for one night.

DIETARY SUPPLEMENTS

As the name indicates, **dietary supplements** are intended to augment the diet. Most contain vitamins, minerals, or plant-based substances (botanicals). Dietary supplements are intended to be taken as a pill, capsule, or liquid. The topic of dietary supplements is one of the most controversial and at times contentious in all of nutrition—an inevitable result when the assorted forces of private enterprise, science, quackery, public health, politics, and the mass media get tangled together. From blatantly fraudulent to alluringly sophisticated, advertisements for dietary supplements are ubiquitous, on television and radio and in magazines and newspapers. The market for dietary supplements is huge; sales exceeded $20 billion in 2004. Literally thousands of different dietary supplements are available. Claims for dietary supplements are highly varied—from treating or preventing a wide array of specific medical conditions (from skin rashes to cancer) to improving sports performance or combating general malaise (low energy, poor appetite, insomnia). Dietary supplements are readily available through many sources, including health food stores, grocery stores, and pharmacies. They are also easily purchased over the phone or on the Internet.

Over half of all American adults use supplements, with the most common being multivitamin/mineral supplements, calcium products, vitamin C, vitamin E, botanicals, and sports nutrition supplements. Over half of all users take two or more supplements on a regular basis. Contrary to what the general populace believes, the federal government *does not evaluate supplements before they are marketed.* In 1994 the dietary supplement industry successfully lobbied Congress to pass legislation favorable to their products—the Dietary Supplement Health and Education Act. The definition of dietary supplement was broadened to include a wide array of products: vitamins, minerals, herbs, botanicals, amino acids, and other constituents and extracts of animal and plant origin. Based on this legislation—which is the law of the land—there is *no requirement for premarket review of dietary supplements* by the Food and Drug Administration (FDA).

Dietary supplements are food products, added to the total diet, that contain vitamins, minerals, herbs, botanicals, amino acids, metabolites, constituents, extracts, or combinations of these ingredients.

In fact, the FDA must prove that a supplement is unsafe *before* it can restrict consumer use. This can be a long uphill battle, as was shown in the case of ephedra, a supplement promoted for weight loss and improved athletic performance. After years of investigation, the FDA found that ephedra use was responsible for five deaths and similar numbers of heart attacks, strokes, and seizures. Clearly, ephedra posed an unreasonable risk. The FDA subsequently banned the sale of all ephedra supplements in 2004. Utah-based Nutraceutical Corporation, one of the largest U.S. supplement companies, went to court, and a Utah judge struck down the FDA ban in 2005. The next step was the U.S. Court of Appeals, which in 2006 ruled in favor of FDA and upheld the ban. The U.S. ban on the sale of dietary supplements that contain ephedra continues today.

This case demonstrates that federal oversight of dietary supplements is limited. Action will be taken only in the most serious cases when a supplement has been shown to be unsafe or dangerous. Questions of effectiveness or truth in advertising are not routinely evaluated. Supplement manufacturers are not supposed to make unsubstantiated health claims, but often do with a caveat in small print. In stark contrast to the limited regulation of dietary supplements, the FDA has stringent approval guidelines for the development of new prescription drugs. For the pharmaceutical industry to get a new drug to market, the drug must be shown to be safe and effective *prior* to its release.

In summary, dietary supplements encompass a wide variety of products. Some products may be beneficial, but many are not. For example, there is evidence to support the use of standard multivitamin/minerals and selected vitamins and minerals for some individuals, particularly those who are not eating a well-balanced diet or have known deficiencies. In general though, it's clearly "buyer beware," since supplements with proven benefits make up only a fraction of the entire dietary supplement market. Examine all advertising with a large dose of skepticism. (See the section on complementary and alternative medicine [CAM] in Chapter 12, "Health Care Fundamentals.") Before buying any dietary supplement, do your research. The Office of Dietary Supplements within the National Institutes of Health provides an excellent consumer Web site: **http://dietary-supplements.info.nih.gov/Health_Information/Health _Information.aspx**

✓ NEED TO KNOW

MyPyramid is a Web-based, consumer-friendly version of the *Dietary Guidelines*. Recommendations in MyPyramid are science-based, yet communicated through practical messages and tools designed to educate and motivate Americans to improve their eating habits and overall health. An understanding of the related topics of food labels, food safety, and dietary supplements is also necessary to be a savvy consumer in today's food wonderland.

News stories on obesity appear almost daily. The Centers for Disease Control and Prevention (CDC) report that obesity rates doubled among American adults between 1980 and 2000. The World Health Organization (WHO) documents similar trends in Canada, Britain, Australia, and other Westernized countries around the world. Based on recent health statistics, obesity is related to over 100,000 deaths per year in the United States alone.

How have we arrived at this current crisis with America's ballooning body weight? In large part, it can be understood as an unintended consequence of major technological advances over the past 50 years. Our 21st-century lifestyles require only minimal levels of physical activity, and our food choices are more plentiful and convenient than ever before. Sedentary living, combined with drive-through fast food and huge portions, has become the norm.

Given these conditions, it's not surprising that most Americans struggle with their weight. Moreover, the body image advertisers promote to girls and women is to be thin while the message targeted at boys and men is to be muscular. Cumulatively, these conflicting factors negatively impact many people. At the one end of the weight continuum are those who are obese, and at the other end are those with eating disorders who are at risk of malnutrition and extreme thinness. Although much less prevalent than obesity, people with eating disorders, including anorexia and bulimia, have been increasing in numbers for several decades. In many cases, these individuals have fallen prey to societal pressures of equating thinness with beauty, success, and self-control.

The key to understanding weight control is the fundamental principle of energy balance—energy intake versus energy expenditure. The basic science and practical aspects of energy balance will serve as the link between our discussion of nutrition in the first part of this chapter and the material to be presented on physical activity in the next chapter.

In the following section, the primary focus is on understanding healthy weight. We start with the questions, What is it, and how is it measured? We will look at selected medical and scientific issues and key resources on obesity and eating disorders and then discuss energy balance. Learning about weight control can help you with your own weight management program and provide insights on weight-related health issues. The best approach to reducing prejudice and dispelling myths about those who are obese or have an eating disorder is to become informed.

WHAT IS A HEALTHY WEIGHT?

A *healthy weight* simply refers to a body weight at which you feel good and physically function at a high level of well-being. Similar terms such as *optimal weight, ideal weight,* and *desirable weight* are also often used, but generally with reference to athletes when the focus is on the best body weight for competing in a particular sport. A healthy weight varies widely from one person to the next based on age and gender as well as body size, shape, and composition. We will limit our discussion of healthy weight to physically mature persons from young adults to those in middle age.

As with most mammals, the male of the species *Homo sapiens* is on average significantly taller, heavier, and leaner than the female. Yet it's important to remember that large variability for height, weight, and leanness exists within each gender as well. Beyond the influence of gender, the basic body shape of a person (stockiness, tallness, roundness) is greatly influenced by heredity. These body characteristics can be assessed by measuring limb and torso dimensions and skinfolds. Individuals with extreme body shapes may be well suited to excel in specific sports—such as horse racing, gymnastics, basketball, football—but may not fare well in a world designed for average-sized persons.

Although measurements of body size and shape can be used as indicators of a healthy weight, the aspect of physique that is most highly related to healthy weight is leanness or, more technically, body composition. The term *body composition* is used to describe the relative amounts of fat weight (adipose tissue) and lean weight (predominantly muscle and bone), and is reported as percent body fat (% fat = fat weight/body weight).

Body Mass Index (BMI)

In recent years, two basic approaches to estimating a healthy weight have become common. The easiest and most popular is to use the **body mass index,** or **BMI.** Often used in population studies, BMI is simply a ratio of body weight to height (kg/m^2). In Table 2.2, find your height (in inches) in the left column and scan across to your weight, then follow the column up to find your BMI. Interpolate as necessary. For example if you are 65" (5'5") tall and weigh 144 lb., your BMI is 24.

Several large epidemiologic studies have found that an increase in BMI is associated with an increase in risk of death. The mortality curve, best described by a J-shaped curve (see Figure 2.5) represents a continuum, which begins to increase at a BMI of 25. The relationship between excess deaths and BMI is similar for men and women and across different racial groups. For a BMI above 25, the chances of dying early increase, mainly due to heart disease and cancer. For a BMI above 30, the chances increase more steeply. Based on this type of evidence, overweight is operationally defined as a BMI of 25 to 29.9, and obesity as 30 or higher. These are the NIH standards (2000) used in surveillance studies that report on the prevalence of overweight and obesity among Americans. The same BMI standards apply to men and women.

An optional additional measurement—waist circumference—is recommended for individuals in the overweight and obese categories (BMI $\geq$ 25)

Body Mass Index, or **BMI,** is a ratio of weight to height (kg/m^2) that is widely used as a measure of healthy weight (18.5–25), overweight (25–29.9), obesity (30 and above), and underweight (less than 18.5).

TABLE 2.2 BODY MASS INDEX (BMI) CHART

BMI	NORMAL						OVERWEIGHT					OBESE									
	19	20	21	22	23	24	25	26	27	28	29	30	31	32	33	34	35	37	39	41	43
Height (inches)											Body Weight (pounds)										
58	91	96	100	105	110	115	119	124	129	134	138	143	148	153	158	162	167	177	186	196	205
59	94	99	104	109	114	119	124	128	133	138	143	148	153	158	163	168	173	183	193	203	212
60	97	102	107	112	118	123	128	133	138	143	148	153	158	163	168	174	179	189	199	209	220
61	100	106	111	116	122	127	132	137	143	148	153	158	164	169	174	180	185	195	206	217	227
62	104	109	115	120	126	131	136	142	147	153	158	164	169	175	180	186	191	202	213	224	235
63	107	113	118	124	130	135	141	146	152	158	163	169	175	180	186	191	197	208	220	231	242
64	110	116	122	128	134	140	145	151	157	163	169	174	180	186	192	197	204	215	227	238	250
65	114	120	126	132	138	144	150	156	162	168	174	180	186	192	198	204	210	222	234	246	258
66	118	124	130	136	142	148	155	161	167	173	179	186	192	198	204	210	216	229	241	253	266
67	121	127	134	140	146	153	159	166	172	178	185	191	198	204	211	217	223	236	249	261	274
68	125	131	138	144	151	158	164	171	177	184	190	197	203	210	216	223	230	243	256	269	282
69	128	135	142	149	155	162	169	176	182	189	196	203	209	216	223	230	236	250	263	277	291
70	132	139	146	153	160	167	174	181	188	195	202	209	216	222	229	236	243	257	271	285	299
71	136	143	150	157	165	172	179	186	193	200	208	215	222	229	236	243	250	265	279	293	308
72	140	147	154	162	169	177	184	191	199	206	213	221	228	235	242	250	258	272	287	302	316
73	144	151	159	166	174	182	189	197	204	212	219	227	235	242	250	257	265	280	295	310	325
74	148	155	163	171	179	186	194	202	210	218	225	233	241	249	256	264	272	287	303	319	334
75	152	160	168	176	184	192	200	208	216	224	232	240	248	256	264	272	279	295	311	327	343
76	156	164	172	180	189	197	205	213	221	230	238	246	254	263	271	279	287	304	320	336	353

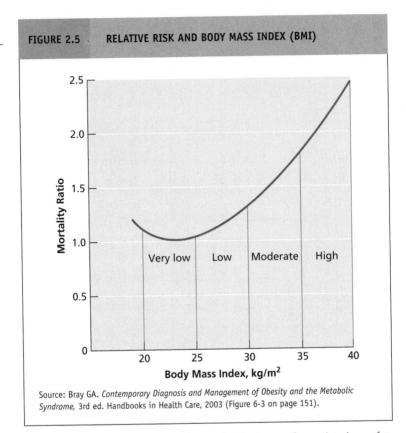

FIGURE 2.5   RELATIVE RISK AND BODY MASS INDEX (BMI)

Source: Bray GA. *Contemporary Diagnosis and Management of Obesity and the Metabolic Syndrome,* 3rd ed. Handbooks in Health Care, 2003 (Figure 6-3 on page 151).

to further assess disease risk. Obviously, the lower the waist circumference for a given BMI, the better—cutoff values are set at 35 in. for women and 40 in. for men.

Body Composition (percent fat)

The second approach is based on the concept of **body composition** in which the body is viewed as consisting of different tissue components. The most common body composition model is a simple two-component one where the body is divided into fat weight (adipose tissue) and lean body weight (the remaining weight, primarily muscle and bone). The body composition approach is widely used in clinical and sports/fitness settings.

In individuals of normal weight, the majority of body fat is stored immediately beneath the skin—in the subcutaneous fat layer—with the remainder

Body composition is the partitioning of body weight into fat (adipose tissue) and lean (primarily muscle and bone) components. Body composition is typically expressed as percent body fat (% fat = fat weight/body weight) and used to recommend a healthy weight range.

TABLE 2.3	BODY COMPOSITION: % FAT GUIDELINES*			
	TOO LEAN	**LEAN**	**MODERATE**	**OVERFAT**
Men	<4	4–12	13–22	>22
Women	<12	12–20	21–30	>30

*Varies by age and goals.

distributed in smaller quantities throughout other tissues and organs. Among obese individuals, large amounts of the excessive body fat can be found within nearly all tissues of the body. Conversely, having too little fat can also lead to an unhealthy state, because fat is an essential component of many tissues (e.g., cell membranes, nervous system). It's estimated that the amount of fat essential for normal physiological function (the lower limit) is equal to about 4 percent of body weight. In women, another 7 to 9 percent of body weight is gender-specific fat (located in breasts and hips) and is necessary to maintain reproductive function, pregnancy, and lactation. In addition to the essential fat (and gender-specific fat in women), another 8 to 10 percent of body weight as fat is considered to be within an acceptable range and normal for body functions such as insulation, protection, and energy storage.

Table 2.3 presents a set of body fat guidelines for adults. These body composition values reflect a general consensus from many studies, although there are in fact no universally accepted norms. Note the different standards for men and women due to differences in gender-specific fat. A healthy body composition for young adult women may range from 12 to 30 percent fat and for young adult men from 4 to 22 percent fat, with the majority of people in these larger ranges falling within the "moderate" subranges. After the age of 30, the norms can be adjusted upward at one percentage point per decade. For example, a 42-year-old man with a body composition of 24 percent would be at the upper end of the moderate range.

The challenge of using the body composition approach is that the measurement of percent fat is not straightforward like BMI where only height and weight are needed. Body composition measurements are categorized as either field-based or lab-based. Common field methods include skinfolds, circumferences, and bioelectric impedance. Field methods provide general estimates of percent fat (error ranges of ± 3–4 percentage points). Results from field methods should be used only as rough approximations. Laboratory measurements such as hydrostatic (or underwater) weighing or dual-energy X-ray absorptiometry (DXA) provide more accurate and reliable values. Although the DXA scan is used mainly for measuring bone mineral density (a measurement of skeletal health) to screen for osteoporosis (low bone density or brittle bones), it is increasingly being used to assess body composition.

Hydrostatic weighing involves submersion in water to determine relative body fatness. In contrast, DXA is an easier procedure for the subject, who merely lies supine on a scanning platform. DXA provides not only a percent fat value but also measures total bone mass. This added information about body composition is valuable as changes in eating and exercise patterns can selectively bring about changes in body fat, muscle mass, and bone mass. DXA scans will increasingly become available to the general public for body composition assessment.

Body Fat Distribution

For people with excessive levels of body fat, the pattern of body fat distribution is another factor to be considered in determining the degree of risk—high or very high—for obesity-related cardiovascular and metabolic diseases. Researchers have shown that upper body fat (abdominal fat) may be more dangerous for long-term health than lower body fat (hips, buttocks). For example, two men—Mr. A and Mr. P—may have the same high BMI of 35 (e.g., 70″, 243 lb.). This puts them well into the obese category. However, since Mr. A has more of an apple shape (upper body fat), he is at a higher health risk compared to Mr. P, who has more of a pear physique (lower body fat). This is the basis for the recommendation to measure waist circumference if BMI is in the overweight or obese categories. Although the apple shape is more common in men and the pear shape in women, both forms of body fat distribution occur within each gender.

Limitations and Interpretation

BMI is calculated using only height and weight. Partly for this reason, it's widely used in public health and is the basis for the CDC population statistics on the incidence and prevalence of overweight and obesity among Americans. As with most simple measures, there are limitations. What are the primary limitations in using BMI?

Since BMI is not a direct measure of body shape (e.g., stockiness vs. roundness) or body composition (leanness vs. overfatness), misclassification can result. Muscle and bone are more dense than fat, so an athlete or muscular person may have a high BMI but not be overfat. Yet, since few adults add muscle and bone after their early 20s, nearly all weight that is gained (from young adulthood on) is adipose tissue. This explains why weight gain during adulthood is such an important predictor of weight-related health.

To illustrate the use and interpretation of BMI and percent fat, let's consider three 30-year old men—a professional football player, a farmer, and a computer programmer—who have identical heights and weights (72″, 221 lb.). The resulting BMI is 30, which is just into the obese category, a category associated with increased risk for multiple chronic diseases. Waist circumferences are 34, 37, and 41 inches respectively. And body composition assessments are 14, 20, and 28 percent fat. It's easy to visualize these three physiques.

Although categorized as obese based solely on their BMI, the football player and farmer are not truly at an increased disease risk as indicated by their normal waist circumferences and percent fat values. They are exceptions. The football player is a muscular, highly-trained, professional athlete, while the

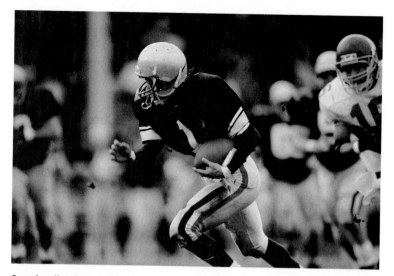

Occasionally when an athlete has more muscle mass than average, his or her BMI may fall in the overweight range. This doesn't mean that person is unhealthy.

farmer also has a relatively large lean weight and is physically conditioned from the routine manual chores he performs in running a farm. Yet most Americans with a BMI of 30 are much more like the computer programmer, who leads a sedentary lifestyle, spending most waking hours sitting. His large waist circumference and high percent fat confirm that he is overfat.

Knowing what each man's weight was at age 20 would provide added insight into interpreting or rating their current weights. However, be assured that as BMI rises to 30 and beyond, it's less and less likely that a person is simply a healthy exception with a large muscle mass, a normal waist circumference, and a healthy percent body fat. Are you at a healthy weight? Use the BMI approach as a first screening. If your BMI is higher than desired, check your waist circumference and perhaps also obtain a body composition assessment. And, remember that both BMI and body composition values are presented as recommended *ranges* for a reason. There is no evidence that a BMI of 21 is healthier than 23 or that a body composition of 20 percent fat for a young adult woman is healthier than 22 percent. Any fine tuning of body weight within recommended ranges depends on individual preferences and circumstances.

THE OBESITY EPIDEMIC

Obesity is a loaded word with many negative connotations. Being referred to as obese or fat is offensive to many people who simply think of themselves as big or large. In a national survey of American adults, only 9 percent said their weight was a problem, even though over half were overweight (Oliver & Lee, 2005). Conversely, judgmental and prejudicial views of the obese by normal-weight individuals are not uncommon. Unless you have firsthand experience coping with excess weight, it's difficult to be sensitive to this

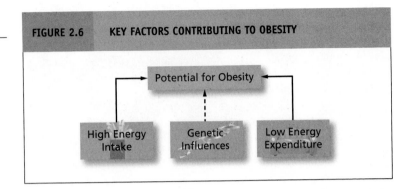

FIGURE 2.6   KEY FACTORS CONTRIBUTING TO OBESITY

issue. In the *Concise Guide,* the term *obesity* is used only in the scientific or medical sense. We encourage you to be tactful when discussing obesity and to dispel unfounded opinions of those who are obese, while at the same time recognizing the serious health consequences of obesity.

Obesity is the consequence of chronic energy imbalance in which the body stores excess energy in the form of adipose tissue. When a person consistently eats more calories than he or she expends, body fat storage will increase. Genetics also plays a role in the likelihood of developing obesity. Children of obese parents have a greater chance of becoming obese themselves than do children of parents who are not obese. As illustrated in Figure 2.6, a person's potential for obesity is associated with high energy intake, low energy expenditure, and genetic predisposition. However, the consensus among experts, based on substantial scientific evidence, is that regulation of body weight is predominantly determined by our eating and physical activity patterns. The underlying principle of energy balance is discussed more fully in a later section. The primary point is that few of us are truly destined to be obese because it's written in our genes.

Public health officials view obesity as an extremely serious epidemic. In 2002, CDC reported that about 30 percent of American adults—3 out of every 10—meet the criteria for obesity (BMI $\geq$ 30). Perhaps even more serious is the fact that 16 percent of children in the USA are obese. This percentage has increased twofold over the last 20 years. If the exponential rise in obesity continues, 99 percent of all American adults will be obese by the year 2053! While this statement seems preposterous to consider and the probability that such a rate will actually ever occur is (hopefully) unlikely, it highlights the phenomenal increase in the number of overweight Americans over the last three decades. This poses a very serious health challenge to our society.

Obesity is the storage of excessive amounts of fat that increases a person's risk for multiple chronic diseases. The accepted definition for obesity is a body mass index (BMI) of 30 or greater.

Obesity and overweight contribute to the development of many medical conditions and diseases. People who are obese have an increased rate of high blood pressure, lipid abnormalities, and diabetes—all factors that increase risk for cardiovascular disease and stroke. People with obesity are at increased risk for cancers, including colon cancer, breast cancer, gall bladder cancer, and uterine cancer. Obesity is associated with arthritis and mobility problems as well as sleep disturbances and breathing problems. Obesity is also linked to problems with childbearing, premature birth, learning disabilities, and other adverse outcomes for infants. Nationwide, obesity accounts for poorer health-related quality of life and higher health care costs than either smoking or problem drinking (Strum, 2002).

If we continue down the same path as we've been on for the past two to three decades, researchers believe that the generation in school now will be the first in American history that will live a shorter life than its parents. Despite the bleak outlook, the tide can turn. Scientists know that obesity can be prevented with a two-pronged approach: (1) the right combination of individual lifestyle behaviors—namely, healthful eating and regular physical activity—and (2) supportive public policies that are accepted by American society. We should each do our part to embrace and promote both aspects for ourselves, our families, and our communities.

EATING DISORDERS

With all the attention on the obesity epidemic, we must not overlook the serious health issues that occur at the other end of the body weight continuum. Extreme dieting to reach a body weight lower and leaner than needed for good health is implicitly promoted by the fashion industry and some sports groups. The National Eating Disorders Association report that the average female model is 5'11" and weighs only 117 lb., which is thinner than 98 percent of American women. Is this idealized female image related to why 80 percent of American women are discontent with how they look? Some individuals—particularly teenage girls and young women—get caught up in the desire to meet unrealistic cultural expectations to be thin or succumb to pressures from family, coaches, or peers.

Eating disorders are one of the key health issues facing young women. More than 90 percent of those with eating disorders are female, and the number of Americans affected by these illnesses has doubled over the past three decades and continues to rise in the United States and worldwide. Eating disorders are a major concern among female athletes, particularly among elite athletes in appearance sports (e.g., gymnastics, diving, figure skating), endurance sports (e.g., distance running, triathlon), and weight-classification sports (e.g., judo). Eating disorders involve serious disturbances in eating

Eating disorders include a spectrum of clinical disorders involving disturbed eating patterns, with the two main types being anorexia nervosa and bulimia nervosa. These disorders are most common in adolescent girls and young women.

behavior, such as extreme reduction of food intake or severe overeating, as well as feelings of distress or excessive concern about body image. More than likely, you have known someone who struggled with an eating disorder. Eating disorders occur across all socioeconomic, ethnic, and cultural groups. Heredity may play a part in why certain people develop eating disorders, but these disorders afflict many people who have no family history.

The exact causes of eating disorders are not clearly understood. However, their characteristics are well known. Eating disorders are complex psychological conditions that may begin with preoccupations about food and weight. But they are often about much more and serve as a way to focus control in one's life. People with eating disorders tend to be perfectionists who suffer from low self-esteem and are extremely critical of themselves and their bodies. They usually "feel fat" and see themselves as overweight, sometimes even despite life-threatening semi-starvation. An intense fear of gaining weight and of being fat may become all consuming. In early stages of these disorders, patients often deny that they have a problem. Eating disorders often coexist with other psychological disorders like depression, anxiety, obsessive-compulsive disorder, and alcohol and drug abuse.

The two main types of eating disorders are anorexia nervosa and bulimia nervosa, commonly referred to as anorexia and bulimia. Anorexia is a dangerous condition in which people can literally starve themselves to death. Anorexia afflicts approximately 1 out of every 100 to 200 girls and young women. Patients with anorexia are usually extremely thin (BMI < 18.5). They don't maintain a normal weight because they refuse to eat, often exercise obsessively, and sometimes force themselves to vomit or use laxatives to lose weight. Severe physical symptoms accompany starvation.

Although less life-threatening, bulimia is more widespread than anorexia, affecting about 1 out of every 30 to 100 girls and young women. Individuals suffering from bulimia follow a routine of secretive, uncontrolled binge eating—ingesting an abnormally large amount of food within a set period of time—followed by behaviors such as vomiting, using a laxative, or fasting to rid the body of food consumed. Individuals with bulimia can be slightly underweight, normal weight, or overweight. Because people with bulimia binge and purge in secret and are not excessively thin or heavy, they can hide the disorder for years. Multiple medical complications develop with repeated and chronic purging behaviors. The bulimia disorder may be constant or occasional, with periods of remission alternating with recurrences of binge eating. Bulimia can and often does occur independently of anorexia.

Eating disorders are not due to a personal failure in one's will or behavior. Rather, they are real psychological illnesses in which maladaptive patterns of eating take on a life of their own. The good news is that anorexia and bulimia are treatable conditions. Treatment teams generally consist of a psychiatrist or psychologist; a physician, who provides general medical care; and a nutritionist. As with most disorders, the earlier the condition is diagnosed, the more likely that treatment will be completely successful. If you know of someone who may have an eating disorder, persuade her or him to get counseling. Few who suffer with eating disorders seek professional help on their own, especially in the early stages. And remember that eating disorders can occur in boys and men (although less commonly) as well as girls and women. For more information on the mental health aspects of eating disorders, see Chapter 7, "Mental Health and Disorders," or refer to the Web sites of the National Eating Disorders Association (**www .nationaleatingdisorders.org**) and the American Psychiatric Association (**www.healthyminds.org/multimedia/eatingdisorders.pdf**).

ENERGY BALANCE: ENERGY INTAKE VS. ENERGY EXPENDITURE

Calories do count. Despite radio and television ads to the contrary, the first law of thermodynamics cannot be broken. Energy is neither created nor destroyed; it only changes forms. Conservation of energy is a law of physics because it always works. Maintaining body weight is fundamentally a balance between energy consumed in the food we eat and energy expended throughout the day based on our body size and level of physical activity. If we eat fewer calories than we expend—known as negative energy balance— then we lose weight. If our energy intake is consistently higher than our energy expenditure—positive energy balance—then we gain weight. This flux in balancing energy intake with energy expenditure is shown in Figure 2.7. **Energy balance** is the essential principle of weight regulation, period.

This is not to say that innate biological variability in energy efficiency (which is the ability to derive energy from food and use it to fuel body processes and activities) does not exist from person to person. Individual differences are present in how we derive and use energy. But in the vast majority of cases, such differences amount to only negligible or very small differences in a person's overall energy balance. Occasionally, medical disorders have been shown to cause obesity; however, these cases are the exception, not the rule.

The principle of energy balance is easy to comprehend but difficult to implement because the modern lifestyle encourages consumption of energy and discourages expenditure of energy. Think of the fast-food menus with portions referred to not just as large but as giant, huge, and enormous or those omnipresent restaurants with the all-you-can-eat buffets. And consider the increase in time spent sitting (at work, at home, and in the car) and the decline in pedestrian-friendly suburbs and cities. (Did you walk or bicycle to school or to the store from your home?) Consequently, to achieve and maintain a healthy weight, we must be vigilant and determined. If we

Energy balance is the relationship between energy input (caloric intake) and energy output (caloric expenditure). If input and output are matched, then a balance occurs and body weight is maintained.

FIGURE 2.7   CONCEPT OF ENERGY BALANCE

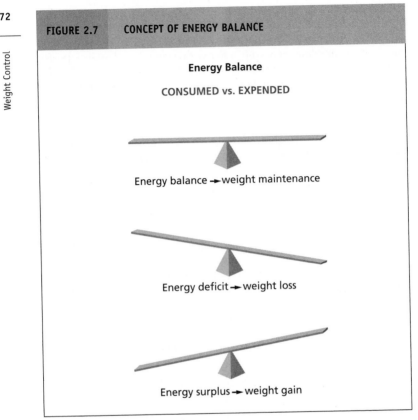

Energy Balance

CONSUMED vs. EXPENDED

Energy balance → weight maintenance

Energy deficit → weight loss

Energy surplus → weight gain

choose to remain intellectually and physically passive, the odds are against us; the calories will add up and pounds will be put on.

On the energy intake side of the equation, vigilance requires a familiarity with the caloric content of the foods and beverages that we consume. (Energy expenditure will be discussed in the following chapter on physical activity.) Knowing, for instance, that a medium piece of fruit (banana, apple, orange) is 50–100 Cal, a small soft drink (12-oz. can) 140 Cal, a small order of French fries about 250 Cal, and a standard fast-food burger (e.g., Big Mac, Whopper) 500–700 Cal is important to understanding the "energy currency" of foods and beverages. If the average American woman needs only 2,000 Cal per day to maintain her weight, then one "value-pack" meal (drink, burger, fries) will provide half the energy she needs for the day! Moreover, how often do we opt to get the larger size of this or that because it's only another dime or quarter? Or how many soft drinks or snacks do we consume throughout the day?

If a person consumes only 100 Cal more than needed every day for a year, this will amount to 36,500 surplus Cal that will be stored as body fat (adipose tissue). Since one pound of body fat is equal to about 3,500 Cal, this small imbalance—only 100 Cal per day—will result in a 10-lb. gain! A slight but steady positive energy balance—less than the energy in a single soft drink, candy bar, or pack of snack crackers each day—can result in a significant weight gain in only a few months. And, conversely, cutting back by the same amount can result in a significant weight (fat) loss.

A more gradual increase in body weight of merely 1–2 lb. a year over many years is even easier to comprehend (an excess 10–20 Cal/day). This seemingly trivial energy imbalance results in the slow but inevitable weight gain that the majority of Americans experience. This process known as creeping obesity is subtle. Several years pass and "suddenly" people notice that they are 5–10 lb. heavier. Continue the process for two to three decades, and the extra poundage becomes substantial.

This is why it's important to periodically consider everything you eat on a typical day and to assess how many calories are contained in those foods and beverages. Refer back and review the individual energy intake results you generated using the MyPyramid Tracker food analysis tool. Interpret the results and plan accordingly. Make it a habit to read food labels. Knowledge of energy intake is a key to being nutrition savvy and achieving energy balance.

Understand, respect, and follow the principle of energy balance, and you will be able to reach and/or maintain a healthy body weight. Due to individual differences in physiology and eating behaviors, doing so will be more difficult for some and easier for others. Regardless though, basic knowledge, vigilance, and action are necessary ingredients for achieving a healthy weight.

✓ NEED TO KNOW

Maintaining a healthy weight in today's society is a challenge. Body mass index (BMI), simply a ratio of weight to height (kg/m²), is a widely used method to define healthy weight. Body composition (% fat) is a more meaningful measurement for evaluating body weight but requires special equipment and expertise. The detrimental health consequences and lower quality of life due to obesity are underestimated by the American public. Although much less prevalent than obesity, eating disorders are also a significant health concern, particularly for teenage girls and young women. Energy balance is a concept fundamental to achieving a healthy weight and to treating weight-related problems.

➤ Translating Knowledge into Action

If it were easy to eat well, we all would be doing it. For most of us, the next step is to translate our newfound nutrition knowledge into positive actions—to improve everyday choices we make about food. This is no small challenge as we live in a society that gobbles up diet books in the search for the one true diet that produces results, whether it is losing body fat, gaining muscle, or removing supposed toxins. Of course, no one true diet exists. This is wishful thinking. At this point, we need to accept the fact that "dieting" is not an effective long-term solution. The dieting approach—"let's try the new X-week diet by celebrity Z"—promotes a temporary mind-set, which is counter to making lasting changes in lifestyle (developing healthier habits). Moreover, most special diets are restrictive, *not* without risk, and seldom successful (not to mention monotonous and illogical—the rice diet, the grapefruit diet, the detox diets).

We must remember that eating is one of our most basic human behaviors. As we eat multiple times every day, it should come as no surprise that we have developed eating habits that are resistant to change. Awareness and the desire to improve are important for change but often not sufficient. As discussed in Chapter 1, if we wish to change a behavior, the likelihood of success is much better if we take the time to develop a plan.

As you map out a plan, consider these behavior-change strategies from the Mayo Clinic for achieving and maintaining a healthy weight. And be aware that these strategies are useful for those who are normal weight or underweight as well as those who plan to shed a few pounds.

1. **Make a commitment.** Be specific about what you are *willing* to do.
2. **Draw on support from others.** Rely on spouse, family, friends, professionals.
3. **Set a realistic goal.** Use the energy balance principle, monitor, be patient.
4. **Learn to enjoy healthier foods.** Explore healthy foods and dishes.
5. **Get active, stay active.** Engage in regular physical activity—more on this in Chapter 3, "Develop a Fitness Program."

The combination of these strategies will assist you in establishing a healthier lifestyle—moving you further along that positive health continuum.

For those who have struggled with weight loss over many years, there is a general perception that almost no one succeeds in long-term maintenance of weight loss. However, this is not true. The National Weight Control Registry estimates that 20 percent or more of overweight and obese people have been able to achieve success (Wing & Hill, 2001). Established in 1994, the National Weight Control Registry enrolls and tracks persons who have been successful not just in losing weight but also in keeping it off. Successful long-term maintenance is defined as intentionally losing at least 10 percent of body weight and keeping it off for at least one year. Based on over 3,000 people in the Registry, three key characteristics are evident. Successful weight maintainers eat a low-fat diet (especially low in saturated fats and *trans* fats), engage in high levels of regular physical activity (about an hour per day), and monitor their food and weight. These findings are real-world evidence that support the *Dietary Guidelines*. If you are overweight or obese, incorporate these practices in your program.

Once you develop a personalized plan, use the following four questions as a final checklist to insure that your plan meets the essential criteria for healthy eating and weight management. Again, these criteria apply equally to those who are normal weight or underweight as well as those who plan to lose excess weight.

1. **Is it nutritionally balanced?**
2. **Is the energy content appropriate?**
3. **Is it based on everyday foods?**
4. **Does it include regular exercise?**

Affirmative answers to these questions dovetail nicely with recommendations of the *Dietary Guidelines*. The following recommendations complete those identified as key by the Dietary Guidelines Advisory Committee.

Recommendations regarding **adequate nutrients within calorie needs:**

- Consume a variety of nutrient-dense foods and beverages within and among the basic food groups while choosing foods that limit the intake of saturated and *trans* fats, cholesterol, added sugars, salt, and alcohol.
- Meet recommended intakes within energy needs by adopting a balanced eating pattern.

Recommendation regarding **physical activity:**

- Engage in regular physical activity and reduce sedentary activities to promote health, psychological well-being, and a healthy body weight.

Recommendations regarding **weight management:**

- To maintain body weight in a healthy range, balance calories from foods and beverages with calories expended.
- To prevent gradual weight gain over time, make small decreases in food and beverage calories and increase physical activity.

If your plan falls short, revisit the basic assumptions and reconsider. Remember that good results depend on a good plan.

In this chapter we reviewed basic nutrition information and dietary guidelines, and we provided tools and strategies for choosing a healthy diet. In the final analysis, eating good food is one of the real pleasures in life. And remember that enjoying good food and healthy eating are fully compatible, so nourish your body with only the best. *Bon appétit.*

✓ NEED TO KNOW

Nutrition is about understanding what types and how much food a person needs and reconciling that with his or her eating habits. The reality is that our eating habits are often well established and not easily changed. To meet this challenge, specific steps can be taken to successfully develop and implement a plan to improve how and what we eat. Using the MyPyramid tools and the *Dietary Guidelines* for guidance, apply proven behavioral strategies to customize a plan that meets *your* needs and circumstances. No one size fits all. Give this plan due attention and integrate healthy eating into your lifestyle.

Nutrition Basics
American Dietetics Association
www.eatright.org
Nutrition Source, Harvard School of Public Health
www.hsph.harvard.edu/nutritionsource
International Food Information Council Foundation
www.ific.org
Center for Science in the Public Interest
www.cspinet.org

Recommendations for Healthy Eating
MyPyramid Food Guidance System
www.mypyramid.gov
Fruits & Veggies—More Matters
www.fruitsandveggiesmatter.gov
Dietary Guidelines for Americans
www.healthierus.gov/dietaryguidelines
Dietary Reference Intakes
www.iom.edu/CMS/3788/21370.aspx

Food Labels
Nutrition Facts Label, FDA
www.cfsan.fda.gov/~dms/foodlab.html

Food Safety
Partnership for Food Safety Education
www.fightbac.org
Food Safety Office, CDC
www.cdc.gov/foodsafety/foods.htm

Dietary Supplements
Office of Dietary Supplements, NIH
http://dietary-supplements.info.nih.gov
Dietary Supplements, FDA
www.cfsan.fda.gov/~dms/supplmnt.html
Herbs at a Glance, NCCAM
http://nccam.nih.gov/health/herbsataglance.htm
Drugs, Supplements, and Herbal Information, Medline Plus
www.nlm.nih.gov/medlineplus/druginformation.html

Healthy Weight
Healthy Weight, CDC
**www.cdc.gov/nccdphp/dnpa/nutrition/nutrition_for_everyone/
healthy_weight/index.htm**
Weight Management Research to Practice Series, CDC
**www.cdc.gov/nccdphp/dnpa/nutrition/health_professionals/
practice/index.htm**

Eating Disorders
National Eating Disorders Association
www.nationaleatingdisorders.org
Let's talk facts about eating disorders, American Psychiatric Association
www.healthyminds.org/multimedia/eatingdisorders.pdf

Knowing the Language

body composition
body mass index (BMI)
Calorie
carbohydrates
dietary supplements
eating disorders
energy balance
fats

foodborne illness
macronutrients
micronutrients
minerals
obesity
protein
vitamins

Understanding the Content

1. What are the six types of nutrients and their roles in the human diet?
2. What is the MyPyramid guide, and how can it be used to tailor your diet?
3. What are three basic rules of food handling that minimize risk of illness?
4. What is body mass index, and how is it used to define overweight and obesity?
5. What is energy intake, and how would you measure it?

Exploring Ideas

1. Why has the prevalence of overweight Americans increased so much over the past two decades?
2. How has the food industry changed its products to provide healthier products to the consumer? Identify three specific examples.
3. Why are so many Americans addicted to trying fad diets? Discuss the possible societal, social, psychological, and behavioral influences.
4. Why are dietary supplements so widely used by Americans? Discuss the positive and negative aspects of dietary supplements.

Adams KF, Schatzkin A, Harris TB, et al. Overweight, obesity, and mortality in a large prospective cohort of persons 50 to 71 years old. *New England Journal of Medicine* 355 (8): 763–778, 2006.

Bray GA. *Contemporary Diagnosis and Management of Obesity and the Metabolic Syndrome* (3rd ed.). Newtown, PA: Handbooks in Health Care, 2003.

Bray GA. Medical consequences of obesity. *Journal of Clinical Endocrinology & Metabolism* 89 (6): 2583–2589, 2004.

Centers for Disease Control and Prevention (CDC). Overweight and Obesity.
www.cdc.gov/nccdphp/dnpa/obesity

Department of Health and Human Services (HHS). Surgeon General's Call to Action to Prevent and Decrease Overweight and Obesity, 2001.
www.surgeongeneral.gov/topics/obesity/

Department of Health and Human Services (HHS) and United States Department of Agriculture (USDA). *Dietary Guidelines for Americans* (6th ed.). Washington DC, U.S. Government Printing Office, Jan. 2005.
www.healthierus.gov/dietaryguidelines

Ellis KJ. Human body composition: In vivo methods. *Physiological Reviews* 80 (2): 649–680, 2000.
http://physrev.physiology.org/cgi/content/full/80/2/649

Flegal KM, Graubard BI, Williamson DF, et al. Excess deaths associated with underweight, overweight, and obesity. *JAMA (Journal of the American Medical Association)* 293 (15): 1861–1867, 2005.

Food and Drug Administration (FDA). FDA Announces Plans to Prohibit Sales of Dietary Supplements Containing Ephedra, 2003.
www.fda.gov/oc/initiatives/ephedra/december2003/

Food and Drug Administration (FDA). How to Understand and Use the Nutrition Facts Label, 2004.
www.cfsan.fda.gov/~dms/foodlab.html

Food and Nutrition Board, Institute of Medicine, National Academy of Sciences. Dietary Reference Intakes, 2006.
www.iom.edu/project.asp?id=4574

Foxhall K. Beginning to begin: Reports from the battle on obesity. *American Journal of Public Health* 96 (12): 2106–2112, 2006.

Hill JO. Understanding and addressing the epidemic of obesity: An energy balance perspective. *Endocrine Reviews* 27 (7): 750–761, 2006.

Hill JO, Wyatt HR, Reed GW, et al. Obesity and the environment: Where do we go from here? *Science* 299: 853–855, 2003.

Kenney WL. Dietary water and sodium requirements for active adults. *Sports Science Exchange* 92, 2004.
www.gssiweb.com/Article_Detail.aspx?articleID=667

Kushi LH, Byers T, Doyle C, et al. American Cancer Society guidelines on nutrition and physical activity for cancer prevention: Reducing the risk of cancer with healthy food choices and physical activity. *CA: Cancer Journal for Clinicians* 56: 254–281, 2006.

Lichtenstein AH, Appel LJ, Brands M, et al. Diet and lifestyle recommendations revision 2006: A scientific statement from the American Heart Association Nutrition Committee. *Circulation* 114: 82–96, 2006.

Mayo Clinic. Weight Loss: 6 Strategies for Success.
www.mayoclinic.com/health/weight-loss/HQ01625

National Eating Disorders Association. General Eating Disorders Information, 2005.
www.nationaleatingdisorders.org/p.asp?WebPage_ID=291

National Heart, Lung, and Blood Institute. The Practical Guide: Identification, Evaluation, and Treatment of Overweight and Obesity in Adults, 2000.
www.nhlbi.nih.gov/guidelines/obesity/practgde.htm

Nestle M. *What to Eat.* New York: Farrar, Straus and Giroux, 2006.

Oliver JE, Lee T. Public opinion and the politics of obesity in America. *Journal of Health Politics, Policy and Law* 30 (5): 923–954, 2005.

Olshansky SJ, Passaro DJ, Hershow RC, et al. A potential decline in life expectancy in the United States in the 21st century. *New England Journal of Medicine* 352 (11): 1138–1145, 2005.

Popkin BM, Armstrong LE, Bray GM, et al. A new proposed guidance system for beverage consumption in the United States. *American Journal of Clinical Nutrition* 83: 529–542, 2006.

Radimer K, Bindewald B, Hughes J, et al. Dietary supplement use by US adults: Data from the National Health and Nutrition Examination Survey, 1999–2000. *American Journal of Epidemiology* 60 (4): 339–349, 2004.

Serdula MK, Khan LK, Dietz WH. Weight loss counseling revisited. *JAMA* 289 (14): 1747–1750, 2003.

Sparling PB. Obesity on campus. *Preventing Chronic Disease* [serial online], July 2007.
www.cdc.gov/pcd/issues/2007/jul/06_0142.htm

Strum R. The effects of obesity, smoking, and drinking on medical problems and costs. *Health Affairs* 21 (2): 245–253, 2002.

Willet WC, Skerrett PJ. *Eat, Drink, and Be Healthy* (updated ed.). New York: Free Press, 2005.

United States Department of Agriculture (USDA) Center for Nutrition Policy and Promotion. MyPyramid, 2005.
www.mypyramid.gov/

Wing RR, Hill JO. Successful weight loss maintenance. *Annual Reviews of Nutrition* 21: 323–341, 2001.

World Health Organization (WHO). Obesity and overweight: Fact sheet, 2006.
www.who.int/mediacentre/factsheets/fs311/en/index.html

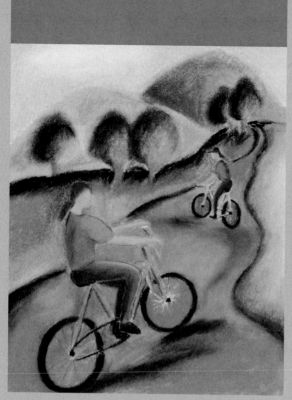

Exercise will make you feel better, function better, look better and live longer.

— STEVEN N. BLAIR,
SENIOR SCIENTIFIC EDITOR,
PHYSICAL ACTIVITY AND HEALTH:
A REPORT OF THE SURGEON GENERAL

Chapter 3

DEVELOP A FITNESS PROGRAM

The main topics in this chapter are health-related physical fitness, responses and adaptations to exercise, and exercise guidelines including national physical activity recommendations to improve health and prevent disease. Strategies are provided to assist you in developing an individualized plan that is enjoyable and sustainable.

Physical Activity, Exercise, and Physical Fitness
PHYSICAL ACTIVITY AND EXERCISE

PHYSICAL FITNESS

How the Body Responds to Exercise
ENERGY PRODUCTION FOR MUSCLE CONTRACTION

CARDIORESPIRATORY FUNCTION AND OXYGEN UPTAKE

ADAPTATIONS TO PHYSICAL TRAINING

Recommendations for Healthy Adults
PRINCIPLES OF EXERCISE TRAINING

CARDIORESPIRATORY FITNESS

MUSCULOSKELETAL FITNESS

PHYSICAL ACTIVITY CONTINUUM

Personalizing an Exercise Program
ENERGY BALANCE: ENERGY EXPENDITURE

DEVELOPING AN EXERCISE PLAN

CONSUMER ISSUES

Establishing the Exercise Habit
IDENTIFYING BARRIERS AND INCENTIVES TO EXERCISE

STRATEGIES FOR INCREASING EXERCISE ADHERENCE

THE HUMAN SPECIES was designed for movement. Until the mid-19th century, humans lived as gatherers, toolmakers, hunters, farmers, and artisans. For 99 percent of human history, physical tasks and manual labor were as much a part of daily life as eating and sleeping. Walking great distances, lifting and carrying loads, working with tools—muscular efforts of all types—were simply part of the everyday world. Our species not only survived but also flourished for several thousand generations prior to the advent of the automobile, television, and the Internet. Then abruptly—within only a few generations—the physical activity demands of work and domestic chores decreased so dramatically as to be nearly nonexistent in present-day urbanized societies.

Without question, the nearly universal adoption of labor-saving technology has brought marvelous advances to nearly all facets of human living. Yet, it's increasingly evident that many of the chronic diseases we face today are associated with the resulting sedentary lifestyle. Physical *inactivity* is a risk factor for heart disease, diabetes, osteoporosis, and colorectal cancer, to name a few. These "diseases of inactivity" begin as early as the second and third decades of life. Moreover, the roots of obesity are at least as much in physical inactivity as in overeating.

From an evolutionary viewpoint, Thomas Rowland, M.D. makes the case that habitual physical activity has a biological basis with a central neural control (not unlike hunger). In young children (and the young of most mammals), movement, which is central to growth and development, is often playful and spontaneous. The joy of movement in children is undeniable. Although the nature of this enjoyment—such as the discovery and mastery aspects—changes from childhood to adulthood, the enjoyment itself need not stop. If this natural drive for physical activity is severely limited, normal physiological function may be disturbed. In modern America, the design of our living spaces restricts physical activity, and most of our leisure pursuits are in fact sedentary. Do our physical environments and social norms subdue our innate biological drives to be physically active?

To be clear, this is not a plea to return to the physical toil that our ancestors endured. Rather, it's a frank reminder that the pendulum has swung too far to the other side. Our bodies were designed and wired for movement, yet we live in an environment where physical activity is no longer needed and in many ways actually discouraged (e.g., fewer sidewalks, more drive-throughs).

Based on extensive evidence, public health researchers have identified regular physical activity as one of the key health behaviors that must be promoted. This is no small challenge. Across the country, rates of participation in fitness and exercise activities decline steadily during the teenage and young adult years—throughout high school, throughout college, and then even more steeply in the years immediately following college.

This widespread decline in physical activity is understandable. In the college setting, considerable time is spent in sedentary behavior (sitting in classes, studying, computer/Internet use). And, in nearly all cases, you are being educated for sedentary occupations. Sedentary patterns are being reinforced and are likely to persist through adult life unless *you* decide otherwise. On the positive side, colleges provide multiple exercise and fitness resources (i.e., extensive facilities, intramurals, sports clubs, credit and noncredit classes) and often a pedestrian- and bicycle-friendly campus. Most students have flexible schedules, making it easier to accommodate fitness and sports activities compared to what lies ahead with full-time jobs following graduation.

If our overall health and functioning are to be optimized, we need to be physically active on a regular basis. Nearly all colleges provide a wide range of exercise and fitness opportunities just waiting to be explored. It's important to note that in addition to the enjoyment and challenge of regular physical activity, exercise can relieve stress, alleviate anxiety and depression, and boost higher-level thinking. These are valuable benefits indeed, especially for college students. The key to reaping the benefits lies with your decision to take a proactive approach.

➤ Physical Activity, Exercise, and Physical Fitness

Terms such as *exercise* and *physical fitness* are probably spoken in every home in America. Although these and related terms actually have very specific meanings, the way in which they are used in everyday conversations varies widely among individuals and across groups. Let's eliminate any possible confusion by setting operational definitions for a few key terms at the onset.

PHYSICAL ACTIVITY AND EXERCISE

We'll begin by defining two core terms: *physical activity* and *exercise*. These have similar but distinct meanings. Then we'll define *intensity* because it is a common descriptor used to characterize physical activity or exercise.

Physical Activity
Physical activity is bodily movement produced by muscle contraction that increases energy expenditure above a resting level. Simply put, *physical activity* refers to moving around using our own muscle power. Physical activity includes all movement whether it is getting out of bed in the

> **Physical activity** is muscular movement of the body that results in significant energy expenditure above the resting metabolism.

morning, getting dressed, preparing a meal, or walking to class. In recent years it has been shown that consistently incorporating physical activity into one's lifestyle (e.g., increasing incidental walking, commuting by foot or bike) can yield significant health benefits, particularly for those who have been sedentary. This active lifestyle approach may be more viable and appealing for many Americans who are not interested in playing sports or working out in a gym.

Exercise

Exercise is a subcategory or type of physical activity. Exercise is physical activity that is planned and structured with the primary purpose of improving or maintaining one or more aspects of our physical capacity, commonly known as physical fitness (which will be defined in the next section). Thus, *exercise* refers to virtually all physical training and sports activities. Sports camps, physical education classes, and basic training in the military are all examples of exercise. Exercising regularly—whether it's training on a sports team or working out at the fitness center—improves health as well as physical capacity and performance.

Intensity

Intensity is arguably the most important characteristic of physical activity or exercise, yet the concept remains fuzzy to many. *Intensity* refers to the physiological or perceptual effort given during a physical activity. Intensity is assessed with objective measurements (e.g., heart rate, energy expenditure) or subjective ratings (e.g., light, moderate, vigorous, all-out). Although intensity may be measured differently from setting to setting (e.g., health club, sports center, medical clinic), heart rate and perceived exertion are two widely used methods for gauging intensity. Both are reviewed in the section "Recommendations for Healthy Adults."

PHYSICAL FITNESS

Physical fitness is a multifaceted concept whose definition has evolved over the past several decades. A generally accepted and enduring definition of physical fitness is "the ability to carry out daily tasks with vigor and alertness, without undue fatigue, and with ample energy to enjoy leisure time pursuits and meet unforeseen emergencies" (Clarke, 1971; Department of Health and Human Services, 2008). A succinct definition from the *Surgeon*

Exercise is structured physical activity that focuses on improving or maintaining physical capacity.

Intensity is the effort associated with physical activity and is typically measured using heart rate or subjective ratings.

Physical fitness is a developed physical capacity that enables people to perform routine physical tasks with vigor, participate in a variety of physical activities, and reduce their risk for multiple, inactivity related chronic diseases.

TABLE 3.1	PHYSICAL FITNESS: HEALTH-RELATED COMPONENTS

Cardiorespiratory (or aerobic) fitness
Musculoskeletal (or muscular) fitness
   Muscular strength
   Muscular endurance
   Flexibility
Body composition

General's Report on Physical Activity and Health is "a set of attributes that people have or achieve that relates to the ability to perform physical activity" (Department of Health and Human Services, 1996). In considering these definitions, three aspects of physical fitness should be noted. First, improved fitness implies an enhanced capacity to perform physical tasks of daily living as well as work-related and leisure-time physical activities. Second, as fitness improves so does physiological well-being, providing protection against numerous inactivity-related diseases. And, third, physical fitness is typically divided into two types or categories—health-related fitness and skill-related fitness—and each type has several components.

Health-related Physical Fitness

Health-related physical fitness includes three fundamental components—cardiorespiratory or aerobic fitness, musculoskeletal or muscular fitness, and body composition (see Table 3.1). The second, musculoskeletal fitness, is in turn composed of three subcomponents—strength, muscular endurance, and flexibility. These terms will be defined and discussed in detail in subsequent sections. For most of you, cardiorespiratory fitness, musculoskeletal fitness, and body composition are familiar concepts because they have long been included in school health and physical education classes.

The physical activity or exercise we engage in to develop health-related physical fitness protects against major threats to our health. Cardiorespiratory fitness lowers risk of dying prematurely, especially from heart disease and stroke. Musculoskeletal fitness increases bone density, muscle mass, and joint health and thereby lowers the risk of osteoporosis, low back pain, and degenerative joint conditions. Maintenance of a healthy weight (body composition) through physical activity and good nutrition protects against obesity, diabetes, and related diseases including heart disease, arthritis, and some cancers. How many of these diseases have you witnessed among family members and friends? As we experience these events firsthand, the connection between physical activity and health becomes more real and less abstract.

Body composition, which partitions body weight into lean tissue (muscle and bone) and fat tissue, prescribes a healthy weight from one's level of relative body fatness (% body fat). This health-related fitness component is plainly dependent on *both* eating patterns and physical activity, much more so than either cardiorespiratory or musculoskeletal fitness. As body composition answers to two masters, it is sometimes discussed under the heading of diet and nutrition and sometimes under exercise and physical fitness. Everyone must eat, but physical activity is largely optional. For that reason, we provide our main discussion of body composition and the importance of healthy weight in Chapter 2, "Choose a Healthy Diet"; see the section on weight control to refresh your understanding of this health-related fitness component.

When considering the health-related fitness components, it's natural to think about the high end of fitness performance. For elite endurance athletes (e.g., Olympic marathoners or Tour de France cyclists) and strength athletes (e.g., world-ranked Olympic weight lifters or power lifters), the focus is necessarily narrow and specialized—to be faster or stronger and have the best performance. The sole aim of the high-level endurance or strength athlete is to train relentlessly to improve performance in a single fitness component; any balance with other fitness components is only an afterthought. Such is the nature of national and international sports competition.

Most elite athletes compete at the highest level for only a few years. Once they retire from competition, their training programs are dramatically scaled down and usually reoriented toward general health and fitness goals. For most of us, training and competing in sports and physically challenging activities are enjoyable leisure-time pastimes, not our livelihood or fulltime pursuit. Thus, we are free to take a balanced approach to our fitness programs. Regardless of our athletic abilities or sports interests, each of us can develop an exercise program that includes the three components of health-related fitness—cardiorespiratory fitness, musculoskeletal fitness, and body composition—in a measured and meaningful way.

Skill-related Physical Fitness
The second type of fitness is skill-related physical fitness. While there are many skill-related components of physical fitness, the best known are agility, speed, coordination, and balance. Skill-related components are associated primarily with sport and motor skill performance and only secondarily with improved health. (This view may be changing because clinicians are increasingly citing the importance of balance to health; loss of balance is the major cause of falls for elderly people.) Among young adults, a finely tuned or specialized physical skill can translate into success in a variety of individual and team sports, from golf and tennis to baseball and basketball.

As many of us know from personal experience, components from both skill-related and health-related fitness intertwine in many sports. Soccer players must develop high levels of cardiorespiratory fitness in combination with soccer-specific skills, and gymnasts require high levels of musculoskeletal fitness to execute their skillful performances. Consider your favorite sports for other examples. As recreational athletes, many of us share a common goal—to develop the right combination of fitness components, both health-related and skill-related, to improve performance in our preferred sport(s).

✓ **NEED TO KNOW**

Physical activity refers to movement due to muscle contraction, which results in an increase in energy expenditure. Exercise is one type of physical activity; it involves planned, structured activity with a focus on physical fitness. *Physical fitness* is a multidimensional concept that relates to a person's ability to perform physical activity. Physical fitness includes both health-related and skill-related components. To counter the development of chronic diseases and to enhance overall quality of life, our personal fitness programs should emphasize the health-related components: cardiorespiratory fitness, musculoskeletal fitness, and body composition.

➤ How the Body Responds to Exercise

The human body transforms the food we eat into our cells and tissues—blood, bone, muscle—along with continuously producing energy to sustain life. To understand how exercise can improve health and fitness, it's necessary to review the basic concept of energy metabolism, or how energy is produced for different types of physical activity.

ENERGY PRODUCTION FOR MUSCLE CONTRACTION

Energy for physical activity is produced in the muscle cells through a complex series of reactions that transforms chemical energy into mechanical energy, resulting in muscle contraction. The most immediate source of energy comes from the high-energy chemical bonds of adenosine triphosphate (ATP). However, ATP—the energy currency of cells—is stored in the muscle in very small amounts and can supply energy for only a few seconds. Only momentary movements such as picking up the phone or turning your head can be accomplished using stored ATP.

As movement is continued or repeated, ATP must be replenished from available macronutrients—primarily carbohydrate (glycogen) and fat. This is when the real work of energy production for muscular activity begins. Energy can be generated to replenish ATP via anaerobic or aerobic pathways. **Anaerobic metabolism** is the production of energy without oxygen present. This pathway of energy production is also relatively short-lived. It can provide a very high-energy output but only for about 30 seconds. Anaerobic metabolism is the predominant pathway for short-term, high-intensity activities such as weight lifting and sprinting. Lactic acid is a byproduct (see the "Breaking It Down" box about lactic acid).

Anaerobic ("without oxygen") **metabolism** refers to biochemical pathways that do not require oxygen to produce energy for muscle contraction.

Among athletes and coaches, it is widely accepted that the buildup of lactic acid in the muscles leads to detrimental effects such as muscle pain, fatigue, and soreness. But scientists have been suspicious of the lactic acid–soreness connection for many years and finally have shown with certainty that it just isn't so. In fact, we now know that a number of the performance limitations and side effects ascribed to lactic acid are simply not true. Let's take a quick look at how the lactic acid story arose.

In the early 1900s, prominent British researchers W. M. Fletcher and F. G. Hopkins found that isolated muscle fibers (from a frog) accumulated large amounts of lactic acid as they fatigued (when stimulated electrically). Following exercise, as the lactic acid dissipated, the muscle fibers recovered and were soon ready to contract again. This finding supported the hypothesis that a buildup of lactic acid causes muscle acidosis, which diminishes force production and in turn leads to fatigue. Good scientists always consider the most obvious or simplest explanation first. And that is what happened in this case. Follow-up studies appeared to support the hypothesis, so this research was readily published and widely disseminated over the next half century.

With better techniques and high-tech tools, our understanding of exercise physiology and energy production has advanced enormously, particularly since the 1970s. George Brooks, Ph.D., a professor at the University of California–Berkeley, led the way in furthering our understanding about lactic acid. For example, his findings show that the body can efficiently use lactic acid as a source of fuel on par with carbohydrates stored in muscle (glycogen) and sugar in blood (glucose). In fact, it appears that lactic acid plays a role in linking the two metabolic cycles—the oxygen-based aerobic pathway and the oxygen-free anaerobic pathway—previously thought to be distinct.

So what is the bottom line on lactic acid? First, lactic acid can serve as an important fuel when athletes work out and compete; lactic acid has an important role in physiological adaptations due to training. Second, although lactic acid may be responsible for some of the discomfort of intense exercise, its role in muscle fatigue remains unclear. The evidence is mixed; some shows lactic acid may prevent fatigue, and some indicates just the opposite. Third, lactic acid does not cause muscle soreness; there is simply no evidence or plausible mechanism. The likely explanation—with substantial evidence to support it—is that the muscle soreness we experience a few days following exercise is due to cellular-level disruption to muscle fibers and surrounding tissue.

Interestingly, these scientific revelations about lactic acid had little impact on how coaches train athletes. Through trial and error, coaches know what works, and to a large degree, this coaching knowledge is independent of understanding the details of human physiology. Since these new scientific insights don't directly affect the actual training of athletes, the misconception persist. As with many aspects of human physiology and performance, the conventional wisdom is often a simplified version of early research and once established in popular thinking becomes difficult to revise or update. As with many questions of human physiology and performance, oversimplifications abound. Now you know the real story about lactic acid, so spread the word and illuminate your friends. Let's set the record straight about lactic acid—it is much more than just a byproduct of intense exercise.

Energy production in the presence of oxygen is called **aerobic metabolism**. This pathway can provide moderate energy output for many hours. Prolonged activities such as distance running, cycling, swimming, and other endurance sports rely on aerobic metabolism for continued energy production. Aerobic metabolism is dependent on the cardiorespiratory system to transport oxygen from the air we breathe to the working muscles, where energy for muscle contraction is released during the oxidation of carbohydrates and fats. Carbon dioxide is a byproduct. The oxygen transport and uptake processes are complex yet efficient.

Only a few types of exercise are purely anaerobic or aerobic. For example, performance in short-duration events such as a 40-yard sprint, high jump, or bench press is essentially completely dependent on the anaerobic pathway. In contrast, performance in events lasting several hours such as running a marathon (26.2 miles) or cycling 50 miles is almost totally dependent on the aerobic pathway, which in turn reflects the capacity of the cardiorespiratory system to transport oxygen to the active muscles. For competitions that are intermediate in duration, such as events lasting 1–10 minutes, both aerobic and anaerobic pathways contribute proportionately, with the relative significance of each depending on the duration. Table 3.2 presents the relative proportions of energy produced from aerobic and anaerobic pathways to perform events of different durations.

Many physical activities and sports are "stop and go," or intermittent in nature. Tennis is a good example. For these activities, both aerobic and anaerobic systems are called on to varying degrees throughout the game. Other factors being similar, the more continuous the activity, the greater the dependence on aerobic metabolism and thus the cardiovascular system. For instance, soccer and basketball, although not pure aerobic activities, are relatively more aerobic than baseball or volleyball.

Aerobic (which means "with oxygen") **metabolism** pertains to biochemical pathways that use oxygen to produce energy for muscle contraction.

TABLE 3.2	CONTRIBUTIONS OF AEROBIC AND ANAEROBIC METABOLISM TO ENERGY OUTPUT DURING MAXIMAL EXERCISE OF DIFFERENT DURATIONS	

DURATION	% ANAEROBIC	% AEROBIC
10 seconds	95	5
30 seconds	85	15
1 minute	70	30
2 minutes	50	50
4 minutes	40	60
8 minutes	30	70
12 minutes	15	85
30 minutes	5	95

Source: Adapted from Astrand PO, Rodahl, K. *Textbook of Work Physiology*. New York: McGraw-Hill, 1977.

CARDIORESPIRATORY FUNCTION AND OXYGEN UPTAKE

Cardiorespiratory function refers to the integration of the heart, lungs, and circulation to transport oxygen in the blood to muscles and other tissues and to remove carbon dioxide, a byproduct of oxidation. Oxygen delivery to the working muscles is paramount to sustain physical activities. To understand the circulation of blood through the body, remember that arteries are vessels carrying blood away from the heart, and veins are vessels carrying blood to the heart (refer to Figure 3.1). As blood circulates through the lungs, hemoglobin in the red blood cells binds oxygen. The freshly oxygenated blood returns to the heart via the pulmonary veins and is pumped to the major parts of the body.

Arteries distribute the oxygen-rich blood to the working muscles, where oxygen is removed (or taken up, thus the term *oxygen uptake*) and used for aerobic metabolism. Carbon dioxide is produced, and the veins return the oxygen-poor, carbon dioxide-rich blood back to the heart and then to the lungs, where carbon dioxide is released in exhaled air and exchanged for oxygen. And the cycle repeats with hemoglobin binding oxygen.

The heart is a special type of muscle (cardiac muscle), and like skeletal muscle, it must have an adequate oxygen supply to continue its work. The coronary arteries branch off the aorta, the main artery from the heart, and back onto the heart's surface. They are responsible for delivering oxygen and nutrients to the heart muscle (myocardium). If these vessels become narrowed with fatty deposits (atherosclerosis), blood flow can become restricted. This can lead to chest pain and heart attack.

Each beat of the heart can be felt as a pulse wherever an artery is close to the surface of the body, such as at the wrist or neck. Heart rate is expressed as beats per minute. The amount of blood ejected with each contraction (beat)

FIGURE 3.1   **FLOW OF BLOOD THROUGH CIRCULATORY SYSTEM, WITH SITES OF O_2/CO_2 EXCHANGE**

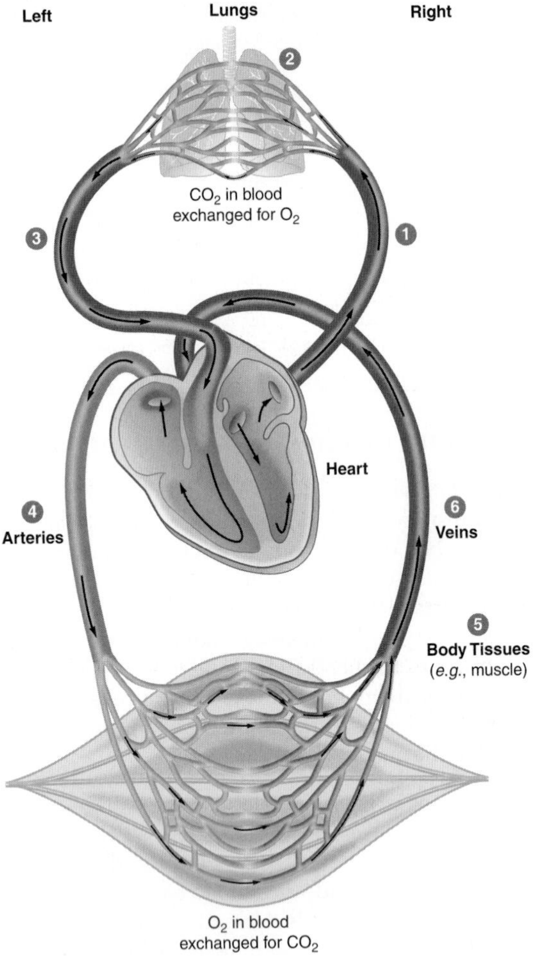

1. Blood rich in CO_2 is pumped from the heart into the lungs through the pulmonary arteries.
2. In the lungs, CO_2 in the blood is exchanged for O_2.
3. The O_2-rich blood is carried back to the heart through the pulmonary veins.
4. This oxygen-rich blood is then pumped from the heart through the aorta to the many tissues and organs of the body.
5. In the tissues, the arteries narrow to tiny capillaries. Here, O_2 in the blood is exchanged for CO_2.
6. The capillaries widen into veins, which carry the CO_2-rich blood back to the heart.

Source: Figure 7 from online tutorial Hemoglobin and the Heme Group. Used with permission of Kit Mao, Ph.D., Department of Chemistry, Washington University, St. Louis.

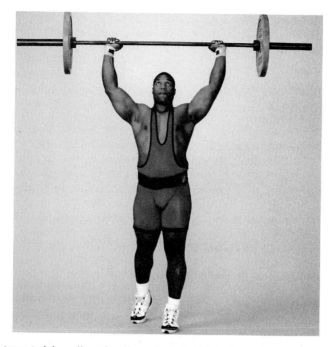

Resistance training relies primarily on the anaerobic pathway, while sports such as running or cycling depend mostly on the aerobic pathway.

of the heart is the stroke volume and is expressed in milliliters per beat. The product of heart rate and stroke volume yields cardiac output, which is the rate of blood flow in liters per minute. Cardiac output is directly proportional to oxygen transport: the greater the rate at which blood is being circulated, the greater the delivery of oxygen to the working muscles.

For most physical activities, the body responds in specific, predictable ways. As exercise begins—for example, going from sitting at your desk to walking across campus—the leg muscles need additional oxygen, so heart rate and stroke volume ramp up to deliver more blood. The elevation in heart rate is directly proportional to the demand for oxygen. Perhaps you are late for a class, so you walk quickly or jog. Again, your heart rate will increase proportionately as your exercise intensity increases. This is why heart rate is a widely used measure of exercise intensity.

In a training or competition, if the exercise is demanding and prolonged, heart rate will continue to increase until the person's **aerobic capacity,** or maximal oxygen uptake, is reached. For example, this is the case for runners,

Aerobic capacity, or maximal oxygen uptake, is the highest amount of oxygen the body can consume during exhaustive exercise. It is considered the single best measure of cardiorespiratory fitness.

cyclists, and triathletes during the final stages of their races. Aerobic capacity refers to one's maximal ability to produce energy aerobically during exhaustive exercise. It can be measured in the lab via a graded exercise test on a treadmill or a stationary bike (cycle ergometer), or it can be estimated from a field test such as a 2-mile run. Aerobic capacity is the single best measure of cardiorespiratory fitness and is the main determinant of endurance performance. This concept plays a central role in individualizing exercise programs and will be discussed in more detail later in this chapter.

For exercise that is focused on musculoskeletal fitness, such as weight training or calisthenics, the demand on the cardiorespiratory system is much less pronounced. As mentioned earlier, the physiological demands of different types of exercise vary widely. At one end of the continuum is cross-country skiing—a total-body form of exercise involving multiple major muscle groups in the legs, trunk, and arms that requires sustained, high-energy output to move one's body weight over a long distance. This type of exercise is clearly aerobic.

At the other end of the continuum is a single-arm bicep curl in which a relatively small muscle is producing force over a distance of only a few feet per repetition. The energy demand on the single muscle can be very high but it is localized. Relative to the entire body, the energy demand to move a dumbbell a short distance is small and short-lived, since multiple repetitions take less than a minute. Consequently, muscular fitness training relies primarily on the anaerobic pathway. The contribution and interaction of aerobic and anaerobic systems vary depending on the duration, continuousness, and type of exercise.

ADAPTATIONS TO PHYSICAL TRAINING

The physiological and performance changes that occur with regular training are collectively termed the **training effect.** A primary adaptation to aerobic exercise is improved oxygen delivery to the muscles. At the level of the lungs, training enhances the exchange of oxygen and carbon dioxide at higher rates. Concurrently, as the heart strengthens, it can eject more blood with each beat. This increase in stroke volume results in the decrease in resting heart rate commonly observed after a few weeks of training. These cumulative pulmonary and cardiovascular changes account for the improved delivery of oxygen to the muscles.

Another fundamental adaptation that improves oxygen uptake and thus energy production takes place within the muscle cells themselves. Most of the cellular changes occur in the cell structure known as the mitochondrion, which is the actual site of aerobic metabolism—the conversion of food to usable energy in the presence of oxygen. Training causes the mitochondria to increase in size and number. The aerobic enzymes, catalysts in the aerobic

The **training effect** is the physiological changes (adaptations) and improved fitness resulting from regular physical training.

pathway of energy production, also increase in quantity. Moreover, endurance is further improved by the enhanced ability of the muscles to use fats
as fuel, sparing muscle carbohydrate stores (glycogen).

Resistance or weight training to improve musculoskeletal fitness can bring
about significant increases in muscle size (hypertrophy), strength, muscular
endurance, and flexibility. Improvements in muscle tone and force production are induced in several ways. A program of resistance training coupled
with flexibility exercises improves blood flow to and neural control of muscle fibers, allowing for more efficient energy production, fiber recruitment,
and muscle recovery. Over the same period, concentrations of anaerobic
and/or aerobic enzymes are increased in the muscle cells, depending on the
energy pathways being challenged. In addition, resistance/flexibility training maintains healthy joints and connective tissues such as tendons, ligaments, and cartilage, and it is protective against musculoskeletal injury.

A balanced exercise program develops or maintains both cardiorespiratory
and musculoskeletal fitness. Such a program improves performance
whether in specific fitness tests, sports competitions, or challenging physical tasks in daily life. A balanced exercise program also yields direct health
benefits modulated through the body's multiple biological systems. Primary health benefits include

- improved metabolism (namely, normalized blood lipids and glucose)
  and lower risk for heart disease and diabetes
- improved body composition and weight control and lower risk for
  obesity
- maintenance of healthy bones, muscles, and joints and lower risk for
  osteoporosis, joint diseases, and low back pain
- improved psychological health and reduced risk for anxiety and
  depression

A dose-response relationship is evident for both cardiorespiratory and musculoskeletal exercise. That is, the more you exercise, the greater the improvements in health and fitness. If a pill could bring about this impressive combination of benefits, it would be hailed as a wonder drug. Moreover, regular
physical activity has few unwanted side effects, and costs are easily minimized. A final point to remember about the training effect: improved fitness
and associated health benefits are reversible and diminish with inactivity.
We can't store up fitness. The key is to establish exercise as a habit.

✓ NEED TO KNOW

Energy for most physical activity is provided via aerobic metabolism, which is
dependent of the cardiorespiratory system to transport oxygen to the working
muscles. Aerobic capacity (maximal oxygen uptake) is the single best measure
of cardiorespiratory fitness. The *training effect* is the physiological adaptations
that occur as a consequence of regular training. A balanced physical activity
program to promote health and fitness includes both cardiorespiratory and
musculoskeletal training.

➤ Recommendations for Healthy Adults

The physical activity recommendations presented in this section focus on the amounts and type of exercise known to improve health. These recommendations are based on the *Physical Activity Guidelines for Americans, 2008* and earlier position from leading scientific and public health organizations including the American College of Sports Medicine, the American Heart Association, and the Centers for Disease Control and Prevention.

For those who lead a sedentary lifestyle, these guidelines provide a reasonable goal. For those who are fit and engage in more advanced training programs, these guidelines serve as a benchmark to check on how balanced your program is. You can glean tips to adjust your current program and gain insights on how to assist a friend in starting or maintaining a program.

First, we'll review the basic principles of exercise training as a prelude to presenting the physical activity recommendations for cardiorespiratory fitness followed by those for musculoskeletal fitness. Then we'll present the physical activity continuum to summarize the recommendations and to illustrate how they fit within the broad spectrum of physical activity levels.

PRINCIPLES OF EXERCISE TRAINING

Exercise training is based on four principles: overload, reversibility, specificity, and individual differences. Consider each principle when planning an exercise program.

Principle of Overload
To improve a physiological system, it must be exposed to a stimulus greater than it is normally accustomed to—such as a faster pace or a heavier weight. This is the fundamental principle upon which all exercise training is based. Repeated exposure over time to progressively greater amounts of exercise results in responsive changes by the lungs, heart, muscle, and connective tissue—structural and functional adaptations from the molecular to the system level. These adaptations include enhanced capacity and efficiency in cardiorespiratory and/or musculoskeletal function. This translates into improved fitness.

Principle of Reversibility
This principle is simply the converse of the principle of overload. When one stops exercising and the training overload is removed, the previously developed physiological systems will over time return to pre-training levels. To maintain fitness, one must continue to exercise. Fitness cannot be stored.

Principle of Specificity
Many training effects are specific to the type of exercise, the particular muscles involved, and the intensity. For example, if the goal is to run a 5-kilometer (5K) race at a seven-minute-per-mile pace, then the principle of specificity suggests that the person should focus on *running* and include training sessions *at the goal pace*. If all training is done at an

eight- to nine-minute-per-mile pace, it will be difficult to shift gears on race day, because the body has not been exposed to the specific demands of running at the faster pace. Moreover, swimming and cycling, although excellent aerobic exercise, will do little to improve running performance because the muscles are used in different ways for each activity. Training specificity is critical for reaching performance goals.

Principle of Individual Differences

There is tremendous variability from one person to the next in both natural fitness level and in the rate of improvement that occurs with exercise training. Due to different genetic endowments, each of us begins at a different point on the fitness continuum. This is no different from variability among individuals in height or hair color. What is not as apparent though is the variability among individuals' responses to a similar training program. A standard exercise dose may be just right for many people but too hard for others and not enough for some. For best results, customize your exercise program as you learn how your body responds. The exercise recommendations that follow should be used as a *guide*. The fine-tuning is left up to each of us individually.

CARDIORESPIRATORY FITNESS

Cardiorespiratory fitness, also known as *aerobic fitness* or *cardiorespiratory endurance,* is the ability of the respiratory and circulatory systems to supply oxygen to the working muscles during sustained physical activity. For most people, being fit or in shape means having good cardiorespiratory fitness. Due to the potent beneficial effect that cardiorespiratory fitness has on lowering chronic disease risk, particularly heart disease, many scientists believe this fitness component is the most important.

The FITT Acronym

Four factors constitute an exercise plan: frequency, intensity, time (duration), and type. Conveniently, the first letters of these four factors form the acronym FITT, which is an easy way to remember them. Recommendations for cardiorespiratory fitness follow.

Frequency: How Often?

The recommended exercise frequency is at least three and up to seven days per week. One should consider frequency relative to both intensity and duration. For example, those who enjoy vigorous exercise should consider training every other day, while those who prefer moderate intensity activity could probably exercise most days of the week (e.g., hard running 3–4 days/week vs. brisk walking 5–6 days/week).

Cardiorespiratory fitness is a health-related component of physical fitness that relates to the ability of the circulatory and respiratory systems to supply oxygen to the working muscles during sustained physical activity.

Exercise intensity should be within 50–85 percent of aerobic capacity, with **moderate intensity** defined as 50–59 percent and **vigorous intensity** as 60–85 percent. For most young adults, a moderate-intensity activity is similar to brisk walking (about 4 mi/hr), and a vigorous-intensity activity is like jogging/running. (A lower threshold of 40 percent of aerobic capacity may be appropriate for older, chronically sedentary people.)

Heart Rate (HR) as a Measure of Intensity. Since oxygen uptake and heart rate are highly correlated, heart rate can be used to gauge intensity. There are several approaches to using heart rate to calculate training zones (ranges). Although it is common to take a straight percentage of a person's estimated maximal heart rate, we prefer the heart rate reserve method because it takes into account resting heart rate and is directly proportional to increases in oxygen uptake (energy expenditure). The heart rate reserve is simply the difference between the resting heart rate (HR_{rest}) and the maximal heart rate (HR_{max}). Maximal heart rate is estimated by subtracting age from 220. To calculate the training heart rate range, determine the lower and upper limits as follows:

$$\text{HR at 50\% intensity} = [(HR_{max} - HR_{rest}) \times 0.50] + HR_{rest}$$

$$\text{HR at 85\% intensity} = [(HR_{max} - HR_{rest}) \times 0.85] + HR_{rest}$$

For example, the heart rate training range (from 50 to 85 percent intensity) for a 20-year-old with a resting heart rate of 70 would be 135–181 beats per minute. As this is a large range, the next step would be to decide whether to train in the moderate or vigorous part of the range. The training heart rate zone for different ages is plotted in Figure 3.2.

How to Measure Heart Rate. Measuring heart rate is easy to learn. Take your pulse on the inside of the wrist (at the radial artery) by placing the tips of your first two fingers about an inch below the base of the thumb. When you feel the pulse, count the beats for 10 seconds and then multiply the 10-second count by six to determine your heart rate in beats per minute. To measure your resting heart rate, check your pulse after sitting quietly for at least 10 minutes or upon waking in the morning. To estimate your exercise heart rate, count your pulse immediately after exercise. Take time to practice so you can reliably measure the higher heart

Moderate-intensity physical activity is brisk walking or similar activities that require 50–59 percent of one's aerobic capacity (equivalent to 50–59 percent of one's heart rate training range using the heart rate reserve method).

Vigorous-intensity physical activity is running and similar sweat-producing activities that require 60–85 percent of one's aerobic capacity (equivalent to 60–85 percent of one's heart rate training range using the heart rate reserve method).

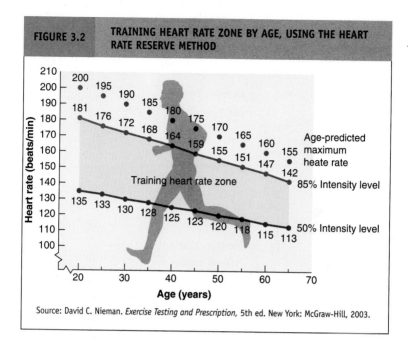

FIGURE 3.2   TRAINING HEART RATE ZONE BY AGE, USING THE HEART RATE RESERVE METHOD

Source: David C. Nieman. *Exercise Testing and Prescription*, 5th ed. New York: McGraw-Hill, 2003.

rates. An option is to use a heart rate monitor that displays heart rate continuously. Heart rate monitors that consist of a chest strap (transmitter) and watch (receiver) are reliable, durable, and relatively inexpensive.

Perceived Exertion as a Measure of Intensity. Another approach for monitoring intensity is to use the **rating of perceived exertion (RPE)** scale developed by Professor Gunnar Borg. This scale links a person's subjective rating of physical exertion to a number between 6 and 20 using verbal descriptors. For example, if the exercise effort feels "very light," the rating would be a 9; "somewhat hard" would be a 13; and "extremely hard" a 19. The RPE scale correlates well with heart rate and is commonly used during exercise testing and exercise class. The scale is useful in teaching people how *hard* or *easy* to work to achieve an appropriate exercise intensity. For most young adults, ratings from 12 to 14 correspond to about 50–60 percent of the heart rate training range (HR reserve method), and ratings from 15 to18 correspond to 60–85 percent.

Exercise intensity is arguably the most important factor in determining the rate of improvement. For motivated people, it's tempting to work

Rating of perceived exertion (RPE) is a subjective measure of how strenuous a physical activity is based on one's overall perception of effort; it is widely used as a measure of exercise intensity. The RPE scale ranges from 6 to 20 with accompanying verbal descriptors (e.g., light, hard).

TABLE 3.3	**RATING OF PERCEIVED EXERTION: BORG RPE SCALE®**

6	No exertion at all
7	Extremely light
8	
9	Very light
10	
11	Light
12	
13	Somewhat hard
14	
15	Hard (heavy)
16	
17	Very hard
18	
19	Extremely hard
20	Maximal exertion

© Gunnar Borg, 1970, 1985, 1998

Instructions to the Borg RPE Scale®

During the work we want you to use this scale to rate your perception of exertion—how heavy and strenuous the exercise feels to you and how tired you are. The perception of exertion is felt mainly as strain and fatigue in your muscles and as breathlessness.

6 "No exertion at all," means you don't feel any exertion whatsoever—no muscle fatigue, no breathlessness or difficulty breathing.

9 "Very light" exertion, such as taking a short walk at your own pace.

13 "Somewhat hard" work, but it still feels OK to continue.

15 "Hard" and tiring, but continuing isn't terribly difficult.

17 "Very hard" means very strenuous work. You can still go on, but you really have to push yourself and you are very tired.

19 "Extremely hard" is for most people the strongest exertion they have ever experienced.

Try to appraise your feeling of exertion and fatigue as spontaneously and as honestly as possible, without thinking about what the actual physical load is. Try not to underestimate and not to overestimate your exertion. It's your own feeling of effort and exertion that is important, not how this compares with other people's. Look at the scale and the expressions and then give a number. Use any number on the scale you like, not just one of those with an explanation next to it.

Any questions?

© Gunnar Borg, 1985, 1998, 2005

out very hard (at high intensities) from the onset of an exercise program with the aim of improving quickly. Yet, exercising too hard without appropriate transition time to build up is generally counterproductive. High-intensity starter programs often lead to prolonged fatigue, extreme soreness, and an increased risk of injury. Forget the crash programs and limit the intensity the first few weeks of a new program.

Time: How Long?

Consensus guidelines recommend engaging in a minimum duration of 20 or 30 minutes depending on intensity. Intensity and duration generally balance each other—the higher the intensity, the shorter the duration, and vice versa. For moderate-intensity aerobic activities like brisk walking, the recommended duration is at least 30 minutes. Durations as short as 10 minutes can be accumulated throughout the day to reach the 30-minute minimum. For vigorous-intensity aerobic activities like running, the duration should be at least 20 minutes. Because of the dose-response relationship between physical activity and health, more is better: 45–60 minutes is preferable and 60–90 minutes may be necessary for weight control (refer to Chapter 2).

Type: Which Activities?

The type or mode of activity should stress the cardiorespiratory, or aerobic, system. Such activities use major muscle groups, are rhythmic, and can be done continuously. The most common aerobic activities are walking, running, cycling, and swimming, but many other activities meet the criteria as well. Most important though is to select an activity that you like. If the activity is not fun or enjoyable, it's unlikely that you will continue. A word of caution for beginning exercisers or older people: avoid high-impact activities like running and aerobic dance as initial choices because of their higher injury rates.

MUSCULOSKELETAL FITNESS

Musculoskeletal fitness, or muscular fitness, is composed of three intertwined elements: muscular strength, muscular endurance, and flexibility. **Muscular strength** is a muscle or muscle group's maximal capacity to exert force against an external resistance—that is, the most weight you can lift one time (e.g., one-repetition maximum, 1RM), such as with the arm curl for the biceps muscle or the leg extension for the quadriceps. **Muscular endurance** is slightly different. It refers to the muscle's ability to sustain a submaximal force or to persist at some relative level—for example, the

---

Musculoskeletal fitness, a health-related component of physical fitness, refers to the combination of muscular strength, muscular endurance, and flexibility.

Muscular strength is the maximal force that a muscle (or muscle group) can exert against a resistance.

Muscular endurance is the ability of a muscle (or muscle group) to apply a submaximal force repeatedly or to sustain a muscular contraction over an extended period.

number of repetitions you can complete at a resistance equal to 50 percent of 1RM. **Flexibility** is the functional range of motion in a joint or group of joints. Flexibility varies from joint to joint and depends on the muscles, tendons, and ligaments at the involved joint or group of joints.

Musculoskeletal fitness is demonstrated in nearly all sports. To varying degrees during a competition, muscles are called on to exert peak force, resist fatigue, and perform well through multiple ranges of motion. Musculoskeletal fitness is certainly related to our health status, too. It enables us to perform demanding physical tasks—both routine and unplanned—that arise in everyday situations as well as helping to combat osteoporosis, low back pain, joint disease, loss of mobility, and frailty.

To develop musculoskeletal fitness, we must engage in some form of **resistance training.** Although it is better known as *strength training* or *weight training, resistance training* is the preferred term for several reasons. First, strength *and* muscular endurance are usually developed in combination. Second, "resistance" can be applied to the muscles using iron weights (dumbbells, barbells, weight stacks), but it can also be accomplished by using muscle- and movement-specific equipment with pneumatic, hydraulic, and computer-controlled resistance, as well as simply body weight (e.g., calisthenics—sit-ups, push-ups, pull-ups). Resistance training coupled with appropriate attention to flexibility exercises is the basis for improving musculoskeletal fitness.

Compared to the hundreds of scientific studies on cardiorespiratory fitness, far fewer have been conducted to determine what constitutes a sufficient (health-promoting) exercise dose for developing strength and muscular endurance. Yet, enough solid research is available to provide guidance with confidence. An adequate evidence base for recommending flexibility exercises is another matter though. Although stretching exercises have proven effectiveness in regaining range of motion during rehabilitation from musculoskeletal injury or surgery, there is little quality research on the health benefits of flexibility for people with no physical limitations. Among the many official statements on physical activity recommendations from scientific organizations, only the American College of Sports Medicine provides commentary and suggestions on flexibility. Although of less overall importance than either aerobic or resistance training, flexibility training is certainly important as a complementary component and should be included as part of a balanced program of physical activity.

Using the FITT acronym's categories, we present recommendations for achieving a healthy level of musculoskeletal fitness.

Flexibility is the range of motion available in a joint (or group of joints).

Resistance training, commonly known as *weight training* or *strength training,* is exercise that develops strength and muscular endurance using free weights, machine weights, body weight (calisthenics), or some combination.

Frequency: How Often?

The recommended training frequency for resistance training is two or more nonconsecutive days per week. Training three days per week will result in greater benefits. The standard practice is to allow two days of rest between resistance training sessions to give muscles time to recover and adapt (e.g., workout on Monday and Wednesday).

Intensity: How Hard Do I Have To Work?

Intensity is a function of the resistance (e.g., amount of weight lifted). The recommendation is to complete at least one set of 8–12 repetitions of 8 to 10 exercises that condition the major muscle groups. Through trial and error, you will learn to select the proper resistance for each exercise—that is, a weight that results in substantial muscle fatigue during the final 1–2 repetitions of the set. In Table 3.4, we provide a sample program of 10 basic exercises.

Time: How Long?

As a practical matter, the time or duration is the length of the entire workout session, which includes the actual time exercising (e.g., lifting weights) and the recovery time between exercises. A duration of 20–30 minutes is a reasonable estimate for the total time needed to complete one set of 8–10 exercises.

Type: Which Activities?

In contrast to training for cardiorespiratory fitness, the options for improving or maintaining muscular fitness are more limited. Such training must involve resistance exercise whether it is traditional weight training, calisthenics, or newer variations of resistance-based exercise. Regardless

TABLE 3.4	STANDARD RESISTANCE EXERCISES AND ASSOCIATED MUSCLE GROUPS
EXERCISE*	**MUSCLE GROUP**
1. Bench press	Chest (pectoralis, triceps)
2. Leg press	Legs, buttocks (quadriceps, gluteals)
3. Shoulder press	Shoulders (deltoids, triceps)
4. Pull down	Back (latissimus dorsi)
5. Arm curl	Front of arm (biceps)
6. Triceps extension	Back of arm (triceps)
7. Front of thigh	Thigh (quadriceps)
8. Leg curl	Back of thigh (hamstrings)
9. Heel raise	Calves (gastrocnemius)
10. Curl-ups	Abdomen (abdominals)

*These or very similar exercises can be done with free weights or on exercise machines. Also, note that all the major muscle groups can be developed with calisthenics (e.g., push-ups, pull-ups, bar-dips, curl-ups, heel-raises, bench stepping with added weight).

of the type of equipment or specific program, the overall goal is the same: to condition all the major muscles, not just a couple specific muscles. Web resources at the end of the chapter provide access to information on a variety of resistance exercises and programs.

To maintain range of motion with the involved joints, flexibility exercises should be included as part of a musculoskeletal training program. Although flexibility training per se is not included in the physical activity position statements of all organizations, it is an accepted component for individual exercise plans. Stretching should focus on muscle/tendons groups at major joints (e.g., ankle, knee, hips, back, neck, shoulder, elbow, wrist). Stretches should be slow and steady (static), maintained at a position of mild discomfort for 15–30 seconds, and repeated three or four times. Refer to the Web resources at the end of the chapter for descriptions and illustrations of flexibility exercises.

PHYSICAL ACTIVITY CONTINUUM

Our level of physical activity can vary greatly along a broad continuum from no physical activity beyond the routine activities of daily living to enormous amounts of training required for high-level sports competition. In Figure 3.3, the physical activity (PA) continuum is depicted as three overlapping spheres representing low, moderate, and high activity levels. Within each sphere, multiple levels exist. During various periods in our lives, we shift among levels within a sphere and from one sphere to another.

Many college students may find themselves in the low-level sphere in which the sedentary lifestyle rules. They engage in few if any physical activities other than those required to get through the day. These students are plainly falling short of achieving recommended levels of physical activity. Some may be taking incremental steps toward incorporating more activity into daily routines (e.g., walking across campus instead of taking the bus), which moves them closer to the next sphere in the continuum.

Those who are achieving recommended levels of physical activity for both cardiorespiratory and muscular fitness are in the middle sphere of the continuum. The recommendations allow wide latitude in developing programs to meet individual needs and preferences. For example, some people prefer vigorous aerobic exercise, while others find moderate-intensity physical activity more to their liking. Similar options exist for meeting recommendations for muscular fitness. Lifting weights and stretching at a fitness center is a popular choice, but others may prefer a home-based program of calisthenics and flexibility exercises. This sphere is expansive and includes those who are expending 800–1,000 Cal per week (e.g., briskly walking two miles per session five days/week) up through those who may be expending twice that amount through a variety of daily activities (e.g., a combination of running, swimming, basketball, and soccer). Approaches are variable:

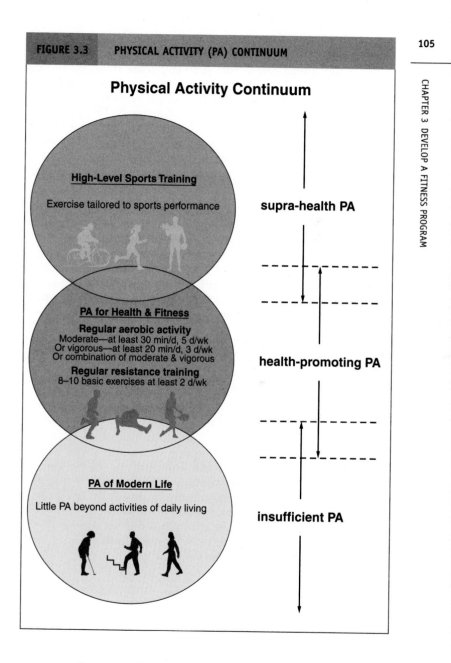

Physical Activity Continuum

High-Level Sports Training

Exercise tailored to sports performance

supra-health PA

PA for Health & Fitness
Regular aerobic activity
Moderate—at least 30 min/d, 5 d/wk
Or vigorous—at least 20 min/d, 3 d/wk
Or combination of moderate & vigorous
Regular resistance training
8–10 basic exercises at least 2 d/wk

health-promoting PA

PA of Modern Life

Little PA beyond activities of daily living

insufficient PA

some may choose lifestyle physical activity such as accumulating multiple 10-minute walks throughout the day, while others opt for structured hour-long exercise classes. Within this middle sphere, regardless of the approach, the greater the total physical activity, the greater will be the health benefits.

The top sphere of the continuum is the realm of high-level exercise and sports training. Many of you have been in this sphere, perhaps as an age group or high school athlete. And some of you are in this sphere now, enjoying the challenge of advanced training on a sports team or for personal fitness. Competing at a high level requires a commitment to training, often several hours a day most days of the week. The goals at this level are performance and recognition rather than just enhanced health. Health benefits derived from training at this level are small compared to health gains achieved from training in the middle sphere. Yet, remember that successful training at this level depends on the fitness base developed in the middle sphere.

Throughout this section, physical activity recommendations have been presented as ranges for frequency, intensity, time, and type of activity. The public health standard—equivalent to 30 minutes of brisk walking at least five days per week—imparts significant health benefits, particularly for those who have been sedentary. If the entire population could achieve this activity threshold, it would significantly improve the nation's health. However, this level of physical activity is the minimal, *not* the optimal— it's the lowest level within the middle sphere. Let's be clear on this point. In general, greater amounts of physical activity result in greater health benefits. People who can maintain an exercise program that is of longer duration and/or more vigorous and encompasses cardiorespiratory and musculoskeletal components (a high level within the middle sphere) will derive greater health benefits as well as improve fitness.

NEED TO KNOW

The physical activity "dose" needed to impart significant health benefits is known. Exercise is prescribed in terms of frequency, intensity, time, and type (FITT) for both aerobic and musculoskeletal conditioning. The basic training principles of overload (and reversibility), specificity, and individual differences can guide you in applying the various exercise recommendations. The physical activity (PA) continuum has three spheres: physical activity of modern life (insufficient PA), physical activity for health and fitness (health-promoting PA), and training for high-level performance (supra-health PA).

➤ Personalizing an Exercise Program

Developing a fitness program involves linking the recommendations to individual goals—such as to improve stamina, gain strength, improve muscle tone, lose body fat, gain muscle mass, control weight, relieve stress, or improve sports performance. What are your goals? Since many exercise goals are related to losing body fat, preventing unwanted weight gain, or gaining muscle mass, we'll review the energy expenditure side of the energy balance equation in this section.

From time to time, each of us are also drawn to new activities or special events but may be wary of the physical demands—perhaps a local 10K road race or a vacation trip centered on downhill skiing, ocean kayaking, mountain biking, or scuba diving. Use this as a goal and devise a fitness plan to prepare accordingly. The more fit you are, the more enjoyable the experience will be, and the more you will be able do. List your main short-term goals and a few long-term goals too. In the latter part of this section, key practical points are shared to help you develop an exercise program that works.

ENERGY BALANCE: ENERGY EXPENDITURE

One of the primary reasons people exercise is for weight control—that is, to help keep a balance between energy intake and energy expenditure. In Chapter 2, the *energy intake* or food consumption side of the energy balance equation was discussed. Now let's take a closer look at the *energy expenditure* side. Understanding how physical activity contributes to energy expenditure is critical to preventing unwanted weight gain and to successful long-term weight management.

Estimating Daily Energy Expenditure

Three factors determine a person's daily energy expenditure: (1) resting metabolic rate, (2) the thermic effect of food, and (3) the amount of physical activity. Resting (or basal) metabolic rate is a function of body size and accounts for the majority of one's daily energy expenditure (about 60–75 percent). Plainly, the larger your mass (the more you weigh), the more energy you need to keep all physiological functions operating at the resting level (e.g., sleeping or sitting quietly).

The *thermic effect of food* refers to the energy associated with digestion. This is that slight but noticeable warm-up many people can feel one or two hours after a large meal. This energy expenditure component is relatively small (5–10 percent) and generally included as part of the resting metabolic rate.

The third factor is the amount of physical activity. This is the only factor which we control. Physical activity is highly variable between people and within an individual. It may account for as little as 25 percent of daily energy expenditure in sedentary folks whose only physical activity is that required by daily living—such as dressing, bathing, and necessary walking. Or physical activity can account for as much as 40 percent or more among highly active people who get an hour or more of exercise every day.

Using Table 3.5, you can estimate your daily energy expenditure using your weight and activity level. As you complete these calculations, you will see how the reference values (printed on nutrition-facts food labels) for the average woman and man—2,000 and 2,500 Cal/day, respectively—were derived.

TABLE 3.5	ESTIMATING DAILY ENERGY EXPENDITURE

Daily Energy Expenditure = Resting Metabolic Rate + Physical Activity
DEE = RMR + PA (All units are expressed in Cal/day)

⇨ Given: **RMR = 1 Cal × hr × kg** (Divide weight in lb by 2.2 to get kg)

Two examples:

121-lb. person: **RMR** = 1 × 24 × (121 / 2.2) = **1,320 Cal/day**
154-lb. person: **RMR** = 1 × 24 × (154 / 2.2) = **1,680 Cal/day**

⇨ To estimate *your* **Resting Metabolic Rate**, enter your weight and calculate:

RMR = 1 × 24 × (____ / 2.2) = _____ Cal/day

⇨ Next, select your average **Physical Activity (PA)** level:

- **Sedentary** (no regular physical activity):   **PA = 25% of DEE**
- **Moderately active** (30 mins/day moderate activity):   **PA = 33% of DEE**
- **Very active** (60 mins/day moderate/vigorous exercise):   **PA = 40% of DEE**

⇨ To estimate **DEE**, divide **RMR** by 1.00 minus **PA** level expressed as a decimal (.25, .33, or .40). See examples below.

Estimate of **Daily Energy Expenditure** for **121-lb.** person who is

- **Sedentary:**   DEE = 1320 / .75 = **1,760 Cal/day**
- **Moderately active:**   DEE = 1320 / .67 = **1,970 Cal/day***
- **Very active:**   DEE = 1320 / .60 = **2,200 Cal/day**

Estimate of **Daily Energy Expenditure** for **154-lb.** person who is

- **Sedentary:**   DEE = 1680 / .75 = **2,240 Cal/day**
- **Moderately active:**   DEE = 1680 / .67 = **2,507 Cal/day***
- **Very active:**   DEE = 1680 / .60 = **2,800 Cal/day**

⇨ To estimate *your* **Daily Energy Expenditure**, enter your **RMR** and divide by the appropriate decimal (.75 for Sedentary, .67 for Moderately active, or .60 for Very active):

DEE = (_____ / ____) = _____ Cal/day

*The daily energy expenditures of 2,000 and 2,500 Cal printed on food labels are based on a moderately active 121-lb. woman and a moderately active 154-lb. man.

Additional Caloric Expenditure through Physical Activity

The recommended target range for energy expenditure is 150–400 Cal per day. This is above the minimal energy expenditure from activities of daily living. The lower end of the range represents a minimal caloric threshold of about 1,000 Cal per week, which equates to the public health physical activity recommendation of 30 minutes of brisk walking five days per week. Based on the positive dose-response relationship between physical activity and health, gradually moving toward the 300–400 Cal per day level is encouraged. Intentional energy expen-

TABLE 3.6   **ENERGY EXPENDITURE FOR INTERMITTENT AND CONTINUOUS ACTIVITIES**

INTERMITTENT ACTIVITIES	CAL EXPENDED IN 30 MINUTES
Resistance training—light	100
Volleyball	100
Golf—walking	150
Resistance training—vigorous	150
Aerobic dance	215
Basketball	220

CONTINUOUS ACTIVITIES	CAL EXPENDED IN 30 MINUTES
Walking at 4 miles/hour	200
Bicycling	245
Swimming	255
Stair climbing	300
Jogging at 6 miles/hour	310
Running at 8 miles/hour	440

These are estimates of total energy expended in 30 minutes for a 154-lb. person. Those who weigh more will expend more, and those who weigh less will expend less. These values are approximations that allow for relative comparison among different activities. Actual calories expended can vary depending on the intensity and continuousness of the activity.

Source: Based on data from B. Ainsworth et al., Compendium of physical activities. *Medicine and Science in Sports and Exercise*, S498–S516, 2000.

diture at 2,000 Cal per week and higher (60–90 minutes per day) has been shown to be successful for both initial weight loss and weight maintenance.

Average calories burned for different types of moderate and vigorous physical activities are shown in Table 3.6. Note that the energy expended during resistance training is quite a bit lower than what is expended for aerobic activities. This should be clear from the earlier discussion on energy pathways and the different energy demands of aerobic training versus muscular fitness training.

A second point to highlight is the trade-off between intensity and duration among aerobic activities. If your primary aim is to expend calories, you have a choice between exercising at a higher intensity for a shorter period of time or longer at a lower intensity. The total energy required to move a mass—in this case, a person's body weight—over a given distance is not substantially affected by the speed at which it occurs. The energy expended by running 2 miles in 15 minutes (about 200 Cal) is only about 10 percent more than is expended by walking the same distance in 30 minutes (about 180 Cal). For a beginning exerciser or a high-BMI person though, the preferable option is to extend duration and go at a moderate pace.

DEVELOPING AN EXERCISE PLAN

It's time to translate the cardiorespiratory and musculoskeletal guidelines into a specific exercise prescription based on your goals. Alternatively, if you are already a regular exerciser, take the time to assess your program in light of the current recommendations. To help with the translation process, consider the following points.

Physical Activity or Exercise?

Most people in their 20s still have moderate to high functional capacities simply due to their youth. Relying solely on moderate-intensity physical activity, such as brisk walking, may not be sufficiently challenging unless you have been very sedentary—in that case, moderate-intensity activity *is* the appropriate choice. The majority of college students report that they *prefer* exercise that is more vigorous whether it's recreational sports, basic fitness training, or a combination.

Since nearly all college students have good-to-excellent sports and exercise facilities available on campus, it's truly a once-in-a-lifetime opportunity to explore different types of classes. The variety of college physical education and campus recreation classes taught by high-caliber instructors is impressive. High school offerings pale in comparison, and your choices following college will be more restricted due to fewer choices, higher cost, and less accessibility and time. Develop an exercise program based on activities and sports you enjoy and, at least once a year, take the plunge and try a new exercise/activity class for a semester.

Initial Screening and Risks of Exercise

For nearly all apparently healthy young adults, it is safe to begin or intensify an exercise program. In fact, some experts contend that you put yourself *at greater risk for medical problems if you remain physically inactive.* However, as a precaution to identify individuals who may need medical clearance, you should take the seven-question Physical Activity Readiness Questionnaire (PAR-Q). This two-page form is available online (**http://www.csep.ca/main.cfm?cid=574&nid=5110**).

Every year a few sudden deaths occur among high school and college athletes during training or competition. There is always immediate speculation as to the cause of death because the official explanation is typically not known for several weeks pending medical tests. At that point, the official cause of death receives only back-page coverage. Nearly all confirmed causes of sudden deaths in young athletes are attributable to cardiac abnormalities, heat stress, drug or supplement use, or a combination of these factors (see the "What Is Your Risk?" box on exercise and sudden death).

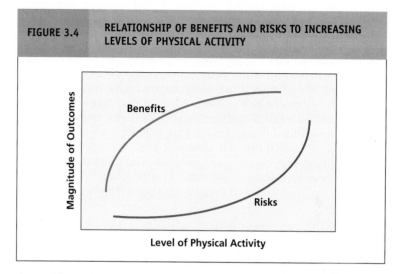

FIGURE 3.4 — RELATIONSHIP OF BENEFITS AND RISKS TO INCREASING LEVELS OF PHYSICAL ACTIVITY

A sensible program of exercise is very safe, especially for young people. The greatest exercise risk for college students is simply overdoing it—too much, too fast. As shown in Figure 3.4, low-to-moderate levels of training impart many benefits with minimal risks. In contrast, as training levels increase beyond those recommended for health and fitness, the benefits diminish while the risks increase. This rise in risk is most notably due to overtraining—exercising too hard, too long, and/or too often. This results in a cumulative overload that exceeds the body's capacity to adapt.

What Is Your Risk? *Exercise and Sudden Death*

During the fitness boom of the 1970s, the safety of exercise was hotly debated. The controversy was widely covered in the popular media because the dissenting views were voiced by well-credentialed physicians. Dr. Thomas Bassler, a California pathologist, contended that training for and completing a marathon (26.2-mile run) provided immunity to death by a heart attack. And he had his followers. To them, exercise was literally a panacea for combating heart disease. Dr. Henry Solomon, a New York City cardiologist, was one of those holding the opposite view—exercise was dangerous to one's health, and the risk of cardiac arrest due to vigorous exercise clearly outweighed any benefits that might be obtained. Interestingly, Bassler's theory and Solomon's view had the same problem. Neither the zealot nor the critic had convincing evidence to support his claims. Most scientists were outraged that such unfounded claims would receive high-profile media coverage.

By the 1990s, medical scientists were studying and comparing both sides— the cardiovascular benefits of regular exercise and the cardiovascular risks (such as sudden death) of an exercise session. Researchers estimated the incidence of exercise-related deaths to be one death annually among 15,000 to 20,000 previously healthy men (Thompson, 2004). Evidence showed that atherosclerosis—the narrowing of the coronary arteries due to fatty deposits—is the primary cause, with the risk being greater for the least active. Predictably, among high school and college athletes, the estimated risk is much lower, at one death per year for every 133,000 male and 770,000 female athletes (Van Camp et al., 1995). Most exercise-related deaths among young athletes are due to inherited cardiac abnormalities, not atherosclerosis. Though tragic, these deaths are rare. This becomes apparent when contrasted to the more common occurrence of dying in a motor vehicle accident, whose rate is one death per year for about every 3,000 young Americans (15 to 24 years of age).

So, is there an increased risk of dying during exercise? Yes, but this risk is quite small, especially among those under 30. A joint report by the American College of Sports Medicine and the American Heart Association put the risk of exercise in perspective, indicating that in most cases the benefits of exercise far outweigh the risks. The small increased risk of sudden death that occurs during exercise is offset by the overall cardioprotection of regular exercise. However, cardioprotection is not immunity. People who regularly engage in moderate to vigorous physical activity are about 50 percent less likely to die of heart disease than those who do not (i.e., relative risk for physical inactivity is 1.9). The bottom line is that physical *inactivity* is a more potent risk factor for disability and death than the transient rise in risk that occurs during an exercise session. Prominent Swedish exercise physiologist and physician Per-Olaf Astrand proposes that people should be required to get their doctor's permission to *not* exercise, because sedentary living is more dangerous to the heart than a physically active lifestyle. (Refer to Chapter 8, "Heart Disease and Stroke," for information on assessing your risk for heart disease.)

Overtraining, commonly results in musculoskeletal injuries or respiratory infections (e.g., common cold, flu). These "breakdowns" are highly treatable with rest, medical management, and common sense.

Initial Fitness Level
One's initial fitness level is the foundation upon which the exercise prescription (frequency, intensity, time, type) is built. If you don't already know your fitness level, consider using standard fitness tests to see where you stand; for example, completing a 1-mile walk or a 2-mile run test to assess cardiorespiratory fitness and using push-up, sit-up, and trunk-flexion tests to assess muscular fitness. A variety of fitness tests with instructions and scoring are available online (**http://www.topendsports.com/testing/tests**). How you rate against normative scores may be of interest.

The true value of assessment though is in using the results as a baseline for tailoring your exercise plan. Be honest in your self-appraisal and set the initial training overload on your current condition. One of the main reasons the exercise recommendations are presented as ranges is to accommodate the wide variability of initial fitness levels.

Equally important is how to gauge the rate of progression for increasing the exercise overload. Rate of progression is dependent on the principle of individual differences in which you learn your dose-response curve through trial and error. Envision an exercise program as having three stages: an initial conditioning stage, which lasts a few weeks; an improvement stage, which can be highly variable in length; and a maintenance stage, which goes on indefinitely. A systematic increase in overload is applied during the second stage. Small, steady increments in the exercise dose (5–15 percent) every week or two is a reasonable rate of progression. Ramping up too quickly is often counterproductive.

Anatomy of the Exercise Session

The format for an exercise session or workout is a warm-up period, the main conditioning phase that involves aerobic and/or muscular training, and a cool-down period. In Figure 3.5, this format is illustrated for a 30-minute aerobic workout in which heart rate is plotted against time. Warm-up facilitates the transition from rest to exercise, and cool-down allows gradual recovery and transition back to the resting level.

When feasible, resistance training and aerobic training should be performed on alternate days, although both activities can be combined into

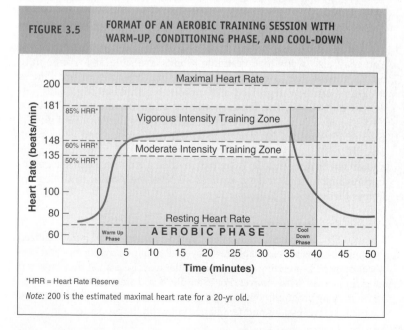

FIGURE 3.5 **FORMAT OF AN AEROBIC TRAINING SESSION WITH WARM-UP, CONDITIONING PHASE, AND COOL-DOWN**

*HRR = Heart Rate Reserve

Note: 200 is the estimated maximal heart rate for a 20-yr old.

the same workout. If combined, the training you wish to emphasize (aerobic or resistance) should be done first. Stretching is typically done during the cool-down, as stretching is more effective when the muscles are warm. However, flexibility exercises are also often included as part of a warm-up and sometimes done at a separate time altogether.

Aerobic, resistance, and flexibility training are the components of a complete fitness program. There is wide latitude in how you choose to mix or blend these activities. For example, participation in sports such as basketball, soccer, and tennis can be a core element of your fitness program or simply be included for competitive and social pleasures. Yet, regardless of the specific sport or fitness activity, it's wise to follow the exercise session format and include a warm-up and a cool-down.

CONSUMER ISSUES

Many consumer issues can arise when developing an exercise program or making a transition from one setting to another (e.g., new school, new job, new living arrangement). Three common topics of interest are fitness centers, personal trainers, and home exercise equipment.

Fitness Centers

Most colleges have good-to-excellent sports facilities for their general student body. Since the 1990s, there has been a nationwide push to upgrade or build new campus recreation centers. Having a state-of-the-art fitness center is increasingly viewed as not just important but necessary. A modern, well-equipped facility also provides an edge with student recruitment. These fitness centers are usually well-staffed, open long hours, and conveniently located. There is often no monthly fee as they are supported from mandatory student fees paid with tuition.

You may also want to investigate what's available at a community health/fitness club as an alternative to using a campus facility. Fitness programs can be categorized as for-profit health clubs (e.g., Bally Fitness, Gold's Gym, LA Fitness), not-for-profit centers (e.g., YMCAs, YWCAs, Jewish Community Centers), and hospital-affiliated fitness centers. Fitness/health clubs vary widely in their size and equipment, breadth and quality of programs and services, and costs. Joining one should not be done lightly. To help in making a wise decision, use guidelines available from trusted sources such as the American College of Sports Medicine and *Consumer Reports*.

Personal Trainers/Expert Instructors

Campus fitness centers usually offer a number of classes and individualized training sessions at reasonable rates by well-qualified instructors and personal trainers. Depending on your particular exercise plan, it may be smart (and fun) to use these services. For example, if you are ready to start a resistance-training program, consider getting a personal trainer to work with you for the first few sessions and familiarize you with the proper technique and use of the resistance-training equipment. Exercise equipment—both resistance and aerobic—can vary widely from one center to another.

A personal trainer provides expert instruction, immediate feedback and motivation. For most people such individual coaching is most helpful. This is particularly true for novices as well as people who have been away from exercise for an extended period or who simply want reassurance and guidance in getting started.

However, be sure to first check out the trainer's qualifications and experience—having a good body is *not* enough! For example, does the trainer have a college degree in the fitness field (e.g., exercise science, kinesiology, physical education) or certification by a nationally recognized organization such as the American College of Sports Medicine or the National Strength and Conditioning Association?

Home Exercise Equipment

For most college students, home exercise equipment is not a pressing consumer issue. Yet, for those considering such a purchase, begin by asking these key questions:

- Will the equipment help me reach my goals?
- Will I really use the equipment regularly?
- Is the equipment well made?
- Do I have room for the equipment?
- Can I afford a quality piece of equipment?

Remember that health-related fitness can be developed without any special equipment. Moreover, high-quality equipment for cardiorespiratory training (e.g., treadmills, stationary bicycles, elliptical trainers) or resistance training is expensive. Refer to *Consumer Reports* and "Web Site Resources" at the end of the chapter for product-testing reviews of exercise equipment, and take your time in making a decision to buy.

NEED TO KNOW

Developing an individualized exercise plan (exercise prescription) involves tailoring the physical activity recommendations to meet your goals, with due consideration of initial fitness level, rate of progression, and available campus resources (i.e., facilities, programs, personal trainers). Selected Web sites listed at the end of the chapter provide additional guidance, expertise, and detail on specific types of exercise training.

➤ Establishing the Exercise Habit

Motivated to lose weight and get in shape, a friend joined a health club several months ago. I asked him how it was going and he said, "Paid my $250 bucks but haven't lost a pound. Guess you actually

Health & the Media A Sport for Every Body

Can you identify these sports legends nattily attired in white tuxedos? This photo by portrait photographer Annie Leibovitz is from a 1987 American Express print ad. Basketball star Wilt Chamberlain towers above champion jockey Willie Shoemaker. Famed LA Lakers player Chamberlain—who once scored 100 points in a game—was 7'1" and weighed over 300 pounds, while Shoemaker—winner of over 9,000 races—was 4'11" and weighed less than 100 pounds. The contrast in body size and dimensions is striking and wondrous. This image should remind us that there is no single ideal form when it comes to sport. Every person can find a sport that matches his or her physique. Clearly, body size does not have to interfere with the innate enjoyment of exercise and one's quest to become physically fit.

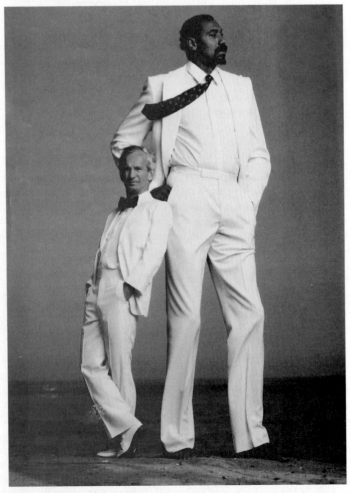

© Annie Leibovitz / Contact Press Images.

have to go and workout!" His comeback quip was a humorous way to describe an unsuccessful effort to begin an exercise program. And he is not by himself. During the last two decades, the year-by-year growth in the number of health clubs mirrored the increase in obesity in the United States with a near perfect correlation (>0.9). Although the growth in health clubs is obviously not causing America's obesity epidemic, it is intriguing that the increase in fitness facilities appears to have no impact on helping Americans reach or maintain a healthy weight. This ironic finding shows that for many, many people facilities alone are not sufficient to make the transition from couch potato to regular exerciser.

When it comes to changing a health behavior, we often have good intentions but poor results. This is especially true regarding exercise because it's voluntary, time consuming, and requires effort. Let's examine some of the factors that influence change in physical activity and consider strategies that may enable you to successfully implement and maintain your exercise program.

IDENTIFYING BARRIERS AND INCENTIVES TO EXERCISE

The large majority of college students report that they enjoy exercise and sports activities, and over 80 percent indicate that they know how to set up a fitness program (Sparling, 2002). Yet, only about one in three engage in recommended levels of exercise (CDC). Why does this large gap exist?

An assessment of self-motivation can be useful in determining likelihood of exercise adherence. Answer the six questions in Table 3.7 and calculate your "dropout" score. Do the results agree with your past exercise experiences?

Also, note that a BMI of 30 or higher is associated with discontinuing exercise. If your self-motivation score or your BMI indicates that you are likely to drop out, view this as a challenge to remain active. Remember these are simple predictors about groups of people, not about each individual within a group. Consider your results in light of insights about modifying your approach to improve consistency with your exercise routine from this point forward.

Readiness to change as described in the stages of change model (see Chapter 1) provides another baseline measure that is useful in translating an exercise plan into action. Most students find themselves in one of the three middle stages—contemplation, preparation, or action. Ten to 15 percent are already in maintenance, and a smaller percentage are in pre-contemplation.

To determine your current stage, select the statement in the following list that best reflects your recent physical activity pattern. Note that *exercise* refers to jogging or similar vigorous activities that lasts at least

TABLE 3.7	ASSESS YOUR SELF-MOTIVATION TO BE A REGULAR EXERCISER

⇨ Read each statement below and circle the number that best describes how you feel.

Very unlike me	Somewhat unlike me	Neither like me nor unlike me	Somewhat like me	Very much like me

• **I get discouraged easily.**

5	4	3	2	1

• **I'm good at making decisions and standing by them**

1	2	3	4	5

• **I seldom if ever let myself down.**

1	2	3	4	5

• **I'm good at keeping promises, especially ones I make to myself.**

1	2	3	4	5

• **If something gets to be too much of an effort, I'm likely to just forget it.**

5	4	3	2	1

• **I'm just not the goal-setting type.**

5	4	3	2	1

⇨ Add the six numbers you circled. A score of 17 or less suggests dropout-prone behavior. The lower the self-motivation score, the more likely it is that you may discontinue a regular exercise program.

Source: Rod K. Dishman, The University of Georgia.

20 minutes at a time, and *walk* refers to brisk walking or similar moderate activities lasting at least 30 minutes at a time.

1. I don't exercise or walk regularly and don't intend to start.
2. I don't exercise or walk regularly, but I have been thinking of starting.
3. I'm trying to begin exercising or walking.
4. I exercise or walk but not on a regular basis (vigorous <3 days/week or moderate exercise <5 days/week).
5. I have been exercising or walking regularly for the last few months (vigorous ≥3 days/week or moderate exercise ≥5 days/week).
6. I have been exercising or walking regularly for more than six months.

If you chose 1, you're in the pre-contemplation stage; 2 is contemplation; 3 is preparation; 4 is action; 5 is maintenance; and 6 is when exercise has become an established behavior. For example, perhaps you are stuck in the preparation stage; you play soccer or run a couple times per week but can't seem to get beyond that. Identifying your current stage can help you see what you need to do to reach the next stage—in this case, to add the third session per week.

There are many barriers to adopting or maintaining an exercise program. Americans often report lack of time and limited access to facilities and equipment. Yet, for most college students these are not significant barriers. In fact, just the opposite—a flexible schedule, fewer family responsibilities and an accessible campus fitness center provide an opportunity. So let's focus on other variables that are more likely to influence exercise adherence. Each can be viewed as a negative or a positive. Consider the following list in relation to your current or planned exercise routine:

- Boring versus enjoyable
- Disapproval versus encouragement by close friends, family
- Injuries, physical limitations versus injury free, no limitations
- Haphazard schedule versus regular routine
- Inadequate instruction versus expert instruction
- Previous experience versus just beginning

The combination of negative factors often outweighs that of positive factors. Consequently, it's important to take stock of key variables and work at turning each negative into a positive whenever possible. Also, despite a sound plan and your best efforts, know that interruptions can occur at all stages. If you have to discontinue exercise for a short time, don't let that stop you from starting again. Relapses are a natural part of the long-term process of establishing a new behavior.

STRATEGIES FOR INCREASING EXERCISE ADHERENCE

The aim is to leverage every feasible strategy to establish exercise as a permanent habit. If we don't, then exercise will frequently lose out to the many other interests that compete for our time. Consider the following practical strategies to tip the scale—the balance between the pros and cons—in the right direction.

- Make exercise fun.
- Schedule your exercise.
- Set specific long-term and short-term goals.
- Keep a log and include periodic testing to monitor your progress.
- Reward yourself for consistency and milestones.
- Minimize injuries by starting out with a moderate program.
- Try something new from time to time.
- Be patient but consistent—remember, the tortoise can beat the hare.
- Exercise to feel better.

Apply as many of these suggestions as possible, especially if you are in the contemplation, preparation, and action stage. Another useful strategy is to exercise with a friend. Although some people prefer to exercise by themselves as a time away from everything and everybody, most of us enjoy the company and camaraderie of exercising with others. Why should all social time with family and friends be centered on eating and other sedentary activities? Physical activity—whether simply a long walk or sports and fitness activities—provides an excellent opportunity to share time together.

The aim of applying behavioral strategies to our physical activity behavior is to make it difficult to *not* exercise. A sensible, individualized program of exercise can directly improve quality of life. Only by engaging in a long-term exercise routine can we experience this health enhancement. The natural consequence is that the value of exercise is elevated and the behavior becomes more ingrained. Eventually, a behavior repeated over months and years becomes a lifelong habit. Follow your individualized plan, apply the most helpful strategies, and with time and commitment you will establish the exercise habit.

✓ **NEED TO KNOW**

Integrating a fitness program into your lifestyle is not just a matter of choice. Becoming a regular exerciser requires a plan and perseverance. By identifying barriers and incentives and applying strategies that fit your situation, you stack the odds in your favor. Exercise empowers living. And it's a metaphor for life. You get out of it what you put into it. Enjoy the good feelings and positive health that come with fitness.

Physical Activity Recommendations

Physical Activity Guidelines for Americans, 2008
  http:www.health.gov/PAguidelines/Report/
ACSM/AHA Physical activity and public health: Updated recommendation for adults (2007)
  http://circ.ahajournals.org/cgi/reprint/CIRCULATIONAHA.107
  .185649
ACSM position stand: Progression models in resistance training for healthy adults (2002)
  www.acsm-msse.org/pt/pt-core/template-journal/msse/media/
  0202.pdf

Examples of Exercise Resources

Resistance exercises from Exercise Prescription on the Net
  www.exrx.net/Lists/Directory.html
Stretching exercises from the Mayo Clinic
  www.mayoclinic.com/health/stretching/SM00043&slide=1
Fitness tests
  www.topendsports.com/testing/tests
Perceived exertion (Borg Rating of Perceived Exertion Scale)
  www.cdc.gov/nccdphp/dnpa/physical/measuring/perceived
  _exertion.htm
Exercise Prescription on the Net
www.exrx.net

Strategies to Increase Physical Activity among the Sedentary

America on the Move
  www.americaonthemove.org
Smallstep (Department of Health & Human Services)
  www.smallstep.gov
Tips on selecting and using fitness facilities and equipment (downloadable brochures)
  www.acsm.org/AM/Template.cfm?Section=Brochures2

General

American College of Sports Medicine (ACSM)
  www.acsm.org
Centers for Disease Control & Prevention (CDC): Physical Activity
  www.cdc.gov/nccdphp/dnpa/physical
Gatorade Sports Science Institute
  www.gssiweb.com
National Strength and Conditioning Association
  www.nsca-lift.org
President's Council on Physical Fitness and Sports Research Digests
  www.fitness.gov/pcpfs_research_digs.htm

Knowing the Language

aerobic capacity
aerobic metabolism
anaerobic metabolism
cardiorespiratory fitness
exercise
flexibility
intensity
moderate intensity
muscular endurance

muscular strength
musculoskeletal fitness
physical activity
physical fitness
rating of perceived exertion
resistance training
training effect
vigorous intensity

Understanding the Content

1. Contrast and define the following terms: *physical activity, exercise,* and *physical fitness.*
2. What are the three primary components of health-related physical fitness? How are they related to our health?
3. What are the minimum levels of aerobic activity and resistance training recommended to improve and maintain health for adults?
4. An exercise session has three phases. Name and describe them and illustrate with an example.

Exploring Ideas

1. Physical activity and health have a dose-response relationship. Explain this concept and comment on the advantages and limitations of prescribing exercise as a medicine.
2. Approximately how many calories should one burn in intentional physical activity (per day or week) to improve and maintain health? Where does this level of energy expenditure fall within the physical activity continuum? Explain.
3. How do the basic principles of exercise training—overload, specificity, and individual differences—relate to tailoring an individual exercise plan? Explain with examples.
4. Most of us enjoy exercise and know it's beneficial. Yet, only a small percentage of Americans exercise regularly. Explain this quandary and suggest strategies to enable folks to become more active.

Selected References

ACSM. ACSM position stand on the recommended quantity and quality of exercise for developing and maintaining cardiorespiratory and muscular fitness, and flexibility in healthy adults. *Medicine and Science in Sports and Exercise* 30 (6): 975–991, 1998.
www.acsm-msse.org/pt/pt-core/template-journal/msse/media/0698a.htm

ACSM/AHA. ACSM/AHA position stand on exercise and acute cardiovascular events: Placing the risks into perspective. *Medicine and Science in Sports and Exercise* 39 (5): 886–897, 2007.
www.acsm-msse.org/pt/pt-core/template-journal/msse/media/0507.pdf

American College of Sports Medicine (ACSM). *ACSM's Guidelines for Exercise Testing and Prescription* (7th ed). Baltimore: Lippincott, Williams & Wilkins, 2006.

American Heart Association (AHA). AHA scientific statement: Exercise and physical activity in the prevention and treatment of atherosclerotic cardiovascular disease. *Circulation* 107: 3109–3116, 2003.
http://circ.ahajournals.org/cgi/content/full/107/24/3109

Anderson B. *Stretching*. Bolinas, CA: Shelter Publications, 2000.

Booth FW, Chakravarthy MV, Gordon SE, et al. Waging war on physical inactivity: Using modern molecular ammunition against an ancient enemy. *Journal of Applied Physiology* 93: 3–30, 2002.

Borg G. *Borg's Perceived Exertion and Pain Scales*. Champaign, IL: Human Kinetics, 1998.

Bouchard C, Blair SN, Haskell WL. *Physical Activity and Health*. Champaign, IL: Human Kinetics, 2007.

Brooks GA, Fahey TD, Baldwin KM. *Exercise Physiology. Human Bioenergetics and Its Applications* (4th ed). New York: McGraw-Hill, 2005.

Brown DW, Brown DR, Heath GW, et al. Associations between physical activity dose and health-related quality of life. *Medicine and Science in Sports and Exercise* 36: 890–896, 2004.

Caspersen CJ, Pereira MA, Curran KM. Changes in physical activity patterns in the United States, by sex and cross-sectional age. *Medicine and Science in Sports and Exercise* 32: 1601–1609, 2000.

Centers for Disease Control and Prevention. Physical activity for everyone.
www.cdc.gov/nccdphp/dnpa/physical/everyone/index.htm

Clarke HH (ed.). Basic understanding of physical fitness. *Physical Fitness Research Digest*. Washington, DC: Presidents Council on Physical Fitness and Sport, July 1971.

Cotman CW, Engesser-Cesar C. Exercise enhances and protects brain function. *Exercise and Sport Science Reviews* 30: 75–79, 2002.

Department of Health and Human Services. *Physical Activity and Health: A Report of the Surgeon General*. Atlanta, GA: Centers for Disease Control and Prevention, 1996.
www.cdc.gov/nccdphp/sgr/sgr.htm

Department of Health and Human Services. *Physical Activity Guidelines for Americans, 2008*.
http:www.health.gov/PAguidelines/Report

Fields KB, Burnworth CM, Delaney M. Should athletes stretch before exercise? *Sport Science Exchange* #104, Gatorade Sports Science Institute, June 2007.
www.gssiweb.com/Article_Detail.aspx?articleid=736

Gladden, LB. Personal communication with PB Sparling on the lactic acid–muscle performance relationship. August 2007.

Haskell WL, Lee I-M, Pate RR, et al. Physical activity and public health: Updated recommendation for adults from the American College of Sports Medicine and the American Heart Association. *Circulation* 116;1081–1093, 2007.
http://circ.ahajournals.org/cgi/reprint/CIRCULATIONAHA.107.185649

Herbert RD, de Noronha M. Stretching to prevent or reduce muscle soreness after exercise. *Cochrane Database of Systematic Reviews* 4: 2007.
http://mrw.interscience.wiley.com/cochrane/clsysrev/articles/CD004577/frame.html

Hill JO, Wyatt HR, Reed GW et al. Obesity and the environment: Where do we go from here? *Science* 299: 853–855, 2003.

Kolata G. Lactic acid is not muscles' foe, it's fuel. *New York Times*, May 16, 2006.

Leslie E, Sparling PB, Owen N. University campus settings and the promotion of physical activity in young adults: Lessons from research in Australia and the USA. *Health Education* 101: 116–125, 2001.

McArdle WD, Katch FI, Katch VL. *Exercise Physiology: Energy, Nutrition, and Human Performance* (6th ed). Baltimore: Lippincott, Williams & Wilkins; 2006.

Powers SK, Howley ET. *Exercise Physiology: Theory and Application to Fitness and Performance* (6th ed). New York: McGraw-Hill, 2006.

Roberts CK, Barnard RJ. Effects of exercise and diet on chronic disease. *Journal of Applied Physiology* 98: 3–30, 2005.

Rowland TW. The biological basis of physical activity. *Medicine & Science in Sports and Exercise* 30 (3): 392–399, 1998.

Sparling PB. College physical education: An unrecognized agent of change in combating inactivity-related diseases. *Perspectives in Biology and Medicine* 46 (4): 579–587, 2003.

Sparling PB, Snow TK. Physical activity patterns in recent college alumni. *Research Quarterly for Exercise and Sport* 73: 200–205, 2002.

Thompson PD. Historical concepts of the athlete's heart. *Medicine & Science in Sports and Exercise* 36: 363–370, 2004.

USDA. Chapter 4: Physical activity. *Dietary Guidelines for Americans* (6th ed.), 2005.
www.health.gov/dietaryguidelines/dga2005/document/html/chapter4.htm

Van Camp SP, Bloor CM, Mueller FO, et al. Nontraumatic sports death in high school and college athletes. *Medicine and Science in Sports and Exercise* 27:641–647, 1995.

Williams MA, Haskell WL, Ades PA, et al. Resistance exercise in individuals with and without cardiovascular disease, 2007 update: A scientific statement from the American Heart Association. *Circulation* 116: 572–584, 2007.
http://circ.ahajournals.org/cgi/reprint/CIRCULATIONAHA.107.185214

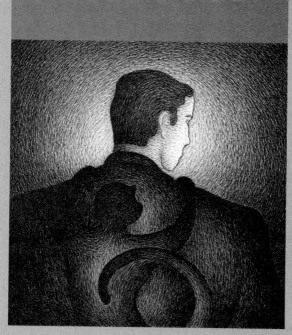

There are people who strictly deprive themselves of each and every eatable, drinkable, and smokeable pleasure which has in any way acquired a shady reputation. They pay this price for health. And health is all they get for it.

— MARK TWAIN

Chapter 4

UNDERSTANDING DRUG USE, MISUSE, AND ABUSE

In Chapter 4 we provide a foundation for an understanding of the principles regarding drug use, misuse, and abuse. The chapter begins with an overview of the scope of drugs in society today and then explains key language and terminology. The chapter moves on to explain various categories of drugs and ends with a discussion of drug testing and drug abuse treatment options. The goal is to provide a grounding in the concepts integral to understanding the risks associated with drugs.

DRUG USE, misuse, and abuse not only alter an individual's body chemistry and perception of reality, but drugs have widespread economic and social costs. Murder, child abuse, drowning, rape, assault, suicide, spousal abuse, and traffic fatalities all too often have improper use of controlled substances as a contributing factor. And substance abuse among young adults is especially common. According to the National Center on Addiction and Substance Abuse at Columbia University (CASA, 2007), college students have higher rates of drug dependence than the general public, with almost 23 percent of them classified as substance dependent. Alcohol abuse is especially common and costly in this age group, with about 30 percent of students meeting the criteria of alcohol abusers. About one in four college students also reports missing classes, falling behind in courses, or doing poorly on school work due to their alcohol consumption. Additionally, each year in the United States among 18- to 24-year-old college students, there are the following alcohol-related incidents (Hingston et al., 2002):

- 1,400 deaths from accidents
- 500,000 injuries
- Over 600,000 physical assaults
- Over 100,000 occasions when students were unsure if they consented to sex
- Over 70,000 sexual assaults
- 400,000 instances of unprotected sex

Instances of drug misuse and abuse among other groups in the United States are also quite high. The United States consumes a whopping 60 percent of the world's supply of illicit drugs. According to the Substance Abuse and Mental Health Services Administration (SAMHSA, 2002), 15.9 million Americans ages 12 and older reported using an illicit drug in the month before they were surveyed. Young-adult males were about twice as likely to abuse drugs as women of the same age group were—15 percent versus 8 percent, respectively. Substance abuse rates shoot up for both men and women when they are unemployed—to 12.5 percent for females and 23 percent for males.

Many Americans mistakenly believe that most drug abusers are minorities; the reality is that the majority of current illicit drug users are white. But even though more white people abuse drugs, fewer are incarcerated for drug offenses compared to other racial groups. Of the 246,100 state prison inmates serving time for drug offenses in 2001, 56 percent were African American, 19 percent were Hispanic, and 23 percent were white.

➤ Drug Administration and Terminology

Drug administration and absorption are key issues that influence safety in drug doses. For any drug to have an effect, it must enter the blood, where it can potentially affect any cell in the body within minutes. There are five types of drug administration:

1. **Oral administration** is when the drug, normally in pill or liquid form, is swallowed and absorbed through the stomach and intestines. This is the most common way to administer drugs, but it is also the most inefficient because of differences in rates of digestion between people.

2. **Parenteral administration** is the injection of a drug with a needle. Types of injection include intravenous (into the vein), intramuscular (into muscle), and subcutaneous (under the skin). The effects of parenteral administration are quick since the drug is absorbed into the bloodstream almost immediately.

3. **Inhalation administration** is when a drug is inhaled into the lungs as a gas or snorted into the nose as a powder. Again, there is an almost immediate effect, as blood vessels in the lungs and nose aid quick absorption.

4. **Rectal administration** is the insertion of suppositories into the rectum. As the suppository melts, the drug enters the many blood vessels that support the lower digestive system.

5. **Transdermal administration** takes place when a drug such as nicotine is contained in an adhesive patch that is affixed to the skin. The drug diffuses into the bloodstream via the skin.

DRUG TERMINOLOGY

It is important to understand some basic drug terminology. **Drug use** refers to taking a drug for its intended purpose, such as swallowing an antihistamine capsule to treat hay fever. **Drug misuse** is the taking of a drug for a reason other than that for which it was intended—for example, taking an antihistamine to feel a "buzz." **Drug abuse** is the chronic, long-term, and consistent taking of a drug for a reason other than the intended use. If someone regularly takes antihistamines to achieve a high, that is considered abuse. These terms can also be applied to alcohol consumption: having a drink to relax is considered

Oral administration is the taking of a drug by mouth in pill or liquid form. **Parenteral administration** refers to injected drugs. **Inhalation administration** is breathing in a drug as a gas or vapor. **Rectal administration** is used for drugs in suppositories that are absorbed through rectal membranes. **Transdermal administration** refers to drugs given through adhesive patches put on the skin.

Drug use is using a drug for its intended purpose. **Drug misuse** is using a drug for a reason other than the intended use. **Drug abuse** is chronically using a drug for a reason other than the intended use.

drug use, drinking enough to get drunk is misuse, and getting drunk regularly, by definition, is considered abuse.

There are also factors beyond the frequency of use that can influence the effect of drugs. **Set** is a powerful variable that refers to a person's expectations regarding how a drug will be experienced. If people believe a drug has a certain effect before they take it—for example, that it causes hallucinations—then there is a good chance that they will experience what they expect while under the influence of the drug. The placebo effect is an example of a set variable. In this case, people take a placebo (sugar pill) rather than a real drug but still display the effect of the drug they thought they took.

The **setting,** or environment in which a drug is taken, also influences the effect. For example, alcohol is a depressant and should induce drowsiness when consumed. If someone drinks in a quiet environment, then the most likely result is sleepiness. But if the same amount of alcohol is consumed in an environment where there is a festive atmosphere and social interaction, chances are that the user will feel stimulated.

Dependence is another important concept related to drug use. **Physical dependence** is when the body learns to require a certain drug in order to function normally. When the drug is removed from the dependent person's body, he or she will have withdrawal symptoms, or physical reactions that can range from a headache to seizures, depending upon the type of drug and the extent of dependence. Withdrawal symptoms eventually subside over time if the drug remains out of the person's system, but they will also subside if the person immediately consumes more of the drug. To become physically dependent, a person usually needs to take a drug for a long period of time. However, drugs such as methamphetamines are capable of reinforcing a craving very quickly, so physical dependence on them can develop in a short period of time.

Psychological dependence is an emotional attachment to a drug that develops in the person taking it. If the user does not take the drug at regular

---

Set is the mental expectation regarding the effects of a drug. The **setting** is the environment in which a drug is consumed, which can influence its effect.

Physical dependence occurs when the body requires a drug, and withdrawal symptoms occur if the drug is not administered and absorbed. **Psychological dependence** is an emotional attachment to a drug.

intervals, then withdrawal symptoms such as anxiety or irritability result. In this case, the drug fulfills an underlying emotional need in the user. Many drugs result in both physical and psychological dependency. For example, a person who usually smokes a cigarette after dinner each night may feel irritable and anxious if he or she is prevented from doing so, even when wearing a patch that prevents nicotine levels from dropping to the point where physical cravings are triggered. Drugs that cause both physical and psychological dependence tend to be the hardest for users to stop taking.

Lastly, there are a few concepts relating to the amount of drugs taken. An **effective dose** of a drug is the amount of the substance it takes to get a desired effect. A **lethal dose** is the amount of drug that will overwhelm the body's systems and result in death.

Normally, effective doses and lethal doses are expressed with respect to the percentage of people experiencing the effect at that dose. For example, if we say the effective dose for 50 percent of people (ED50) for a certain drug is 10mg, that means that 50 percent of people will experience the desired therapeutic effect after taking 10mg. But it also indicates that the other 50 percent of people will need more or less of the drug to achieve the intended effect. The same concept holds true for lethal dose—the amount of a drug that may cause one person to die may even be an effective dose for another person.

The effect of different doses varies depending on body mass and underlying health, as well as tolerance. **Tolerance** is a condition that occurs

---

✓ **NEED TO KNOW**

Drugs can be administered orally, transdermally, rectally, and parenterally, as well as via inhalation. Taking a drug for its intended purpose is called *drug use*. *Drug misuse* is the taking of a drug for a reason other than the one for which it was intended, and *drug abuse* is the chronic, long-term, and consistent taking of a drug for a reason other than the intended use. Set and setting are perhaps as important in determining a drug's effect as the actual physical action of the drug itself because mental expectations and environment influence one's behavior.

Effective dose is the dose necessary to produce a desired effect. **Lethal dose** is the dose capable of causing the user's death. **Tolerance** is a condition in which a person needs an increased amount of a drug to achieve the desired effect.

when a drug is taken repeatedly over time and the effects at the original dose diminish. To get the same original effect, the user must take increasingly larger doses. A person who has established a tolerance has probably taken the drug over a long period of time, and the body has adapted to certain blood levels of the drug.

CLASSIFYING DRUGS

In the United States, the Drug Enforcement Agency (DEA) is in charge of regulation and classification of controlled substances. It "schedules" drugs according to five categories (I, II, III, IV, and V) that describe effects, legal availability, and potential for abuse, as well as the legal penalties for distributing or using a drug incorrectly. (See Figure 4.1.) The drug schedule weighs the negative risks and effects of various drugs against their possible beneficial uses and then assigns penalties and use parameters accordingly. Drugs with the fewest accepted medical uses and the most negative or dangerous effects are often banned outright and carry the highest penalties for improper trafficking and distribution. Drugs that are dangerous under most circumstances but still have therapeutic medical uses are made available only under strict controls and with high penalties for misuse or improper possession. At the other end of the scheduling spectrum are drugs deemed as having little chance for misuse, abuse, and dependency. These drugs are more readily available, and the penalties for abuse tend to be lower. (See Figure 4.2 on page 134 for detailed information on penalties.)

According to the DEA, Schedule I drugs are the ones with the highest potential for abuse and dependency and are not currently acceptable for medical use. Examples of Schedule I drugs include heroin, marijuana, and LSD. Possessing or taking these drugs is banned outright in the United States. The government also considers Schedule II drugs highly addictive, but these drugs have widely accepted medical uses. Examples of Schedule II substances include morphine, cocaine, and methamphetamines.

Schedule III drugs have common uses in medical treatment, and they include anabolic steroids, most barbiturates, and the anti-nausea drug Marinol. Like Schedule I and II drugs, these drugs are addictive, and they may cause moderate physical or high psychological dependence.

Finally, Schedules IV and V drugs have medical uses but low potential for abuse and the risk of only limited physical or psychological dependence. The anti-anxiety drug Xanax and the sedative barbital are examples of Schedule IV drugs. Mixtures having small amounts of codeine, such as a prescription cough syrup or Tylenol 3, are examples of Schedule V drugs.

FIGURE 4.1   DRUG SCHEDULES AND LEGAL PENALTIES

A new class of substances was created by the Anti-Drug Abuse Act of 1986. Controlled substance analogues are substances which are not controlled substances, but may be found in the illicit traffic. They are structurally or pharmacologically similar to Schedule I or II controlled substances and

SCHEDULE I

◇ The drug or other substance has a high potential for abuse.

◇ The drug or other substance has no currently accepted medical use in treatment in the United States.

◇ There is a lack of accepted safety for use of the drug or other substance under medical supervision.

◇ Examples of Schedule I substances include heroin, lysergic acid diethylamide (LSD), marijuana, and methaqualone.

SCHEDULE II

◇ The drug or other substance has a high potential for abuse.

◇ The drug or other substance has a currently accepted medical use in treatment in the United States or a currently accepted medical use with severe restrictions.

◇ Abuse of the drug or other substance may lead to severe psychological or physical dependence.

◇ Examples of Schedule II substances include morphine, phencyclidine (PCP), cocaine, methadone, and methamphetamine.

SCHEDULE III

◇ The drug or other substance has less potential for abuse than the drugs or other substances in schedules I and II.

◇ The drug or other substance has a currently accepted medical use in treatment in the United States.

Source: Drug Enforcement Administration, *Drugs of Abuse,* 2005 (**www.justice.gov/dea/pubs/abuse/1-csa.htm#Analogues**).

have no legitimate medical use. A substance which meets the definition of a controlled substance analogue and is intended for human consumption is treated under the Controlled Substances Act (CSA) as if it were a controlled substance in Schedule I. [21 U.S.C.802(32), 21 U.S.C.813]

- Abuse of the drug or other substance may lead to moderate or low physical dependence or high psychological dependence.

- Anabolic steroids, codeine and hydrocodone with aspirin or Tylenol®, and some barbiturates are examples of Schedule III substances.

SCHEDULE IV

- The drug or other substance has a low potential for abuse relative to the drugs or other substances in Schedule III.

- The drug or other substance has a currently accepted medical use in treatment in the United States.

- Abuse of the drug or other substance may lead to limited physical dependence or psychological dependence relative to the drugs or other substances in Schedule III.

- Examples of drugs included in schedule IV are Darvon®, Talwin®, Equanil®, Valium®, and Xanax®.

SCHEDULE V

- The drug or other substance has a low potential for abuse relative to the drugs or other substances in Schedule IV.

- The drug or other substance has a currently accepted medical use in treatment in the United States.

- Abuse of the drug or other substances may lead to limited physical dependence or psychological dependence relative to the drugs or other substances in Schedule IV.

- Cough medicines with codeine are examples of Schedule V drugs.

FIGURE 4.2 PENALTIES FOR DRUG POSSESSION AND TRAFFICKING

DRUG/SCHEDULE	QUANTITY	PENALTIES	QUANTITY	PENALTIES
Cocaine (Schedule II)	500–4999 gms mixture	**First Offense:** Not less than 5 years, and not more than 40 years. If death or serious injury, not less than 20 years or more than life. Fine of not more than $2 million if an individual, $5 million if not an individual.	5 kgs or more mixture	**First Offense:** Not less than 10 years, and not more than life. If death or serious injury, not less than 20 years or more than life. Fine of not more than $4 million if an individual , $10 million if not an individual.
Cocaine Base (Schedule II)	5–49 gms mixture		50 gms or more mixture	
Fentanyl (Schedule II)	40–399 gms mixture		400 gms or more mixture	
Fentanyl Analogue (Schedule I)	10–99 gms mixture		100 gms or more mixture	
Heroin (Schedule I)	100–999 gms mixture	**Second Offense:** Not less than 10 years, and not more than life. If death or serious injury, life imprisonment. Fine of not more than $4 million if an individual, $10 million if not an individual.	1 kg or more mixture	**Second Offense:** Not less than 20 years, and not more than life. If death or serious injury, life imprisonment. Fine of not more than $8 million if an individual, $20 million if not an individual.
LSD (Schedule I)	1–9 gms mixture		10 gms or more mixture	
Methamphetamine (Schedule II)	5–49 gms pure or 50–499 gms mixture		50 gms or more pure or 500 gms or more mixture	**2 or More Prior Offenses:** Life imprisonment.
PCP (Schedule II)	10–99 gms pure or 100–999 gms mixture		100 gms or more pure or 1 kg or more mixture	

DRUG/SCHEDULE	QUANTITY	PENALTIES
Other Schedule I and II drugs (and any drug product containing Gamma Hydroxybutyric Acid)	Any amount	**First Offense:** Not more than 20 years. If death or serious injury, not less than 20 years, or more than life. Fine $1 million if an individual, $5 million if not an individual. **Second Offense:** Not less than 30 years. If death or serious injury, not less than life. Fine $2 million if an individual, $10 million if not an individual.
Other Schedule III drugs	Any amount	**First Offense:** Not more than 5 years. Fine not more than $250,000 if an individual, $1 million if not an individual. **Second Offense:** Not more than 10 years. Fine of not more than $500,000 if an individual, $2 million if not an individual.
Flunitrazepam (Schedule IV)	30–999 mgs	

DRUG	QUANTITY	
All other Schedule IV drugs	Any amount	**First Offense:** Not more than 3 years. Fine not more than $250,000 if an individual, $1 million if not an individual. **Second Offense:** Not more than 6 years. Fine not more than $500,000 if an individual, $2 million if not an individual.
All other Schedule V drugs	Any amount	**First Offense:** Not more than 1 year. Fine not more than $100,000 if an individual, $250,000 million if not an individual. **Second Offense:** Not more than 2 year. Fine of not more than $200,000 if an individual, $500,000 million if not an individual.

FEDERAL TRAFFICKING PENALTIES—MARIJUANA

DRUG	QUANTITY	
Marijuana	1,000 kg or more mixture, or 1,000 or more plants	**First Offense:** Not less than 10 years, not more than life. If death or serious injury, not less than 20 years, not more than life. Fine not more than $4 million if an individual, $10 million if other than an individual. **Second Offense:** Not less than 20 years, not more than life. If death or serious injury, mandatory life. Fine not more than $8 million if an individual, $20 million if other than an individual.
Marijuana	100–999 kg mixture, or 100–999 plants	**First Offense:** Not less than 5 years, not more than 40 years. If death or serious injury, not less than 20 years, not more than life. Fine not more than $2 million if an individual, $5 million if other than an individual. **Second Offense:** Not less than 10 years, not more than life. If death or serious injury, mandatory life. Fine not more than $4 million if an individual, $10 million if other than an individual.
Marijuana Hashish	More than 10 kg hashish, or 50–99 kg mixture; More than 1 kg of hashish oil, or 50–99 plants	**First Offense:** Not more than 20 years. If death or serious injury, not less than 20 years, not more than life. Fine not more than $1 million if an individual, $5 million if other than an individual. **Second Offense:** Not more than 30 years. If death or serious injury, mandatory life. Fine of not more than $2 million if an individual, $10 million if other than an individual.
Marijuana Hashish Hashish Oil	Less than 50 kg mixture, or 1–49 plants; 10 kg or less; 1 kg or less	**First Offense:** Not more than 5 years. Fine not more than $250,000 if an individual, $1 million if not an individual. **Second Offense:** Not more than 10 years. Fine of $500,000 if an individual, $2 million if other than an individual.

Source: Drug Enforcement Administration (DEA).

What Is Your Risk?

It has been said that if a person can't go without using a recreational drug for 30 days then he or she has a drug problem. There probably is some truth to the statement. Humans are creatures capable of rationalization, and rather than admit we have a problem with smoking, drinking, or drugs, it is often easier to tell ourselves, "I can quit any time I want."

So how do you know if you are at risk of having a problem with drug misuse or abuse? Take a look at the following questions and answer them honestly:

1. On many occasions I have used more drugs, or used them longer, than I originally intended.
2. I have tried (or wanted to try) to control my drug use.
3. I spend a great deal of time trying to obtain drugs, using them, or recovering from them.
4. During times when I was (or should have been) at work, school, or home, I have frequently been intoxicated or experiencing withdrawal symptoms.
5. I give up important social or work activities in order to use drugs in a group or by myself.
6. I realize my drug use causes ongoing physical/psychological/social problems in my life, but I use them anyway.
7. Sometimes I have to use more of a particular drug than before in order to achieve the effect I want.
8. There are times when I experienced withdrawal symptoms after I stop using drugs.
9. There have been times when I used drugs in order to avoid withdrawal symptoms.

Source: DSM-IV, American Psychiatric Association, 1995.

These questions address mainly the issues of tolerance and control—both key variables in defining dependence and abuse. If you answered yes to any of the above questions, it indicates a higher risk of a drug problem and time to begin to think about talking with someone regarding your drug use.

✓ NEED TO KNOW

There are two types of drug dependence: physical and psychological. Effective and lethal doses of drugs can vary according to many factors, including body mass and tolerance. Tolerance of a drug can develop over time, requiring larger doses to achieve the desired effect. The government regulates the selling and taking of all drugs and classifies use and penalties under a system of "schedules." Penalties regarding unlawful use and trafficking of controlled substances are severe and aggressively prosecuted by state and federal governments.

Now we will turn to the second way drugs are classified—by their effect—and discuss some of the major types of drugs that medical professionals and regulators are concerned with today.

➤ Depressants

Depressants are drugs that decrease or slow down body processes. These drugs include opioids, sedative-hypnotics, and the number-one drug of use, misuse, and abuse in the United States—alcohol.

ALCOHOL

The major forms of alcoholic beverages are beer, wine, and distilled liquor. Generally beer has a 3–6 percent concentration of ethyl alcohol, wines have 10–14 percent, and distilled liquors such as rum and scotch have 35–40 percent. In terms of standard serving sizes, a can or bottle of beer is usually 12 ounces, a glass of wine is 4 ounces, and a mixed drink contains one shot (1–1.5 ounces, depending on the proof of the liquor). It is interesting to note that although the concentration of alcohol in each type of beverage is different, the standard size adjusts total volume so that in the end, one serving of beer, wine, or liquor each contains one-half of an ounce of ethyl alcohol. This guide can be a handy measure for monitoring your alcohol consumption. Just be aware that certain mixed drinks such as margaritas and Long Island iced teas contain more than one shot of alcohol, so they count as more than one serving.

Because alcohol is a liquid, it quickly absorbs into the bloodstream, where it moves on to affect the nervous, circulatory, endocrine, and digestive systems. The higher the dose, the greater the effect. In the central nervous system, alcohol's depressant effect is most noticeable in the cerebrum, cerebellum, and medulla areas of the brain. Alcohol affects memory, awareness, and reasoning—collectively, these are what we call *judgment*—and it diminishes balance and coordination. Heart rate and breathing are also slowed. With smaller doses of alcohol, such as 1–2 drinks in an hour, the main effect felt is relaxation—hence alcohol's reputation as the social lubricant. With high doses, such as 7–8 drinks in one hour, the user would have impaired judgment, impaired movement, and balance, and decreased heart rate and breathing. With extremely high doses of alcohol, say 15–20 drinks in one hour, loss of consciousness and death can result because in addition to the continuing depression of the cerebrum and cerebellum, the medulla is being depressed to a point where it no longer instructs the heart to beat or the lungs to breathe. (See Figure 4.3.)

Alcohol causes blood vessels to expand, so the drinker feels very warm and sweats. The more alcohol in the system, the longer the vessels will dilate and the longer one will feel uncomfortably warm or hot. Alcohol also increases urination, so it is easy to become dehydrated while drinking too much alcohol.

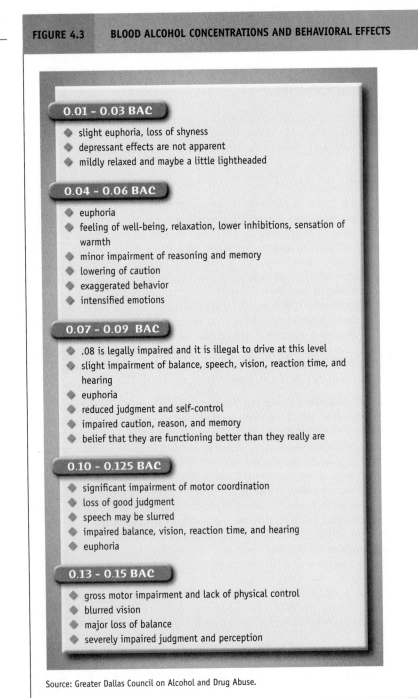

FIGURE 4.3   **BLOOD ALCOHOL CONCENTRATIONS AND BEHAVIORAL EFFECTS**

0.01 – 0.03 BAC

- slight euphoria, loss of shyness
- depressant effects are not apparent
- mildly relaxed and maybe a little lightheaded

0.04 – 0.06 BAC

- euphoria
- feeling of well-being, relaxation, lower inhibitions, sensation of warmth
- minor impairment of reasoning and memory
- lowering of caution
- exaggerated behavior
- intensified emotions

0.07 – 0.09 BAC

- .08 is legally impaired and it is illegal to drive at this level
- slight impairment of balance, speech, vision, reaction time, and hearing
- euphoria
- reduced judgment and self-control
- impaired caution, reason, and memory
- belief that they are functioning better than they really are

0.10 – 0.125 BAC

- significant impairment of motor coordination
- loss of good judgment
- speech may be slurred
- impaired balance, vision, reaction time, and hearing
- euphoria

0.13 – 0.15 BAC

- gross motor impairment and lack of physical control
- blurred vision
- major loss of balance
- severely impaired judgment and perception

Source: Greater Dallas Council on Alcohol and Drug Abuse.

- reduced euphoria
- dysphoria (anxiety, restlessness) beginning to appear

0.16 - 0.19 BAC

- dysphoria predominant
- nausea may appear
- drinker has the appearance of "sloppy drunk"

0.20 BAC

- feeling dazed, confused, and otherwise disoriented
- may need help to stand or walk
- if injured, may not feel the pain
- nausea and vomiting
- impaired gag reflex—drinker can choke if they vomit
- blackouts—drinker may not remember what has happened

0.25 BAC

- severely impaired mental, physical, and sensory functions
- increased risk of asphyxiation from choking on vomit
- increased risk of serious injury by falls or other unintentional accidents

0.30 BAC

- stupor
- little comprehension of where they are
- may pass out suddenly and be difficult to awaken

0.35 BAC

- level of surgical anesthesia
- coma is possible

0.40+BAC

- onset of coma
- possible death due to respiratory arrest

The digestive system is affected in two ways. First, alcohol is a gastric irritant that causes food to move through the system quicker, so there is poor absorption of nutrients, and constipation, diarrhea, or both can result. People who have digestive problems such as ulcers or gastric reflux should abstain or significantly limit drinking and never drink on an empty stomach. Second, alcohol also affects the liver, which is chiefly responsible for breaking down alcohol in the body in a process called *oxidation*. The liver oxidizes the amount of alcohol in a standard size drink (half an ounce) in about one hour. Oxidizing alcohol is hard on the liver, and prolonged excessive drinking will damage it. But most experts agree that 1–2 drinks per day won't cause a negative impact on the liver of an otherwise healthy person.

Blood Alcohol Level

The effects of alcohol are directly related to the amount of alcohol in the blood, referred to as *blood alcohol level* (BAL) or *blood alcohol concentration* (BAC). Figure 4.3 shows the effects of alcohol at selected blood alcohol concentrations.

The higher the level of alcohol in the blood, the greater the effect: from relaxation (.01) to death (.40). Four variables influence blood alcohol concentration: (1) the amount of alcohol consumed in a given time period, (2) the weight of the drinker, (3) the gender of the drinker, and (4) the amount of food in the stomach. Figures 4.4 and 4.5 bring together the first three variables. Here we can see that blood alcohol levels are influenced by the amount consumed as well as the weight and gender of the drinker. When they consume the same number of drinks, a person who weighs less will have a higher BAL than a person who weighs more. In addition, if a man and a woman consume the same number of drinks and they also weigh the same, the woman will still

FIGURE 4.4   BLOOD ALCOHOL CONCENTRATION ESTIMATE FOR MEN

Drinks[a]	Body Weight in Pounds								Influence[b]
	100	120	140	160	180	200	220	240	
1	.04	.03	.02	.02	.02	.02	.02	.02	Possibly Impaired
2	.08	.06	.05	.05	.04	.04	.03	.03	
3	.11	.09	.08	.07	.06	.06	.05	.05	Impaired
4	.15	.12	.11	.09	.08	.08	.07	.06	
5	.19	.16	.13	.12	.11	.09	.09	.09	DUI
6	.23	.19	.16	.14	.13	.11	.10	.09	
7	.26	.22	.19	.16	.15	.13	.12	.11	
8	.30	.25	.21	.19	.17	.15	.14	.13	
9	.34	.28	.24	.21	.19	.17	.15	.14	
10	.38	.31	.27	.23	.21	.19	.17	.16	

[a]One drink is 1.25 oz. of 80-proof liquor, 12 oz. of beer, or 5 oz. of wine.
[b]Subtract .01 for each hour of drinking.

Source: Greater Dallas Council on Alcohol and Drug Abuse.

FIGURE 4.5 BLOOD ALCOHOL CONCENTRATION ESTIMATE FOR WOMEN

Drinks[a]	Body Weight in Pounds							
	90	100	120	140	160	180	200	220
1	.05	.05	.04	.03	.03	.03	.02	.02
2	.10	.09	.08	.07	.06	.05	.05	.04
3	.15	.14	.11	.10	.09	.08	.07	.06
4	.20	.18	.15	.13	.11	.10	.09	.08
5	.25	.23	.19	.16	.14	.13	.11	.10
6	.30	.27	.23	.19	.17	.15	.14	.12
7	.35	.27	.23	.19	.17	.15	.14	.12
8	.40	.36	.30	.26	.23	.20	.18	.17
9	.45	.41	.34	.29	.26	.23	.20	.19
10	.51	.45	.38	.32	.28	.25	.23	.21

Influence[b]
- Possibly Impaired
- Impaired
- DUI

[a]One drink is 1.25 oz. of 80-proof liquor, 12 oz. of beer, or 5 oz. of wine.
[b]Subtract .01 for each hour of drinking.

Source: Greater Dallas Council on Alcohol and Drug Abuse.

have a higher blood alcohol level than the man. This is because women normally have less of a digestive enzyme called *gastric acetaldehyde*, and as a result they digest less alcohol than men. Another reason is that women have a lower percentage of body water than men. Because of enzyme and body water differences, women absorb more alcohol than men.

As a general rule, an average-size man's BAL will rise approximately .025 per drink per hour. An average-size woman's BAL will rise approximately .030 per drink per hour. The liver oxidizes one drink each hour, so BAL will drop .025 per drink per hour for both genders. This is a general approximation of oxidation rates, including the fact that women tend to process alcohol in their system more slowly than men. A more precise, individualized measure can be obtained with a breathalyzer, a machine that analyzes alcohol content when a person exhales into it. The concentration of alcohol in the breath is an excellent indication of the concentration of alcohol in the blood, and it is legally defensible, as in the case of a Driving Under the Influence (DUI) legal charge.

Alcohol-related Problems

Alcohol is a caustic substance that over time can lead to debilitating conditions such as deterioration of the heart muscle and cirrhosis of the liver. But perhaps the most common alcohol-related problem is the headache, nausea, dehydration, and lightheadedness collectively referred to as a *hangover*. A number of factors come into play with a hangover. The expansion of cerebral blood vessels can cause the headache. Furthermore, the first step in the liver's breaking down of alcohol produces a toxic chemical that, in abundance, can also cause nausea and headache. Finally, the dehydration that comes with excessive drinking can also cause symptoms such as headache, nausea, and lightheadedness.

Health & the Media Alcohol Advertising and Behavior

It has been reported that by age 18 the typical American youth has seen or heard over 100,000 alcohol advertisements on television, in print, and on the radio. Billions of dollars are spent each year on alcohol advertising. In a 2006 *Archives of Pediatrics and Adolescent Medicine* study, researchers reported that underage youth viewed, on average, 23 alcohol ads per month. The study also found that such advertising contributes to an increase in drinking among underage youth, and that for each additional dollar per capita spent on alcohol advertising in a local advertising market, young people drank 3 percent more. Does alcohol advertising work? The short answer is yes.

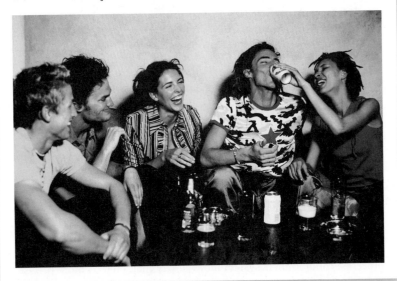

Hangovers are for the most part self-limiting—their symptoms pass after the body oxidizes the alcohol and systems have cycled back to normal. There is no cure for a hangover except time. Hangover symptoms can be treated, but one must be careful, because certain common over-the-counter medications, such as acetaminophen (Tylenol) and ibuprofen (Advil), can interact with alcohol and damage the liver. People who take too much pain reliever medication after a hangover can experience profound liver problems, including liver failure.

Another alcohol-related problem is drinking and driving. Driving Under the Influence **(DUI)** or Driving While Intoxicated **(DWI)** are the

DUI stands for "driving under the influence." **DWI** stands for "driving while intoxicated."

most common legal terms describing one who is driving after having consumed alcohol. "Under the influence" and "while intoxicated" are defined as driving while having a .08 BAL or above. If you recall (see Figures 4.4 and 4.5), it doesn't take a huge amount of alcohol to reach a .08 level, and people with a high tolerance may not even appear to have been drinking but have a .08 BAL. However, tolerance is individual and subjective, but the laws governing drinking are fairly universal and black and white. A .08 BAL can impair judgment and driving reflexes in most people, so it is now the main criteria for a DUI or DWI conviction in almost all states.

In most states conviction of a DUI or DWI is a Class I misdemeanor, which means that the person will have a criminal record forever. Conviction can also mean that the person will not be eligible for certain occupations, especially those that require a security clearance, since these organizations will not hire someone with a criminal record. Also, car insurance premiums can increase 200–400 percent (assuming that the driving record other than the DUI or DWI is good) for 2–3 years. Finally, legal representation, fines, and court costs can total thousands of dollars. Thomas von Hermet of the Thomas Jefferson Area (Virginia) Community Criminal Justice Board estimated that the financial costs of a DUI could be as high as $20,000. A DUI/DWI is a serious offense with lifelong implications.

Another alcohol-related problem is drinking while under the legal age of consumption, which is 21 years old in all 50 states. The fake ID is a popular way for underage people to misrepresent their age and be allowed to purchase alcohol and attend nightclubs or parties where alcohol is served. Possessing a fake ID is legally considered fraud and depending on the context of use, it can result in a Class I misdemeanor conviction and criminal record for life. To compound matters, a fake ID Class I misdemeanor can be considered a "crime of moral turpitude," which means that the person convicted is a dishonest person who committed fraud. Many employers, organizations, and segments of the general population view this as a character flaw with far-reaching implications. So the legal and societal penalties related to fake ID convictions can be surprisingly harsh.

High-risk Drinking

In recent years much attention has been directed at what is termed **binge drinking,** which is defined as four or more drinks for a female and five or more drinks for a male in one setting. There is no time limit inherent in binge drinking, although some researchers attach a two-hour period for consumption of these drinks. Binge drinking is a concern on college campuses, but

Binge drinking is having four drinks in one occasion for a woman and five drinks for a man.

what is of more concern is consumption of even higher amounts of alcohol in a short period of time, which is referred to as "high-risk drinking."

Much high risk drinking is done in a game context, such as the "power hour"—21 shots in an hour during a 21st birthday celebration. As blood alcohol levels rise, judgment gets more impaired, personal safety can be compromised, and blood alcohol content can rise to lethal levels. High-risk drinking is certainly a problem. However, high-risk drinking can range being episodic (for festive events) to something done by an inexperienced underage drinker with limited access to alcohol.

Problem drinking, in a clinical context, usually refers to alcohol abuse and alcohol dependence. *Alcoholism*, although a commonly used term, is not typically used in clinical contexts. **Alcohol abuse** is defined as "continued drinking despite recurring social, interpersonal, and legal problems." **Alcohol dependence** is predicated on the presence or absence of tolerance and withdrawal symptoms. How would one know if he or she is a normal drinker or a problem drinker heading toward alcohol abuse, alcohol dependence, or both? Answers to the series of questions in Figure 4.6 on page 146 can provide an idea if there is potentially a problem. If there is a problem, help can be found.

Help for Problem Drinkers

A typical model for assisting a problem drinker involves three steps: detoxification, counseling, and support groups. Detoxification is a medically supervised effort that removes the alcohol from a person's system and helps reduce the related cravings. It is important that the detoxification be medically supervised because of potentially serious withdrawal symptoms, including tremors, rapid heart beat, confusion, nausea, anxiety, and convulsions. Medications can be used to help limit the severity of symptoms.

Once detoxification is over, people should undergo counseling to deal with the issues that drove them to use alcohol in the first place. Counseling can be individual, family, or group. The counseling effort also focuses on coping skills other than the use of alcohol. In addition, emotional support is also important to help people stay clean and sober. Without this, it is more likely that the user will relapse. Support groups are made up of people who are also trying to stay clean and sober. In every community there are numerous support groups that meet daily, and in these groups people hold each other accountable in the effort to stay clean and sober. Perhaps the best example of a support group is Alcoholic Anonymous (AA).

Alcohol abuse is continued drinking despite recurring social, interpersonal, and legal problems. **Alcohol dependence** is predicated on the presence of withdrawal symptoms.

✓ **NEED TO KNOW**

The amount of alcohol in a standard size drink is the same in a glass of wine, a shot of liquor, or a glass of beer. Nothing can be done to speed up the oxidation of alcohol by the liver. Women digest alcohol slower than men, so even if they weigh the same, women will have a higher blood alcohol level than men after the same number of drinks. It takes women longer than men to rid their body of alcohol due to differences in levels of certain digestive enzymes between men and women. Taking too many pain relievers (such as Tylenol or Advil) after drinking heavily can lead to liver damage. Excessive alcohol consumption is a high-risk behavior that can have disastrous consequences. DUI and fake ID convictions are economically costly and have lifelong implications in regard to security clearances for certain jobs. Finally, help for problem drinkers usually involves three steps: medically supervised detoxification, counseling, and support groups.

OPIOIDS

Another class of depressant drugs is called *opioids*. This name refers to natural products of crude opium, semi-synthetic products containing some natural crude opium, and synthetic opiates, which react in the body in the same manner as opiates but are made without natural products. Collectively opioids are a very important class of drugs due to their effectiveness at treating pain. But they also have a high potential for dependence and abuse, and their use is highly regulated. The range of effects includes euphoria, including a dreamlike state of significant relaxation; drowsiness; respiratory depression; nausea; and constipation.

Crude opium is a product of a poppy that grows wild in Asia and other parts of the world. For centuries opium was used to treat pain, diarrhea, and coughs. It was also used recreationally to induce euphoria or a sense of well-being. In the early 1800s, morphine, the active ingredient in crude opium, was isolated, and later that century heroin, a semi-synthetic drug, was also created. Codeine, another active ingredient in crude opium, was isolated in the 1930s. All of these opiates were used medically for decades. There were originally no laws regarding their sale or use, and it was not until the Civil War, when thousands became morphine addicts after receiving drugs for treatment of war injuries, that the downsides to opiates became widely known in the United States. In the early 1900s the government passed the first legislation to control distribution and use of opium, morphine, heroin, and other drugs referred to as *narcotics*.

Heroin is a Schedule I narcotic, meaning it is illegal and considered to have no medical use. It continues to be widely abused, causing many personal and societal problems. Most heroin addicts do not live long because the habit is expensive and they often have to turn to crime to pay for drugs. Further, heroin addicts often share needles and eventually expose themselves to bloodborne infections such as HIV and hepatitis.

FIGURE 4.6   MICHIGAN ALCOHOLISM SCREENING TEST (MAST)

Directions: Circle "yes" or "no" for each question. The scoring key is at the end.

1. Do you feel you are a normal drinker? ("normal" = drink as much or less than most other people)
   YES   NO

2. Have you ever awakened the morning after some drinking the night before and found that you could not remember a part of the evening?
   YES   NO

3. Does any near relative or close friend ever worry or complain about your drinking?
   YES   NO

4. Can you stop drinking without difficulty after one or two drinks?
   YES   NO

5. Do you ever feel guilty about your drinking?
   YES   NO

6. Have you ever attended a meeting of Alcoholics Anonymous (AA)?
   YES   NO

7. Have you ever gotten into physical fights when drinking?
   YES   NO

8. Has drinking ever created problems between you and a near relative or close friend?
   YES   NO

9. Has any family member or close friend gone to anyone for help about your drinking?
   YES   NO

10. Have you ever lost friends because of your drinking?
    YES   NO

11. Have you ever gotten into trouble at work because of drinking?
    YES   NO

12. Have you ever lost a job because of drinking?
    YES   NO

13. Have you ever neglected your obligations, your family, or your work for two or more days in a row because you were drinking?
    YES   NO

14. Do you drink before noon fairly often?
    YES   NO

15. Have you ever been told you have liver trouble such as cirrhosis?
    YES   NO

16. After heavy drinking have you ever had delirium tremens (D.T.'s), severe shaking, or auditory (hearing) hallucinations?
YES   NO

17. Have you ever gone to anyone for help about your drinking?
YES   NO

18. Have you ever been hospitalized because of drinking?
YES   NO

19. Has your drinking ever resulted in your being hospitalized in a psychiatric ward?
YES   NO

20. Have you ever gone to a doctor, social worker, member of the clergy, or mental health clinic for help with any emotional problem in which drinking was part of the problem?
YES   NO

21. Have you been arrested more than once for driving under the influence of alcohol?
YES   NO

22. Have you ever been arrested, even for a few hours, because of other behavior while drinking?
YES   NO

Scoring for the MAST Test

Please score one point if you answered the following:
1. No
2. Yes
3. Yes
4. No
5. Yes
6. Yes
7 through 22:   Yes

Add up the points, and compare your score to the following score card:

0–2	No apparent problem
3–5	Early or middle problem drinker
6 or more	Problem drinker

Sources: Selzer, M.L. (1971) *The Michigan Alcoholism Screening Test: The quest for a new diagnostic Instrument.* American Journal of Psychiatry. 127, 1653–1658. National Council on Alcoholism and Drug Dependenc of the San Fernando Valley, Inc.

Many other semi-synthetic opioids have medical uses, so they are listed as Schedule II narcotics. These include Demerol, Dilaudid, and Darvon. In recent years two other opioids, methadone and Oxycontin, have received much publicity.

Methadone is primarily used in heroin rehabilitation. So-called methadone maintenance is designed to determine the stabilization dose of methadone necessary to eliminate the craving for heroin. Once that dosage is reached, the heroin addict can undergo both personal and vocational counseling in order to reintegrate back into society as a productive member. Methadone maintenance is controversial, mostly because one drug (methadone) is substituted for another (heroin). There is conflict between the view that drug addiction is a poor life choice (a "disorder of the will") and that it is a disease. However, the two views do intersect. At first, the person is making a choice to modify his or her mood (an act of the will), but after time, if tolerance, physical dependence, and psychological dependence are established, the user has little control, and stopping the drug will lead to withdrawal symptoms requiring medical intervention. There is no easy answer to this conflict, as both views of addiction have merit.

A more recent controversy involves the drug **Oxycontin,** a time-released opioid normally prescribed to people in significant pain, such as cancer patients. It is a powerful opioid, and like many powerful drugs, has become a popular illicit drug because of the high it can produce. Patients taking Oxycontin must be monitored closely because of the potential problems of drug interactions, tolerance, and dependence and the possibility of dosages reaching a lethal level. Recreational abuse of Oxycontin has particularly been a problem in Appalachia (southwest Virginia and eastern Kentucky), where it is has been referred to as "Hillbilly Heroin."

SEDATIVE HYPNOTICS

Sedative-hypnotic drugs are a category of depressants normally used to induce sedation and sleep (hypnotic). There drugs are medically prescribed and include barbiturates, which are classified as ultra-short, intermediate, and long-acting. Ultra-short barbiturates such as thiopental are used to induce anesthesia; intermediate ones such as Seconal are used to induce sleep; and long-acting ones such as butalbital and phenobarbital are used to treat headaches and prevent seizures, respectively. Of the three types of barbiturates, the intermediate drugs have been the most problematic, since at one point they were popularly used to treat insomnia. Seconal dependence can occur fairly rapidly, and Seconal combined

---

Oxycontin is a time-released opioid similar to morphine and extremely potent.

Sedative-hypnotic drugs are capable of producing sedation and sleep.

with alcohol can be toxic and result in death. Further, withdrawal from barbiturates can cause serious problems and even be life-threatening.

Nonbarbiturate sedative hypnotics also exist. Meprobamate (Miltown) has the same effect as an intermediate barbiturate, but the risk of dependence is not as serious. With the introduction of minor tranquilizers in the 1960s, there has been less need for barbiturates and nonbarbiturates as sedative-hypnotics.

INHALANTS

Inhalants are solvents and solutions that are used in hair spray, gasoline, paint, glue, and other commonly used items. *Huffing* is the term used to describe use of inhalants. The effects from huffing include euphoria, light-headedness, and lack of coordination. The chemicals in the solvents can interfere with the amount of oxygen reaching the brain and other tissues, resulting in a condition called *hypoxia*, a dangerously low level of oxygen. Inhalant use can introduce toxic levels of the solvent into the system, and brain damage can result.

Nitrous oxide, or "laughing gas," is a popular inhalant. Nitrous oxide is used medically as an anesthetic. Inhaling nitrous oxide results in relaxation and a loosening of inhibitions often resulting in uncontrolled laughter. The amount of nitrous oxide administered for medical purposes must be closely monitored. Recreational users find items such as CO_2 cartridges containing nitrous oxide used in baking and inhale the nitrous oxide right from the cartridge. This is extremely dangerous because of the freezing temperature in the cartridge. Frostbite of the nose and lung damage from freezing can result.

> **NEED TO KNOW**
>
> Other depressants include opioids, sedative-hypnotics, and inhalants. Drugs in the opioid category including morphine, codeine, Vicodin, and Oxycontin. These drugs are powerful and have a high potential for abuse. Sedative hypnotics is a broad category of depressants with a wide variety of uses ranging from anesthesia to prevention of seizures. Inhalants also have medical uses but like other depressants, they can be abused, especially by adolescents who have easy access to glue, household chemicals, and other common substances that when inhaled can deprive the brain of oxygen and induce a euphoric effect.

➤ Stimulants

Stimulants are a large category that includes powerful drugs such as cocaine, crack, and amphetamines and milder cerebral stimulants such as nicotine and caffeine. *Speed* is a term used to describe stimulants, particularly amphetamines. All stimulants have the capability to increase functional activity of the nervous system. This can have a significant effect on thought processes to the point where thinking becomes so scrambled that it is difficult for people to focus their thoughts because they are so "wired." Sometimes this can serve as a catalyst for creativity, such as in stand-up comedy, but it can also lead to a split from reality involving the personality called a *psychosis*.

COCAINE AND CRACK

Cocaine is a drug found in the leaves of the coca bush, which grows wild in parts of Bolivia, Colombia, and Peru. Ancient civilizations such as the

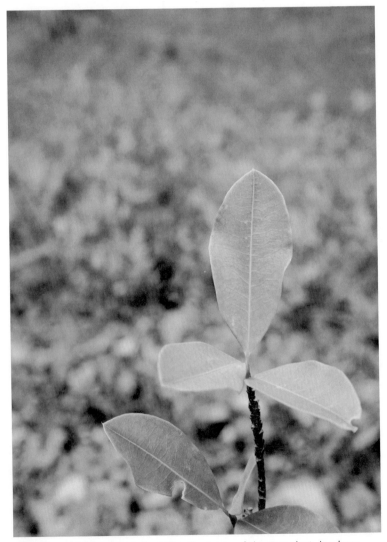

Cocaine, a stimulant drug derived from the leaves of the coca plant, has been used by humans for at least one thousand years.

Incas integrated cocaine into their culture through chewing coca leaves for the stimulant effect. Cocaine also has local anesthetic properties. What the common pick-me-ups caffeine and nicotine are to current society, cocaine was to the ancient Incas.

Cocaine has an interesting history that includes Sigmund Freud, who at first espoused the use of cocaine to treat morphine addiction, then renounced it as a scourge when he became addicted himself. The fictional detective Sherlock Holmes is known for his "7 percent solution," the special formula he used in preparing his cocaine. Inventor John Pemberton used cocaine in his original formula for Coca-Cola. In low doses cocaine can increase heart rate and blood pressure, decrease fatigue, and increase mental alertness and sociability. But in high doses it can cause dizziness, blurred vision, and tremors, as well as repress heart enzymes and cause convulsions and death. The cocaine experience is short-lived. After snorting it, users experience a euphoric high for 15–30 minutes. After that they "crash," becoming light-headed and nauseated. The only ways for the user to resolve the experience are to wait out the crash or to snort more cocaine to alleviate it. Snorting more cocaine will reinforce the craving—this is why cocaine is considered so addictive.

Recreational use of cocaine ebbs and flows in popularity. When it was extremely popular to abuse in the 1980s, a new, purer form called *crack* was created. Crack is about ten times more powerful than regular cocaine, in terms of both its euphoric high and the painful crash afterwards. As such, it is even more addictive than cocaine.

Interestingly, cocaine is not a Schedule I drug. The DEA placed it in Schedule II because it is a powerful local anesthetic used to numb the eyes or nasal passages for surgery.

AMPHETAMINES

Amphetamines are powerful prescription stimulants used to treat narcolepsy, low blood pressure, and attention-deficit/hyperactivity disorder (ADHD). Amphetamines are similar to cocaine in experience, but their effect lasts much longer, up to 10 or more hours. The crash from amphetamine use is also more prolonged. Because amphetamines have such as long duration, they are popularly taken to help people stay awake for long periods of time. Some students use them to stay awake all night to cram for an exam, and some truck drivers use them to drive for longer periods of time. Unfortunately, the effects of the amphetamines can be scary and even life threatening. Extreme restlessness, anxiety, confusion, paranoia, high blood pressure, convulsions, and cardiac arrest can result from excessive doses or extended use.

In a medically supervised context, amphetamines improve quality of life. Attention-deficit/hyperactivity disorder (ADHD) is a case in point. The stimulant Ritalin is prescribed for children, but adults who are diagnosed with ADHD can also be prescribed the drug. In ADHD the attention span is short, and the person has difficulty concentrating and is easily distracted. Learning is compromised. How Ritalin works is not entirely clear, and it does seem like a paradox that a hyperactive person would find relief from a prescription stimulant, but true ADHD patients receive tremendous benefit from Ritalin. They can take the drug without experiencing euphoria. People who take Ritalin who do not have ADHD will experience an amphetamine high, though. For that reason, Ritalin has become a drug of abuse in non-ADHD populations.

In recent years a form of amphetamine called *methamphetamine* has become a serious problem, especially in communities where the rave culture is prominent. Methamphetamine use has increased in popularity. There was a 50 percent increase in emergency room visits between 1995–2002 due to methamphetamine-related emergencies. In its oral form, the drug is often called "speed" or "meth," and in smokeable form, "ice" or "crystal." Both forms are normally made in illegal laboratories from ingredients in common over-the-counter drug products such as appetite suppressants, decongestants, and allergy products. Methamphetamines generally have a much more intense effect on the nervous system than prescription amphetamines, and the addictive potential is more profound.

Methamphetamines are extremely dangerous, and increased use can result in delusions and hallucinations, as well has heart problems. Smoking methamphetamine allows the administration and absorption to be quicker than taking it in tablet form, and the effects are more intense because the drug is getting to the brain quicker. The long-term effects of methamphetamine use include aggressive and violent behavior, weight loss, and psychosis. In addition to these effects, people who smoke methamphetamines can develop "meth mouth" when the teeth become destroyed and look like they are rotting away.

NICOTINE

Nicotine is another naturally occurring stimulant. Found in tobacco, nicotine is highly addictive. Once absorbed into the blood, it exerts a cerebral stimulant effect that is both pleasurable and short-lived. The smoker must inhale again and again to obtain more of the pleasurable feeling, and over time that produces cravings and addiction. Unfortunately, in addition to the nicotine, a smoker inhales tars and carbon monoxide, which starve tissue of oxygen. This is why smokers are at higher risk of both cancer and heart disease. The health hazards associated with any form of tobacco use are documented and well known. And for the approximately 29 percent of the population who smokes, tobacco use is an expensive habit. A pack-a-day cigarette habit will cost most smokers well over $1,000 each year.

In addition to the health hazards associated with smoking, those who are exposed to cigarette smoke are also at risk for health problems. Second-hand smoke (the smoke that people around a smoker inhale) contains carbon monoxide and carcinogens and can cause heart disease or even cancer in nonsmokers who spend large amounts of time in the company of smokers.

Getting dependent to nicotine is easy. Quitting tobacco use is hard. The withdrawal symptoms of nicotine include headache, nervousness, fatigue, poor concentration, and sleep disturbances. But users who have a desire to quit have numerous options. First, there is the classic "cold turkey" withdrawal, whereby the user quits tobacco, overcomes the withdrawal symptoms, and stays tobacco free. Second, there are gums that contain nicotine. They provide enough of the drug to reduce the craving for tobacco gradually. Third, there are nicotine patches, which release the drug into the blood at a steady rate through the skin and reduce the craving for nicotine. Finally, there are prescription medications such as Zyban that also will reduce the craving for nicotine.

CAFFEINE

Caffeine is the most common cerebral stimulant. It is found in coffee, chocolate, tea, soft drinks, and many over-the-counter drugs from analgesics to weight-loss products. The highest amounts of caffeine are found in coffee, where the dose can range from 30–40 mg per cup for instant coffee to 150 mg per cup for drip coffee. In soft drinks the caffeine can range from 30 mg in a 12-oz. can of Pepsi to 75 mg in extra-caffeinated drinks like Jolt Cola. Other energy drinks contain 120 mg or more.

Ingesting caffeine results in a higher level of alertness and mild euphoria. A dose of caffeine can exert this effect for about an hour and then it gradually wears off. People can become dependent on caffeine, and this can lead to a craving. The most common withdrawal effect is a headache.

Sometimes caffeine users over-caffeinate themselves and induce a state of **caffeinism.** The symptoms include tremors, restlessness, agitation, confusion, light-headedness, and anxiety. Abstaining from coffee for a few hours will cause the symptoms to subside. Although it is not pleasant, caffeinism is not generally harmful or dangerous. However, people should be aware that caffeine is rather caustic and can aggravate ulcers and acid reflux disease, so people who have digestive problems should not use it. People with anxiety disorders and women who are pregnant should also avoid excessive caffeine in their diets.

Caffeinism is an outcome of an excessive dose of caffeine.

➤ Hallucinogens

Hallucinogens are a category of drugs capable of inducing hallucinations, which is a perception of sights, sounds, physical senses (touch), or taste with no basis in reality. Similar to a hallucination is a delusion—a misinterpretation of something real. For example, a person who looks at a car and sees a dog instead of the vehicle is having a delusion, while a person seeing a car when nothing is there is having a hallucination.

LSD

LSD was accidentally discovered in the late 1930s when a Swiss chemist was working with ergot, a fungus that grows on rye, in an attempt to find a cure for migraine headaches. LSD proved not to have any headache-relief properties despite numerous experiments to find a medical use for the drug. In the 1960s LSD became popular as a part of the counterculture movement. It is a colorless, odorless, and tasteless drug. A small dose, called a "microdot," can induce an 8- to 12-hour psychoactive experience that includes hallucinations. This experience can be framed by anxiety, and the beginning, several hours of hallucinations, can be followed by several hours of depression. Like any other drug, the intensity of these effects varies.

There has been no documentation of physiological damage among LSD users. However, some users have experienced a post-hallucinogenic sensory disorder and have hallucinations years after using LSD. Also, during the hallucinogenic phase of the LSD experience, safety can be compromised if the false perception involves a potentially dangerous situation. For example, a person could be unaware of their surroundings and walk in front of oncoming traffic or fall out of a window. Like cocaine, LSD popularity ebbs and flows. Much of the current LSD use is tied to rave culture.

PSILOCYBIN

Psilocybin is a hallucinogenic drug found in *teonanacatl*, a type of mushroom native to the United States and Mexico. The term *schrooms* is sometimes used for these psilocybin-containing mushrooms. Schrooms are usually eaten, and the effects can last from 3 to 8 hours. Small doses of psilocybin induce a tranquil euphoric state, and higher dosages can induce hallucinations. The schroom experience is similar to LSD, but normally not nearly as intense or potent.

MESCALINE

Mescaline is a hallucinogenic drug found in peyote, a growth or "button" found on a small cactus that grows in Mexico and the southwestern United States. Mescaline produces a total psychoactive experience for about 10 hours, with hallucinations lasting about 2 hours. Although not a very powerful hallucinogen, mescaline can still pack a punch depending on the size and frequency of doses. Unlike many other hallucinogens, mescaline has medical uses; it is prescribed as a respiratory stimulant and as a treatment for heart problems.

PCP AND KETAMINE

Phencyclidine (PCP) was originally developed as a dissociative anesthetic (one capable of keeping patients awake but pain free during surgery and other procedures). The early trials of PCP as an anesthetic found it to be effective, but the patients experienced mood swings, hallucinations, and displayed violent behavior, all symptoms that indicated a narrow margin of safety, so the FDA never approved PCP for human use. However, it was approved for use as a veterinary anesthetic and tranquilizer. Consequently, it was easy to divert to human populations.

The effects of PCP are very unpredictable, causing some experts to characterize PCP as the most dangerous illicit drug. It can induce profound mood swings, delusions, violent primal behavior, and hallucinations. This experience can last for hours, and users may endanger themselves and others while under the influence. To complicate matters, when users are hurt, they do not feel the pain because of PCP's anesthetic properties. So users can continue violent and destructive behavior for much longer than would be possible for anyone who is not under the influence of PCP.

Like PCP, ketamine is a dissociative anesthetic and is used in veterinary medicine. Not as powerful as PCP, ketamine is also used as an anesthetic for humans. It can induce a PCP-like experience, and when used illicitly, it is sometimes called "Special K." Often ketamine is marketed as PCP.

✓ **NEED TO KNOW**

Hallucinogens are powerful drugs with unpredictable effects. PCP and ketamine are particularly dangerous due to the unpredictable, sometimes violent behavior they can cause users to exhibit.

➤ Marijuana

Marijuana is the name for products from the cannabis plant that are dried and prepared for smoking. Cannabis has been referred to as a weed because it does grow wild in many areas of the world. A resin called tetrahydrocannabinol (THC) is the chief agent responsible for the physical and psychological effects associated with marijuana.

FORMS AND EFFECTS OF MARIJUANA

How cannabis impacts someone relates to the concentration of THC in the final product. Ganja, the tops and leaves of the cannabis plant, generally contains 3–5 percent concentration THC. Sinsemilla, or "without seeds," refers to a form of marijuana with an 8–10 percent concentration of THC. Hashish is a more concentrated form that is usually smoked in small, square blocks and contains a 14–16 percent THC concentration. Finally, the most potent form is hash oil, which can contain up to 60 percent THC. Hash oil will induce an LSD-like experience. The other forms of marijuana are less potent and can induce significant sedation and possibly delusions but not hallucinations.

Because smoking is the chief method of administration, the effects are felt almost immediately. The psychological effects of THC include relaxation, relief from anxiety, euphoria, laughter, and if the concentration of THC is high enough, impaired judgment and short-term memory. Physical effects of marijuana include dry mouth, increased appetite, bloodshot eyes, coughing, and decreased muscle coordination. Often the effects of marijuana are compared to alcohol, particularly by those who want to see marijuana legalized. Long-term effects of marijuana use include the development of amotivational syndrome, impaired immunity, respiratory problems, and increased cancer risk.

Physical dependence and tolerance to marijuana have not been shown. Psychological dependence can be related to anything, so it is safe to say that users can become psychologically dependent on marijuana.

MARIJUANA'S SAFETY AND THE QUESTION OF LEGALIZATION

Due to its common illicit use since the 1960s, some people feel that using marijuana in moderation is as safe as alcohol or cigarettes and ought to be legalized. Just how safe is marijuana use?

Although THC and alcohol may both be used for relaxation, alcohol is not smoked, so the method of administration is not comparable. Smoking marijuana puts one at risk of the same kinds of conditions that cigarette smokers are at risk for, including heart disease and cancer. **Cannabinoids** are

---

Cannabinoids are tars in cannabis and marijuana, some of which are carcinogenic.

tars in cannabis, many of which are cancer causing. Further, marijuana smoke, like cigarette smoke, contains high levels of carbon monoxide. Thus tissues become oxygen starved when marijuana is used. The dangers that may come with marijuana smoke have not been studied as closely as the dangers of cigarette smoke, so the long-term impact of marijuana use is not as well understood. See the Breaking It Down box "Should More Drugs Be Legalized?" for more information on the legalization controversy.

Breaking It Down Should More Drugs Be Legalized?

The United States spends billions of dollars on drug regulations, prohibitions, and enforcement. High-profile people such as former Secretary of State George Shultz and the late Nobel laureate Milton Friedman have stated that making drugs illegal leads by default to the involvement of organized crime. If drugs were legal, the argument goes, the government could control sales and tax the products. This would generate large amounts of revenue now lost to the government because they cannot currently track illegal sales. Further, if drugs were legal, organized crime might be reduced because people seeking drugs could do so legally. Without the involvement of organized crime in drug trafficking, there might be fewer homicides and other types of violent crime surrounding drug use and sales. There would also be fewer incarcerations and possibly fewer health problems such as overdoses, because if the government enforced quality control of drugs, people would be able to ascertain the exact substance they had and know the safer dose levels. Finally, most of those who favor legalizing some or all drugs feel that drug use is a personal choice and should not be subject to government interference.

In contrast, opponents of legalizing some or all drugs, such as Lee P. Brown, director and spokesperson of the Office of National Drug Control Policy and Drug Enforcement, argue that legalization of drugs is immoral. People who are against legalizing drugs also tend to believe that the stiff penalties for drug use deter many from trying drugs in the first place, and that saves lives. Opponents feel legalization would only increase social problems like addiction and the violent crimes that are committed by people under the influence.

Although the idea of legalizing heroin or cocaine is not widely accepted in the United States, a growing number of Americans seem to feel that the classification of marijuana as a Schedule I drug should be changed. They point out that Marinol, an anti-nausea drug used by cancer patients, is derived from marijuana, so the government's claim that marijuana is a Schedule I drug without any accepted medical uses is inconsistent and incorrect. Many states—including California, Alaska, Colorado, Hawaii, Maine, Montana, Nevada, New Mexico, Oregon, Rhone Island, Vermont, and Washington—have passed laws in the past decade that remove state-level penalties for possessing or growing marijuana if it is intended to be used as a treatment for depression, chronic pain from illnesses such as cancer, or for the treatment of glaucoma. Furthermore, another ten states (plus the District of Columbia) have statutes that symbolically support the idea of medical marijuana use but do not specifically provide users protections under state laws.

Despite widespread public support for medical marijuana use, the Bush administration maintained a desire for federal prosecution of anyone possessing marijuana for any reason. Opponents of legalization claim that the pro-legalization camp is disingenuous about its motives and simply wants to relax the bans and make the recreational use of marijuana easier for everyone. Opponents point out that although the psychological effects of THC are similar to alcohol, the long-term effects of chronic use of marijuana are more similar to smoking cigarettes. Marijuana smoke has high levels of carbon monoxide and carcinogenic tars. Collectively these substances can starve the tissues of oxygen, leading to cardiovascular disease as well as cancer. So significant health risks are associated with marijuana. Further, marijuana dependence does occur in some people, and marijuana can impair driving performance.

There seems to be more controversy and less support for the total legalization of marijuana because opinions on its general safety vary and there may be wisdom in restricting recreational use. But continuing the ban on medical use of marijuana is much more up in the air. If a new presidential administration comes to power with different goals, federal prosecution of medical marijuana cases might be stopped. States with pro-medical use statutes would find the atmosphere surrounding marijuana use to be quite different.

NEED TO KNOW

Marijuana is a popular recreational drug. The concentration of THC in the marijuana induces the psychoactive effect. The higher the concentration of THC, the more intense the effect. Street-grade marijuana today is much more powerful than it was in the 1960s and 1970s. Use of marijuana carries health risks that are similar to the health risks associated with smoking. The common comparison to alcohol holds true only for THC ingested in some way other than smoking.

➤ Psychotherapeutic Drugs

Psychotherapeutic drugs treat mental and emotional problems that range from anxiety to depression. For many, this category of drugs represents a medical miracle—these substances can enable users to continue with their life in a healthful way and be free from symptoms of mental illness.

Further, the effectiveness of these drugs confirms the biological basis of anxiety and depression, which previously had been subject to debate. The most common psychotherapeutic drugs include antidepressants, minor tranquilizers, and major tranquilizers.

ANTIDEPRESSANTS

Clinical depression has a biological basis. Abnormalities in the level of neurotransmitters, specifically serotonin, can result in depression. Antidepressants as a category of drugs have improved the lives of millions of people because they "adjust" the neurotransmitters to a point where depression is prevented. The most common antidepressants today are a category called selective serotonin reuptake inhibitors **(SSRIs).** These drugs allow serotonin to stay in the synapse longer and prevent depression. Examples of SSRIs include Prozac, Zoloft, and Paxil.

A person diagnosed with depression and who is prescribed an antidepressant should see some improvement within just a few weeks. The hopelessness and despair should be significantly lessened. This improvement should give the person a clearer perspective on life and life's events.

Not only are antidepressants popular in treating depression, but some such as Paxil are popular in treating generalized anxiety feelings, including fear, over-worry, over-concern, and panic. And since antidepressants influence neurotransmitters, they are often prescribed for conditions other than depression. Many people are able to prevent migraine headaches with antidepressants, and many people with chronic pain feel antidepressants decrease the intensity of pain they regularly experience.

Long term use of antidepressants appears to be safe. On occasion a news article has focused on a bad side effect with Prozac or Zoloft, but upon further evaluation, there has not been enough evidence to pull the drug off the market. This doesn't mean that it won't eventually happen; it just means the problem that was observed could not be related to the use of antidepressants, or the effect happens in such a small number of users that closer patient monitoring is needed rather than pulling the drug from the market.

MINOR TRANQUILIZERS

Minor tranquilizers have been referred to as "anti-anxiety drugs." **Benzodiazepines** are the most commonly prescribed minor tranquilizers and

An **SSRI** is a selective serotonin reuptake inhibitor, which is used to treat depression.

Benzodiazepines are minor tranquilizers and include drugs such as Xanax, Valium, and Tranxene.

include such drugs as Valium, Xanax, and Tranxene. These drugs are designed for short-term medication of anxiety and insomnia. They should not be used long term. If long term medication is needed for anxiety, most physicians will cycle the person through the SSRIs to determine which one works best.

Minor tranquilizers are generally taken in pill form. The effects last a short time, and tolerance to these drugs can build quickly. When taken in conjunction with alcohol, the effect can be toxic.

MAJOR TRANQUILIZERS

Major tranquilizers are termed "anti-psychotic drugs" because they can be effective in medicating people with serious conditions such as schizophrenia. Drugs from a category of major tranquilizers called phenothiazines, such as Thorazine, have made a positive difference in the lives of millions. Before the introduction of phenothiazines, most people who suffered from schizophrenia had to be institutionalized.

Lithium is another major tranquilizer. It is used to treat serious bipolar disorder, which has also been called "manic depression." The benefits of major tranquilizers far outweigh the side effects.

DATE RAPE DRUGS

The common scenario for a date rape begins with a man dropping a drug into a woman's drink. About 20 minutes after consuming the drugged beverage, the woman feels light-headed and wants to go home. The man who put the drug in her drink assists her, but his motive is to rape her. Shortly after the onset of symptoms, she lapses into unconsciousness or dissociates herself from the environment, meaning that she is awake but not processing environmental stimuli. In this state, he rapes her, and later when she is conscious, she has no memory because the drug has induced amnesia.

A drug commonly used in date rapes is Rohypnol, a minor tranquilizer from the benzodiazepine group. Rohypnol is similar to Valium but ten times more powerful. Rohypnol is illegal in the United States but is available in many other countries, so there are multiple sources for the drug.

Another date rape drug is gamma-hydroxybutyrate, or GHB. GHB was originally developed as a dissociative anesthetic, and like PCP, it was found to have negative side effects and so was never marketed. The precursor to GHB contains chemicals commonly used by bodybuilders, so smart chemists can purchase these chemicals at health food stores and cook up GHB. The effects of GHB include significant muscle relaxation, nausea, vomiting, and amnesia. A high dose can cause hallucinations, respiratory distress, seizures, and possible coma. When combined with alcohol, the effects are enhanced and potentially life-threatening.

✓ **NEED TO KNOW**

It is easy for a drug such as Rohypnol or GHB to be put into a drink. Always make sure that there is no possibility for someone to add something to a drink. Trust your instincts—if you feel unusually or excessively drowsy or light-headed after a drink, then be sure to have friends take you home.

➤ Designer and Club Drugs

Designer drugs and club drugs are not categories of drugs like stimulants. **Designer drugs** are those made a certain way, and **club drugs** are those used in nightclubs or raves. Designer drugs are chemical analogues—that is, drugs that are very similar chemically to another drug but not exactly the same.

For example, fentanyl is a pain reliever more powerful than morphine. In many cities, the heroin that is marketed is actually a designer drug derived from fentanyl that is processed to look like heroin. Just about any drug distributed in the illegal market could be a designer drug.

A more common designer drug is the amphetamine analogue called Ecstasy. Its effect is similar to an amphetamine in that it increases heart rate and respiration. Some users experience mild distortions of perception, interpreted as a tranquil effect, which often progresses to a feeling of trust in their social interactions. This has led to Ecstasy being referred to as the "love drug."

There have been two waves of Ecstasy popularity—one in the mid-1980s and one currently. After the wave of use in the mid-1980s, the drug was discovered to destroy serotonergic neurons, those neurons that produce serotonin, and brain damage can result. For this reason, Ecstasy is considered a dangerous drug.

In addition to its negative effect on neurons, Ecstasy can throw off the body's thermostat, resulting in dehydration and, potentially, cardiac arrest. People do die from Ecstasy use because of this. Ecstasy users trying to game the system have been known to "front load" their water, or drink gallons of water before or immediately after consuming Ecstasy, so that they will not become dehydrated. This behavior can also be life-threatening because it can produce a condition called hyponatremia, in which too much water causes tissues to swell. In extreme cases death can result.

Designer drugs are chemical analogues of other drugs. **Club drugs** are powerful drugs used in the nightclub scene or raves.

Ecstasy is also considered a club drug. Other club drugs include LSD, "shrooms," and marijuana. These are drugs that have long-lasting effects, are used in club or rave settings, and are used to maximize the club or rave experience.

✓ **NEED TO KNOW**

Ecstasy is an extremely powerful chemical. It destroys nerve cells and disrupts the body thermostat, resulting in extreme dehydration. People under the influence of Ecstasy don't feel thirsty yet they need fluids. This loss of fluids can result in a heart attack. Some users recognize this and drink excessive amounts of water before experiencing the effects of Ecstasy. This also has some dangers because consuming excessive amounts of water can cause body tissues to swell, and if swelling occurs in the brain, brain damage or death can result.

➤ Drug Testing and Drug Treatment

Drug testing is a common practice to determine if a person has used certain drugs. The most common drugs tested for are opiates, cocaine, amphetamines, marijuana, Ecstasy, and barbiturates. Traces of these substances remain in urine for varying times after use. The typical window of time for a person's urine sample to test positive after use of opiates, cocaine, amphetamines, ecstasy, and barbiturates is 24–48 hours. Marijuana can be detected for one week up to two months, depending on frequency of use, because THC is stored in the fat and released slowly.

DRUG TESTING PROTOCOLS AND PROCEDURES

There are three major drug testing protocols: random, for cause, and condition of employment. Random drug tests can be carried out at any time without a particular reason or suspicion. Most random drug screens are done in professions with a strong public-good emphasis where the employees should be drug-free, such as medicine, law enforcement, airlines, and the military. For-cause drug tests are given to employees because a problem or incident at work provokes suspicion of substance abuse. Drug testing as a condition of employment is done to screen out drug-using candidates before they are hired.

A urine test is the most common procedure in testing for drugs. It is simple and inexpensive. The urine sample is divided into two separate samples. The first one is subjected to an **immunoassay** test, where antibodies react to the drug being tested for. If the person tests positive, the second sample is subjected to a confirmation test, such as gas chromatography or mass spectrometry. This confirmation test is expensive, but it is precise in

Immunoassay is the most basic drug test used as a part of the urine screen.

terms of confirming the immunoassay. There is also a possibility of a false positive, so the confirmation test is very important.

Another test for drugs in the system uses hair samples. Not currently as popular as urine, the hair-sample test for drugs adds another dimension to testing because a drug is contained in the hair for a long time after ingestion, whereas urine tests only detect what has been in the system for a short period.

FALSE POSITIVES AND FALSE NEGATIVES

Drug testing is usually very accurate. However, some substances can interfere with the tests and make the results inaccurate. When a person

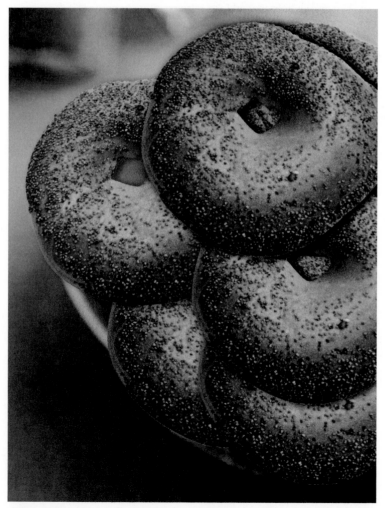

Certain foods such as the poppy seeds on bagels or over-the-counter drugs such as Benadryl can cause false-positive results in certain drug tests.

tests positive to a drug but has not used it, this is called a "false positive." Benadryl, a common antihistamine, can cause a false positive for amphetamines. Ibuprofen, an over-the-counter analgesic, can cause a false positive for marijuana. Poppy seeds can cause a false positive for opiates. This is why the confirmation test is so important. A gas chromatography or mass spectrometry will be able to determine if the person used Benadryl or amphetamines.

When a person has used a drug and tests negative, this is called a "false negative." Generally a false negative results when the urine has been adulterated with a chemical that can deceive the immunoassay. Many products are sold in counterculture magazines and on the Internet that claim a false negative will result if the product is ingested before a drug test. The most common way for a false negative to occur is if the urine is diluted to a point where the immunoassay cannot react to the drug.

STANDARD DRUG TREATMENT MODEL

The standard treatment model for substance dependence is detoxification, counseling, and support groups. This model was discussed earlier in the chapter with respect to treatment for alcohol dependence. The components are similar no matter what drug dependence is being treated. What is important for treatment is a three-pronged approach: medical detoxification, psychological counseling, and support groups that give reinforcement for staying clean and sober. If all three elements are not in place, then a person will be at high risk for relapse.

Unfortunately too few drug treatment programs are available in the United States. Many more resources are allocated to law enforcement than to treatment. Beyond the physical and mental difficulties of breaking from addictive behaviors, the cost of treatment is also a major hurdle. People who want to become clean and sober but who don't have good health insurance can find treatment and recovery a difficult road to navigate.

NEED TO KNOW

Drugs can circulate through the body for long periods of time. Most drugs have about a 24- to 48-hour window of being detectable in the system. Marijuana (THC) is different—it is stored in the fat and slowly released into the blood. So THC can be detected for much longer periods of time—weeks or months depending on the extent of use. Drug testing will be a part of everyone's future whether it be a condition of employment or health insurance.

CASA—The National Center on Addiction and Substance Abuse at Centers for Disease Control
www.cdc.gov
Columbia University
www.casacolumbia.org
DanceSafe—Promoting Health and Safety Within the Rave and Night-club Community
www.dancesafe.org
Drug Enforcement Administration
www.usdoj.gov/dea/index.htm
Drug Policy Alliance
www.drugpolicy.org
National Clearinghouse for Alcohol and Drug Information
http://ncadi.samhsa.gov/
National Institute on Drug Abuse
www.nida.nih.gov
National Organization for the Legalization of Marijuana
www.norml.org
Office of National Drug Control Policy: Media Campaign
www.mediacampaign.org
Substance Abuse and Mental Health Administration
www.samhsa.gov

Knowing the Language

Alcohol abuse
Alcohol dependence
Benzodiazepine
Club drugs
Designer drugs
Drug abuse
Drug misuse
Drug use
False negative

False positive
Immunoassay
Interfering substances
Physical dependence
Psychological dependence
Set
Setting
Tolerance

Understanding the Content

1. Distinguish between the different methods of drug administration and absorption.
2. Define the following terms: *drug use, drug misuse, drug abuse, set, setting, physical dependence, psychological dependence,* and *tolerance.*
3. Describe the effects of alcohol on the cerebrum, cerebellum, and medulla.

4. What are the differences between the different forms of marijuana?
5. What are the major dangers in designer and club drugs?
6. Describe the components of the standard drug treatment model.

Exploring Ideas

1. Use of alcohol, including underage drinking, is considered a "rite of passage" in college. At age 18, one can legally vote and serve in the military. Should the drinking age be lowered to 18? Why or why not?
2. How does someone know they may have a drug problem? What kinds of signs and symptoms should they look for?
3. Some professionals feel that the more punitive the measures, the more compliant people will be with the law. With that in mind, should college students be randomly drug tested to determine the extent of drug use in this population?

Selected References

Centers for Disease Control. Alcohol attributable deaths and years of potential life lost—United States, 2001. *Morbidity and Mortality Weekly* 53 (37): 866–870, September 24, 2004.

Drug Enforcement Administration. Drug Schedules. **www.usdoj.gov/dea/pubs/scheduling.html**

Drug Enforcement Administration. Federal Trafficking Penalties. **www.usdoj.gov/dea/agency/penalties.htm**

Engs RC, Diebold BA, Hansen DJ. The drinking patterns and problems of a national sample of college students, 1994. *Journal of Alcohol and Drug Education* 41 (3):13–33, 1996.

Esteban, MA, Schafer, W. Confronting college student drinking: A campus case study. *California Journal of Health Promotion* 3 (1): 1–55, 2005.

Harrison, PM, Allen, JB. *Bureau of Justice Statistics: Prisoners in 2002.* Washington, DC: U.S. Dept. of Justice, July 2003, p. 10.

Hingston RW, Heeren T, Zakocs RC, Kopstein A, Sechsler H. Magnitude of alcohol-related mortality and morbidity among U.S. college students ages 18–24. *Journal of Studies on Alcohol* 63 (2): 136–144, 2002.

Kinney, J, Leaton, G. *Loosening the Grip: A Handbook of Alcohol Information* (7th ed.). New York: McGraw-Hill, 2003.

Maxwell, JC. *Patterns of Club Drug Use in the U.S., 2004.* Austin, TX: Center for Excellence in Drug Epidemiology, 2004.

National Center on Addiction and Substance Abuse at Columbia University (CASA). *Wasting the Best and Brightest.* New York: Columbia, March 15, 2007.

National Institute on Drug Abuse. *Community Drug Alert Bulletin (Club Drugs).* Bethesda, MD: National Institute on Drug Abuse, May 2004.

National Institute on Drug Abuse. *Methamphetamine Abuse and Addiction*. Research Report Series. Bethesda, MD: National Institute on Drug Abuse, September 2006.

Office of Applied Studies, Substance Abuse and Mental Health Services Administration. Substance use among past year Ecstasy users. *The NSDUH Report*, April 29, 2005.

Office of Applied Studies, Substance Abuse and Mental Health Services Administration. *Prevalence of Substance Use Among Racial and Ethnic Subgroups in the U.S.*, 2005.
www.drugabusestatistics.samhsa.gov/NHSDA/Ethnic/ethn1006.htm

Office of National Drug Control Policy. *Drug Data Summary*. Rockville, MD: Drug Policy Information Clearinghouse, March 2003.

Presley CA, Meilman PW, Cashin JR. *Alcohol and Drugs on American College Campuses: Use, Consequences, and Perceptions of the Campus Environment*, Vol IV: 1992–1994. Carbondale, IL: Core Institute, Southern Illinois University, 1996.

Presley CA, Meilman PW, Cashin JR, Lyerla R. *Alcohol and Drugs on American College Campuses: Use, Consequences, and Perceptions of the Campus Environment*, Vol III: 1991–1993. Carbondale, IL: Core Institute, Southern Illinois University, 1996.

Rosenthal, E. San Francisco's medical clubs. *Heads* 5 (2): 38–41, 2005.

Ruhm CJ. Alcohol policies and highway vehicle fatalities. *Journal of Health Economics* 15 (4): 435–454, 1996.

Snyder, LB, Milici, FF, Slater, H, Sun, H, Strizhakova, Y. Effects of alcohol advertising exposure on drinking among youth. *Archives of Pediatrics and Adolescent Medicine*: 2006.

Substance Abuse and Mental Health Services Administration (SAMHSA). *Results from the 2001 National Household Survey on Drug Abuse*. Rockville, MD: SAMHSA, September 2002.

U.S. Department of Health and Human Services. *Alcohol Alert, Economic Perspectives in Alcoholism Research*. Rockville, MD: U.S. Department of Health and Human Services, 2001.

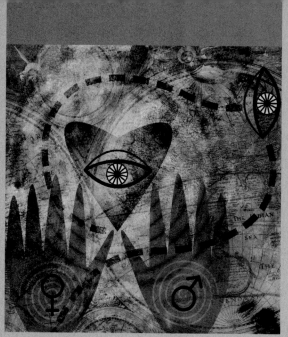

Familiarity breeds
contempt—and
children.

— MARK TWAIN

Chapter 5

RESPECT SEXUALITY

In Chapter 5, we cover a wide variety of topics related to both
the physical and psychosocial aspects of human sexuality.
Probably no other topic is as misunderstood as sexuality, from
the details of reproductive anatomy to the range of behaviors.
Most misunderstandings result from questionable sources of
sexuality information. Friends, family, and media often communicate incomplete or incorrect information, and ignorance
about the facts can lead to high-risk decisions. This chapter
reviews the basics of sexual anatomy, reproduction, and contraception. It also discusses selected aspects of sexual dysfunction, sexual identity, sexual behavior, and relationships.

Female and Male: Genetics and Hormones
>
> THE FEMALE REPRODUCTIVE SYSTEM
>
> THE MALE REPRODUCTIVE SYSTEM
>
> DISORDERS

Conception, Pregnancy, and Childbirth
>
> FIRST TRIMESTER
>
> SECOND TRIMESTER
>
> THIRD TRIMESTER
>
> LABOR AND CHILDBIRTH
>
> COMPLICATIONS OF PREGNANCY AND CHILDBIRTH

Contraception
>
> HORMONAL METHODS
>
> BARRIER METHODS
>
> SURGICAL METHODS
>
> NATURAL METHODS
>
> EMERGENCY CONTRACEPTION
>
> TERMINATION OF PREGNANCY
>
> THE ABORTION CONTROVERSY
>
> LEGAL HISTORY OF ABORTION

Sexual Behavior
>
> THE HUMAN SEXUAL RESPONSE MODEL
>
> SEXUAL DYSFUNCTION

Gender Identity and Sexual Orientation

Healthy Relationships
>
> COMMITTED RELATIONSHIPS AND MARRIAGE
>
> HEALTHY AND UNHEALTHY RELATIONSHIPS
>
> COMMUNICATION AND CONFLICT RESOLUTION SKILLS

CONCEPTION, PREGNANCY, AND CHILDBIRTH are integral forces in the world. Having some control over births is central to control of property, wealth, and lineage—in other words, power—for both individuals and societies. Before contraception existed, the only way to control births was to discourage certain segments of the population, such as the very young and the unmarried, from having sex. Abstinence was the only reliable birth control. Relatedly, the main activity of women was child rearing, and families tended to be large.

The rules by which society operated changed with the development of reliable contraception methods in the 20th century. Especially after the birth control pill became widely available in the 1970s, consequences for various behaviors became different. In turn, so did the behaviors of many Americans. People could engage in sexual activity without a baby being a near-automatic part of the relationship. Women could delay reproduction, have fewer children, or avoid motherhood altogether. This created opportunities for women to enter educational, professional, and social circles that had once been exclusive to men. This so-called sexual revolution in the late 20th century sometimes encouraged good outcomes, such as more equality among men and women, but it also contributed to new challenges, such as the rise of AIDS and other STIs.

Today sexuality is defined as much more than just fertility. It is something that begins before birth and continues throughout life, influencing and shaping relationships at every age. In addition to anatomy, physiology, sexual development, and reproduction, sexuality includes sexual orientation, gender identity, and people's values and beliefs regarding these issues. To make good decisions regarding health and relationships, adults must be educated in the full range of these issues.

➤ Female and Male: Genetics and Hormones

Healthy people are born with 46 chromosomes arranged in 23 pairs. It is the 23rd pair of chromosomes that determines sex—females have an XX pair, and males have an XY pair. Sexual development is genetically programmed to occur when children reach the age of twelve or thirteen, and signs of maturation begin well before that. During puberty, the reproductive system matures, secondary sex characteristics appear, and masculine and feminine body features become refined.

Chemical messengers called **hormones** bring about puberty and rule sexuality. The most important sexual hormones are estrogen, progesterone, and testosterone. **Estrogen** controls female secondary sex characteristics such as breast development and also plays a part in menstruation and ovulation.

> **Hormones** are chemical messengers. **Estrogen** is a female hormone responsible for female secondary sex characteristics.

FIGURE 5.1   FEMALE REPRODUCTIVE SYSTEM

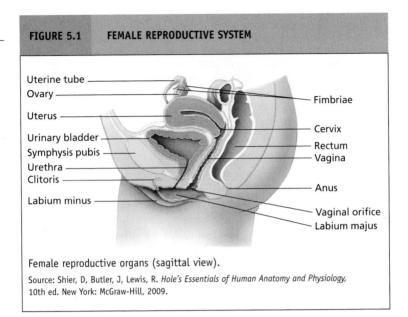

Uterine tube
Ovary
Uterus
Urinary bladder
Symphysis pubis
Urethra
Clitoris
Labium minus

Fimbriae
Cervix
Rectum
Vagina
Anus
Vaginal orifice
Labium majus

Female reproductive organs (sagittal view).

Source: Shier, D, Butler, J, Lewis, R. *Hole's Essentials of Human Anatomy and Physiology,*
10th ed. New York: McGraw-Hill, 2009.

Progesterone builds up the endometrial tissue lining a woman's uterus, a key step of the female fertility cycle. In males, **testosterone** is responsible for both primary and secondary sex characteristics, such as a deepening voice and sperm production. We tend to classify estrogen as female and testosterone as male, but women actually have small amounts of testosterone in their bodies and men have small amounts of estrogen. In addition to being important for secondary sex characteristics, estrogen and testosterone are necessary for brain functions, including the sex drive.

THE FEMALE REPRODUCTIVE SYSTEM

The female reproductive system includes both internal and external organs (see Figure 5.1). The internal organs are the ovaries, fallopian tubes, uterus, cervix, vagina, clitoris, and Bartholin's glands. The **ovaries** are the female reproductive glands that produce ova (eggs), the female sex cells. They also produce estrogen and progesterone. When an ovary releases an egg, it is swept into the nearby **fallopian tube,** where fertilization can take place, if the egg meets up with a sperm cell.

Progesterone is a female hormone responsible for the development of endometrial tissue. **Testosterone** is a male hormone responsible for male secondary sex characteristics.

Ovaries are glands that produce ova and the hormones estrogen and progesterone. **Fallopian tubes** are the structures into which a ripe ovum is released and where it is fertilized by a sperm.

Whether fertilized or not, an egg travels down the fallopian tube and ends up in the **uterus,** an elastic, muscular organ designed to stretch to accommodate a growing baby. At the bottom of the uterus is a round, thick muscle called the **cervix.** The cervix connects the uterus to the **vagina,** where sperm are deposited during intercourse. The vagina is also the route through which a woman's endometrial tissue sloughs off during menstruation, and it is the canal through which a baby enters the world during birth.

The external female genitalia, collectively referred to as the *vulva,* include the clitoris, labia majora, labia minora, and Bartholin's glands. The **clitoris** contains a dense nerve network that when stimulated results in an orgasm, the heightened pleasurable sensation that is the climax, or culmination, of sexual stimulation. The labia majora and labia minora are folds of tissues that cover the opening to the vagina. The Bartholin's glands, located inside the labia minora, secrete a lubricating substance during sexual arousal that results less skin friction during intercourse.

The menstrual cycle (or fertility cycle) is typically about 28 days long (see Figure 5.2). The first day of the menstrual cycle, or "period," is usually counted as day 1, with the menstrual period lasting about five days. After menstruation ends, the pituitary gland secretes follicle-stimulating hormone (FSH), which causes an ovum to ripen in an ovary. FSH also signals the ovary to secrete more progesterone, so the endometrial tissue in the uterus builds up in preparation for a potential pregnancy. The ovum reaches maturity around halfway through the cycle (approximately day 14), and at that point the pituitary gland secretes luteinizing hormone (LH), signaling the ovary to release the ripe egg into the fallopian tube. This is called **ovulation.**

An egg in a fallopian tube can survive 48–72 hours. If the ovum is not fertilized by a sperm during that time, it will break down and be reabsorbed into the body. At day 28 of the cycle, a new period begins.

Some women experience physical and emotional discomfort before menses, referred to as premenstrual syndrome (PMS). Common PMS symptoms include acne, breast swelling and tenderness, bloating, headache, backache, tension, irritability, and anxiety or depression. If a woman is bothered by these symptoms, her physician may prescribe synthetic estrogen or progesterone to provide relief.

The **uterus** is the organ in which a fertilized ovum implants and develops into a baby. The **cervix** is the neck of the uterus, opening into the vagina. The **vagina** is the passage between the cervix and the external sex organs and the female structure for sexual intercourse; it is also referred to as the *birth canal.*

The **clitoris** is composed of a dense nerve network and is important in female arousal and orgasm.

Ovulation is the release of a mature or ripe ovum.

FIGURE 5.2   MENSTRUATION HORMONES

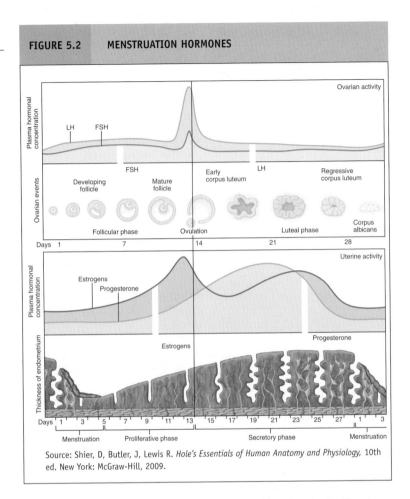

Source: Shier, D, Butler, J, Lewis R. *Hole's Essentials of Human Anatomy and Physiology*, 10th ed. New York: McGraw-Hill, 2009.

If fertilization occurs, cell division begins immediately. The fertilized egg leaves the fallopian tube and implants in the endometrial tissue in the uterus (see Figure 5.3).

Females usually become fertile around age thirteen, when they get their first period. Women usually lose the ability to get pregnant in their late 40s or 50s. **Menopause** is the term for the process by which ovaries stop releasing eggs and monthly periods end. Menopause is a gradual process, but as the ovaries produce less and less progesterone and estrogen, many physical and emotional symptoms can occur as the body adjusts to the changes. Common symptoms include hot flashes, irritability, loss of libido, depression, muscle aches, and sleep problems.

Menopause is the cessation of the menstrual cycle.

FIGURE 5.3   FERTILIZATION

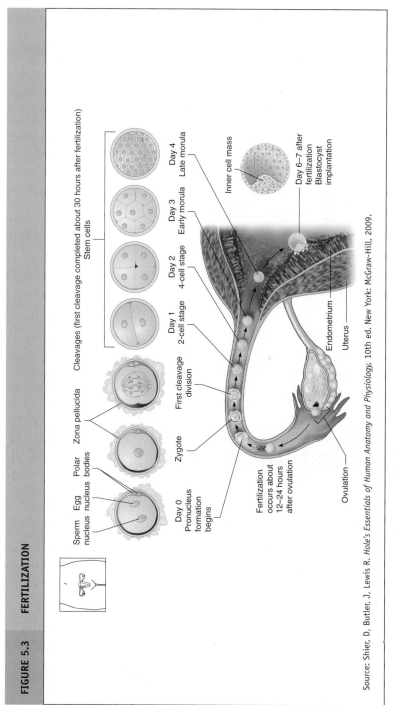

Source: Shier, D, Butler, J, Lewis R. *Hole's Essentials of Human Anatomy and Physiology*. 10th ed. New York: McGraw-Hill, 2009.

| FIGURE 5.4 | MALE REPRODUCTIVE SYSTEM |

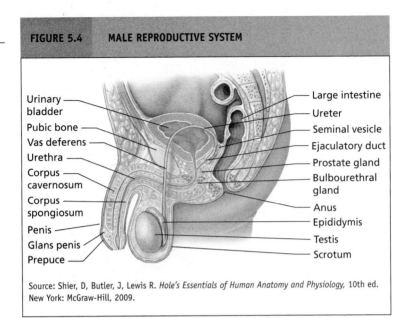

Source: Shier, D, Butler, J, Lewis R. *Hole's Essentials of Human Anatomy and Physiology,* 10th ed. New York: McGraw-Hill, 2009.

THE MALE REPRODUCTIVE SYSTEM

Like the female system, the male reproductive system includes both internal and external organs (see Figure 5.4). The internal organs are the testes, vas deferens, bulbourethral glands, prostate gland, urethra, and the glans penis. The external organs are the penis and the scrotum.

Testes are glands that produce sperm, the male sex cells, and the hormone testosterone. Surrounding the testes is a sac of skin called the **scrotum.** The scrotum not only protects the testes but also maintains a lower-than-core-body temperature in the organs inside it, which is important for healthy sperm production.

After sperm are produced in the testes, they move to the **vas deferens,** where sperm are stored and provided with a route to the urethra, where during orgasm they will be ejaculated. As sperm travel down the vas deferens, they collect fluids from three major glands: the **seminal vesicles,** the **bulbourethral glands,** and the **prostate gland.** The seminal vesicles

---

Testes are glands that produce sperm and the hormone testosterone. The **scrotum** is the sac of skin that protects the testes.

Vas deferens are structures that receive sperm from the testes and provide a route for the movement of sperm. **Seminal vesicles** secrete a nutritive substance so that sperm can survive. The **prostate gland** secretes an alkaline substance that neutralizes the acid medium normally present in the vagina.

secrete a nutritive substance so that sperm can thrive. The **bulbourethral**
glands (also called *Cowper's glands*) secrete a lubricating substance that is
believed to lubricate the urethra to facilitate the passage of sperm. The
prostate gland secretes an alkaline substance that neutralizes the acidic
environment in the vagina. Collectively, secretions from all these glands
and the sperm are referred to as *semen*.

The urethra in males is located in the penis and transports both urine and
semen, though not at the same time. (In females, the urethra is not part of
the reproductive system; its sole purpose is to carry urine from the
bladder.) The penis is the male external reproductive organ that contains
the majority of the urethra. The head of the penis (or **glans penis**) has a
dense nerve network that when stimulated can result in orgasm, inducing
the involuntary ejaculation of semen.

During sexual activity, sperm move from the testes to the vas deferens
and then pass through the seminal vesicles, bulbourethral glands, and
prostate gland. The semen travels down the urethra and if orgasm occurs,
it is ejaculated. If ejaculation occurs during vaginal intercourse, sperm in
the semen will attempt to move up through the cervix, uterus, and
fallopian tubes. If the sperm comes into contact with a mature ovum in
the fallopian tubes, then fertilization can occur.

DISORDERS

A variety of common disorders can affect both the female and the male
reproductive systems. Effects of these disorders can range from mild discomfort to infertility.

Female Disorders

Several fairly common irregularities can affect female fertility. **Menorrhagia**
is heavy menstrual bleeding, or an excess flow of endometrial tissue. It is
often caused by hormonal imbalances and can be treated with synthetic
estrogen and/or progesterone (in the form of birth control pills). Less often
it is caused by uterine fibroids, which are benign tumors of the uterus.

Amenorrhea is the absence of menstruation. If the woman is not pregnant or breastfeeding, amenorrhea is usually caused by stress, being extremely underweight, or having an extremely low percentage of body fat.

The **bulbourethral glands** secrete a lubricating substance to help sperm pass
through the urethra.

The **glans penis** is the head of the penis and is a dense nerve network and the
focal point for orgasm.

Menorrhagia is excessive menstruation.

Amenorrhea is the absence of menstruation.

FIGURE 5.5   HERNIA

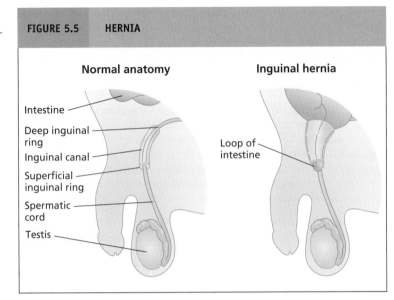

Normal anatomy · Inguinal hernia

Intestine · Deep inguinal ring · Inguinal canal · Superficial inguinal ring · Spermatic cord · Testis · Loop of intestine

Excessive exercise and participation in rigorous sports can lead to amenorrhea, as can eating disorders such as anorexia nervosa.

Dysmenorrhea is painful menstruation, characterized by severe cramping. It can be caused by high levels of body chemicals called *prostaglandins;* when this is the case, symptoms can often be relieved simply with ibuprofen. It can also have other causes, including endometriosis, a condition where endometrial tissue becomes implanted in the abdominal cavity outside the uterus; ectopic pregnancy, when a fertilized egg implants in the wrong location in the uterus or in the fallopian tube or ovary; and pelvic inflammatory disease (PID), a widespread infection of tissue in the pelvic area.

Menstrual problems require a physician's evaluation, and once the cause is identified, there are usually interventions available to treat the condition. Medical interventions can range from occasional use of pain relievers or taking birth control pills (which tend to make women's periods lighter) to, in severe cases, a surgery called *dilation and curettage* (D&C), which removes the endometrial tissue from the uterus.

Male Disorders
Several disorders for males are also relatively common. A hernia is a protrusion of an organ through a structure that contains it. Hernias can result from too much pressure or straining when lifting heavy objects. An inguinal hernia occurs when a loop of intestine has broken through the abdominal wall located above the scrotum (called the *inguinal wall;* see Figure 5.5).

Dysmenorrhea is painful menstruation.

Hernias can be serious because the intestinal loop can push its way into the scrotum, causing a bowel constriction or even sterility. Physicians conducting physical exams on male patients typically will place the index finger up under the pubic bone in the top part of the scrotum and ask the patient to cough. The coughing usually can exert enough pressure for the physician to feel if a hernia exists. Sometimes surgery is needed to pull the loop of intestine back to where it belongs and suture the damaged inguinal wall.

Prostate problems are most common in older males, but infections such as STIs can cause prostate problems in younger men. If the prostate becomes infected, a man may have difficulty urinating or have a continual urge to urinate. The prostate is checked through a digital rectal exam whereby the physician inserts a finger into the rectum and feels the prostate for enlargement and for growths.

In addition to some prostate problems, STIs can also cause pelvic inflammatory disease (PID) or infertility. Many of these problems are discussed in Chapter 11.

✔ **NEED TO KNOW**

Hormones are chemical messengers that represent the most basic language of sexuality. The female hormones include estrogen and progesterone. Estrogen and progesterone are the major hormones produced by the ovaries and are responsible for secondary sex characteristics in females. Testosterone is the major hormone produced by the testes and is responsible for secondary sex characteristics in males. Secondary sex characteristics begin to develop during puberty. The female and male reproductive systems are different in structure but similar in function: production of hormones and of female ova or male sperm. Some common problems in the reproductive systems are menstrual problems such as dysmenorrhea, menorrhagia, and amenorrhea in females and hernia and prostate problems in males. Medical interventions are available to treat these problems.

➤ Conception, Pregnancy, and Childbirth

Pregnancies typically last about 40 weeks and are divided into three phases of about three months (13 weeks) each, referred to as **trimesters.**

FIRST TRIMESTER

The first trimester lasts 12–13 weeks. During most of the first trimester the ball of rapidly dividing cells is referred to as an **embryo.** From the

Trimesters are the three phases of pregnancy, each about three months long.

An **embryo** is an unborn baby from conception through the eighth or ninth week of pregnancy.

tenth week onward, the unborn baby is called a **fetus.** Formation of all the vital organs, including the brain and spinal cord, occurs in the first trimester. The heart begins to beat, arms and legs grow, and the face and gender of the baby become distinguishable. In addition to the anatomical development, an organ called the placenta grows. Placentas allow unborn babies to obtain oxygen and nutrients and exchange waste products with their mother. At the end of the first trimester the baby is about 2–4 inches long and weighs 1–2 ounces.

SECOND TRIMESTER

Weeks 14–26 are the second trimester of pregnancy. The organs that formed in the first trimester become more specialized and functional. The baby can swallow and digest, has waking and sleeping periods, and moves. Hair grows. At the end of the second trimester the baby is about 15 inches long and weighs 2–2½ pounds.

THIRD TRIMESTER

Weeks 27–40 are the final phase of pregnancy. During this period the fetus grows rapidly. Toward the end of the trimester the baby begins to change position in preparation for birth. Fetal lungs mature to the point that they will be ready to breathe air after birth, when the placenta stops providing oxygen. At birth an average baby weighs about 7–8 pounds and measures over 14 inches long.

LABOR AND CHILDBIRTH

The third trimester culminates in labor, which has three stages. During the first stage, strong uterine contractions cause the cervix to thin and open and also cause the baby to move lower into the mother's pelvis. The contractions may cause the amniotic sac that surrounds the baby with fluid to break, an event sometimes referred to as "the water breaking." During the second stage of labor, the mother pushes the baby out the birth canal. Once delivered, the baby's umbilical cord, which connects the child to the placenta, is cut and the baby starts breathing on its own for the first time. Finally, the placenta detaches and is pushed out the birth canal by the mother in the third stage of labor.

Most babies are born head first, but in some cases the baby is in a breech position, meaning its feet or buttocks come down the birth canal first. Breech births are risky because the baby can get stuck in the birth canal or have its umbilical cord pinched, cutting off oxygen to the baby. A breech birth requires the aid of a skilled physician or a certified nurse-midwife to ensure that neither the mother's nor the baby's health are

A **fetus** is an unborn baby from about the 10th week of pregnancy to birth.

compromised during the birth process. If the baby or mother is believed to be in jeopardy, a physician may opt to deliver the baby by caesarian section (C section). In this procedure, the baby is surgically removed from the uterus through an incision in the mother's abdomen.

COMPLICATIONS OF PREGNANCY AND CHILDBIRTH

Although most pregnancies culminate in the birth of a healthy baby, complications can sometimes occur. For instance, gestational diabetes is a form of diabetes that occurs only during pregnancy. The pregnancy affects the woman's pancreas, which produces insulin, so that levels of blood sugar become uncontrolled. The condition can occur during the second half of pregnancy and is usually treated with insulin. (For more information on diabetes, see Chapter 10.) Urinary tract infections are also common during pregnancy, and if undiagnosed and untreated, they can cause premature labor.

When a fertilized egg implants in a location other than the uterus, such as in the fallopian tube or on the ovary itself, the result is an **ectopic pregnancy.** In some cases, the body rejects the embryo and the pregnancy ends naturally, but in other cases the embryo may rupture the fallopian tube, causing life-threatening problems, including massive hemorrhaging. The embryo and sometimes the fallopian tube need to be removed surgically to save the mother's life.

Normally placentas develop above the cervix inside the uterus, but occasionally a placenta will cover the cervix as it grows. This condition is called *placenta previa,* and it can cause severe bleeding beginning at the end of the second trimester. Treatment for placenta previa can range from bed rest during pregnancy to blood transfusions. Vaginal delivery is considered too dangerous due to risk of hemorrhaging. So, if someone has placenta previa at the end of pregnancy, the baby will be delivered via C section.

Placental abruption occurs when the placenta separates from the uterine wall before delivery, potentially depriving the baby of oxygen. Once the condition is diagnosed, depending on its severity, the treatment can include bed rest, hospitalization, or a caesarian section.

Preeclampsia is a condition characterized by high blood pressure, edema (the swelling of tissue from excess fluid), headaches, dizziness, vision problems, and stomach pain in the pregnant woman. It can also cause fetal distress and even fetal death. If not treated, preeclampsia can progress to eclampsia, which is characterized by seizures, coma, and sometimes death. If preeclampsia is severe enough, labor may be induced or an emergency C section may be performed to protect both mother and baby.

Ectopic pregnancy occurs when a fertilized egg implants somewhere other than the uterus, usually in a fallopian tube.

Premature labor is labor that occurs before 37 weeks of gestation. If premature labor cannot be stopped with bed rest and other means, medications may be prescribed to stop the contractions.

Postpartum depression is normally a mild depression that occurs three days to two weeks after delivery. Most times the depression ends naturally; however, there are some extreme cases where the depression requires counseling and medication.

Miscarriage is the expulsion of the embryo or fetus from the uterus before the middle of the second trimester. In most cases, a miscarriage is due to a problem with a lack of progesterone being produced during the first and second trimesters. During the first and second trimesters of pregnancy, significant amounts of progesterone are produced until the placenta matures. However, if the production of progesterone decreases before the placenta is mature, then a miscarriage can result.

➤ Contraception

Unless you are actively trying to have a baby or would not object to an unexpected pregnancy, it is very important to use contraception whenever you engage in sexual activity. Table 5.1 presents a more in depth presentation of each of the contraceptive methods by type, failure rates, risk, availability and convenience.

HORMONAL METHODS

Hormonal contraceptives such as injections, implants, birth control pills, and the contraceptive patch or ring are made from estrogen and/or progesterone (sometimes called by its synthetic form, progestin). These contraceptives biologically simulate pregnancy in the woman's body, thus suppressing ovulation. In addition, some of the hormonal methods thicken cervical mucus, which impedes the movement of sperm. Hormonal methods of contraception are very effective, with a failure rate of only 1–3 percent. In the United States they are available only by prescription. Usually a physician conducts a comprehensive physical evaluation to ensure that the woman does not have risk factors that would rule out their use.

Birth control pills come in a variety of dosages and strengths and are taken either daily or for three weeks each month, depending on the type

---

Hormonal contraceptives introduce progestin and/or estrogen into a woman's body in order to suppress ovulation.

The **birth control pill,** commonly known as "the pill," is a hormonal method of contraception in pill form.

TABLE 5.1   CONTRACEPTIVE DEVICES AND APPROACHES BY TYPE, FAILURE RATE, RISKS, AND AVAILABILITY

TYPE OF CONTRACEPTIVE	DESCRIPTION	FAILURE RATE (number of pregnancies expected per 100 women per year)	SOME RISKS	PROTECTION FROM SEXUALLY TRANSMITTED DISEASES (STDs)	AVAILABILITY
Male Condom Latex/Polyurethane	A sheath placed over the erect penis blocking the passage of sperm.	11	Irritation and allergic reactions (less likely with polyurethane)	Except for abstinence, latex condoms are the best protection against STDs, including gonorrhea and AIDS.	Nonprescription
Female Condom	A lubricated polyurethane sheath shaped similarly to the male condom. The closed end has a flexible ring that is inserted in the vagina.	21	Irritation and allergic reactions	May give some STD protection; not as effective as latex condom.	Nonprescription
Diaphragm with Spermicide	A dome-shaped rubber disk with a flexible rim that covers the cervix so that sperm cannot reach the uterus. A spermicide is applied to the diaphragm before insertion.	17	Irritation and allergic reactions, urinary tract infection. Risk of Toxic Shock Syndrome, a rare but serious infection, when kept in place longer than recommended.	None	Prescription
Spermicide Alone	A foam, cream, jelly, film, suppository, or tablet that contains nonoxynol-9, a sperm-killing chemical.	20–50 (studies have shown varying effectiveness rates)	Irritation and allergic reactions, urinary tract infections	None	Nonprescription

(Continued)

TABLE 5.1   CONTRACEPTIVE DEVICES AND APPROACHES BY TYPE, FAILURE RATE, RISKS, AND AVAILABILITY (continued)

TYPE OF CONTRACEPTIVE	DESCRIPTION	FAILURE RATE (number of pregnancies expected per 100 women per year)	SOME RISKS	PROTECTION FROM SEXUALLY TRANSMITTED DISEASES (STDs)	AVAILABILITY
Oral Contraceptives—combined pill –Progestin-only minipill –91 day Regimen (Seasonale)	A pill that suppresses ovulation by the combined actions of the hormones estrogen and progestin. A chewable form was approved in November 2003.	1–2	Dizziness; nausea; changes in menstruation, mood, and weight; rarely cardiovascular disease, including high blood pressure, blood clots, heart attack, and strokes	None	Prescription
Patch (Ortho Evra)	Skin patch worn on the lower abdomen, buttocks, or upper body that releases the hormones progestin and estrogen into the bloodstream.	1–2 Appears to be less effective in women weighing more than 198 pounds.	Similar to oral contraceptives—combined pill	None	Prescription
Vaginal Contraceptive Ring (NuvaRing)	A flexible ring about 2 inches in diameter that is inserted into the vagina and releases the hormones progestin and estrogen.	1–2	Vaginal discharge, vaginitis, irritation. Similar to oral contraceptives—combined pill	None	Prescription
Post-Coital Contraceptives (Preven and Plan B)	Pills containing either progestin alone or progestin plus estrogen	Almost 80 percent reduction in risk of pregnancy for a single act of unprotected sex	Nausea, vomiting, abdominal pain, fatigue, headache	None	Prescription

Type	How it works	Estimated failure rate (%)	Some risks	STDs protection	How to get
Injection –Depo-Provera –Lunelle	An injectable progestin that inhibits ovulation, prevents sperm from reaching the egg, and prevents the fertilized egg from implanting in the uterus.	less than 1	Irregular bleeding, weight gain, breast tenderness, headaches	None	Prescription
IUD (Intrauterine Device)	A T-shaped device inserted into the uterus by a health professional.	less than 1	Cramps, bleeding, pelvic inflammatory disease, infertility, perforation of uterus	None	Prescription
Periodic Abstinence	To deliberately refrain from having sexual intercourse during times when pregnancy is more likely.	20	None	None	Instructions from health care provider
Transabdominal Surgical Sterilization—female –Falope Ring, –Hulka Clip, –Filshie Clip or –Essure System	The woman's fallopian tubes are blocked so the egg and sperm can't meet in the fallopian tube, preventing conception.	less than 1	Pain, bleeding, infection, other postsurgical complications, ectopic (tubal) pregnancy.	None	Surgery
Surgical Sterilization—male	Sealing, tying, or cutting a man's vas deferens so that the sperm can't travel from the testicles to the penis.	less than 1	Pain, bleeding, infection, other postsurgical complications	None	Surgery

Failure rates are based on information from clinical trials submitted to the U.S. Food and Drug Administration (FDA) during product reviews. This number represents the percentage of women who become pregnant during the first year using a birth control method. For methods that the FDA does not review, such as periodic abstinence, numbers are estimated from published literature. For comparison, about 85 out of 100 sexually active women who wish to have a child and do not use contraception become pregnant within one year of first trying to conceive.

Source: Food and Drug Administration 12/03

of pill. Side effects include high blood pressure, headaches, diabetes, elevated cholesterol levels, and blood clots.

Contraceptive implants are surgically placed under the skin of the upper arm. The implants contain progestin and can suppress ovulation for up to five years. Implanon, consisting of a single capsule and providing protection for three years, was approved by the FDA in 2006 and is now available.

Injectable contraceptives are administered via a shot in the arm or buttocks and provide protection for approximately 14 weeks. The best known injectable is **Depo-Provera,** but others are under development. Each injection is effective for three months.

The vaginal ring is a flexible plastic ring that contains low levels of hormones. It is inserted into the vagina and left in place around the cervix for approximately three weeks and then removed for one week for menstruation. A new ring is inserted every month.

The contraceptive patch contains hormones that slowly absorb into the body through the skin. The patch can be placed on the buttocks, upper arm, or upper torso and is changed once a week for three weeks and then not worn one week during menstruation.

Hormonal methods of contraception have the advantage of providing long-term, highly effective protection against pregnancy with little effort on the part of the woman. However, hormonal methods are not for all women because some of the side effects mentioned earlier can be significant and result in medical emergencies.

BARRIER METHODS

Barrier methods of contraception include the intrauterine device (IUD), condom, sponge, diaphragm, and cervical cap. These methods work by blocking sperm from traveling through the cervix and into the uterus and fallopian tubes. Some of the barrier methods, such as the sponge, diaphragm, and cervical cap, also use a chemical that kills sperm (spermicide), making them even more effective.

An **IUD** is a small, T-shaped, plastic or copper device that is inserted into the uterus by a physician. Depending upon the type, the IUD can be left in place from one to ten years. It works as a physical barrier to sperm and also changes

Contraceptive implants, such as Implanon, are surgically inserted under the skin and can provide hormonal contraception for up to five years.

Depo-Provera is a hormonal method of contraception delivered in an injection.

An **IUD** (intrauterine device) is a barrier method of contraception in which a small plastic or copper unit is placed in the uterus and functions as a barrier to the movement of sperm.

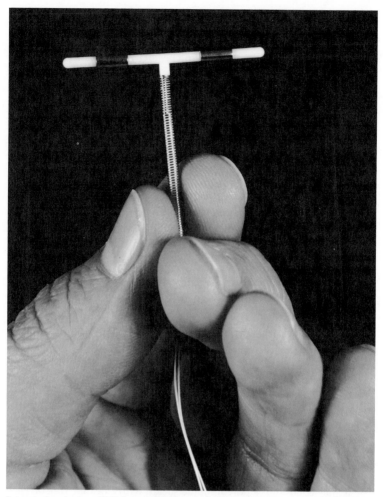

Intrauterine devices (IUDs) must be placed in a woman's uterus by a trained medical professional. It can remain in place and provide highly reliable contraception from anywhere from one to ten years.

the hormonal environment in the uterus and fallopian tubes, inhibiting the movement of sperm. The effectiveness of the IUD as a contraceptive method is high, with a failure rate of only 4–5 percent. Some relatively rare side effects of IUDs include uterine perforations, cramping, and heavy bleeding.

A **diaphragm** is a thick, flexible concave rubber structure with a hard but flexible outer ring. It is inserted into the vagina and placed over the

A **diaphragm** is a concave latex "cup" that is inserted into the vagina and serves as barrier method of contraception.

cervix, forming a barrier to sperm. A small amount of spermicide is placed in the diaphragm and around the rim to kill any sperm that penetrate the physical barrier. For maximum effectiveness, the diaphragm must be inserted before intercourse and be left in place for six hours afterwards. The failure rate for the diaphragm ranges from 6 to 8 percent. If the diaphragm is left in place for an extended period of time, there is a small risk of toxic shock syndrome, a dangerous bacterial infection.

The **cervical cap** is a small, flexible cap that is inserted into the vagina and placed over the cervix to form a barrier to sperm. Like the diaphragm, it is used with spermicide. FemCap, the only type of cervical cap currently available, is a silicone cup with a brim to hold spermicide and a strap over the dome for easier removal. Because it is smaller, the cervical cap can be more difficult to insert than the diaphragm is, but it can be left in place for longer—up to 48 hours. The failure rate can be as high as 18 percent. As with the diaphragm, there is a slight risk of toxic shock syndrome if the cervical cap is left in place too long.

Condoms are the most common and popular type of barrier contraception because they do not require a prescription, are available in many stores, and are fairly inexpensive and simple to use. Condoms are made and marketed for both males and females, but the more popular ones are male condoms.

The male condom is a tightly rolled latex sheath that is worn by unrolling it down over an erect penis. During intercourse, semen is ejaculated into the condom, thus preventing sperm from entering the vagina. The failure rate is approximately 15 percent. Male condoms not only help prevent pregnancy, but they also provide protection against sexually transmitted infections (STIs). They are available in a wide variety of brands, colors, and styles, with and without lubricants and spermicides. Condoms that contain the spermicide Nonoxynol-9 (N-9) in some cases have been found to increase tissue irritation, which can increase the likelihood of STI transmission. (See this chapter's Breaking It Down, "Nonoxynol-9's Downfall?").

The female condom is a polyurethane sheath with a flexible ring on each end. The ring on the closed end is inserted into the back of the vagina and the other ring remains outside the vagina. During intercourse, the sheath creates a barrier to sperm. The failure rate for female condoms is 13 percent, slightly less than that for male condoms.

Spermicides are chemicals marketed in many forms: gels, foams, suppositories, and jellies. These chemicals are inserted into the vagina before intercourse. In theory, when sperm are ejaculated into the vagina, the

---

The **cervical cap** is similar to the diaphragm but smaller.

Condoms are latex devices that either cover the penis (male condom) or line the vagina (female condom) and serve as a barrier to sperm.

Spermicides are chemicals that kill sperm.

spermicide kills them. To be effective, the spermicide should be placed in the vagina one hour before intercourse, and if intercourse is repeated, more spermicide should be used. The failure rate is 20–30 percent.

Combining barrier methods can significantly decreases failure rate. For example, use of both spermicides and condoms can be 95 percent effective in preventing pregnancies.

Breaking It Down Nonoxynol-9's Downfall?

Nonoxynol-9 (N9) has been used as a spermicide since the early 1980s. Because N-9 had a demonstrated an ability to kill HIV in a laboratory setting, condoms containing N-9 were recommended as one of the key public health interventions to prevent the spread of HIV/AIDS. For about 15 years most public health prevention messages emphasized use of condoms containing N-9. But now studies have found that N-9 is not only ineffective at stopping the spread of HIV, but it has actually increased risk of disease transmission. How could this have occurred?

The problem originated because officials and product manufacturers made a critical error: they assumed that if N-9 killed HIV in the laboratory, it automatically must be effective in real-world situations involving sex. Unfortunately, this proved untrue. The evidence against the effectiveness of N-9 was highlighted in a 2000 study of N-9 use among sex workers in South Africa and Thailand. A chief finding of this study was that the incidence of HIV was higher among women using N-9 than among those using a similar product without N-9. Even worse, some people who used N-9 frequently had problems with tissue damage. This led the Centers for Disease Control and the World Health Organization to the following conclusions:

- N-9 is ineffective at killing the HIV virus and other STIs.
- When used vaginally multiple times a day, N-9 can cause genital lesions that may increase a woman's risk of acquiring HIV.
- Condoms lubricated with a small amount of N-9 are no more effective in preventing pregnancy than are lubricated condoms without N-9.

The case against N-9 was so strong that major condom manufacturers like Johnson & Johnson discontinued production of condoms containing N-9. The Planned Parenthood Federation of America also recommended that production of condoms containing N-9 be stopped.

N-9's plunge in popularity reflects an important principle in science and health. When new information from scientific studies discredits a "sound" prevention approach, then industry and society respond, and in this case

(Continued)

they responded appropriately. It also shows how important it is for us to keep our health knowledge current. "Best practices" in all areas of health continue to evolve. What may have been the gold standard in treatment last decade could turn out to be less than optimal as scientific evidence builds up.

SURGICAL METHODS

Vasectomy for men and tubal ligation for women are the two most common surgical methods of contraception. Neither procedure should have an effect on sex drive.

The **vasectomy** is a simple surgical procedure in which the vas deferens in each testis is cut and the exposed ends are sealed by cauterization (burning with special instruments). After cauterization the exposed end is folded back and tied. Sperm are still produced and released but are not able to progress past the cauterized, tied end of the vas deferens. The vasectomy takes about 20–30 minutes and can be done in a physician's office under local anesthesia.

Tubal ligation is usually done in a surgical facility under general anesthesia, but the principle is similar. An incision is made in the lower abdomen, and the fallopian tubes are cut, cauterized, and tied back. Mature ova are still produced and menstruation still occurs, but the egg that is released into the fallopian tube will travel only as far as the cauterized, tied end of the fallopian tube.

Vasectomy and tubal ligation should be considered permanent. Although the procedures can be reversed in some cases, there is no guarantee that reversal will be successful.

NATURAL METHODS

Of course, the most "natural" method of birth control of all—complete abstinence from sexual intercourse—is also the most effective. But another **natural method** of birth control that is used by some sexually active women is referred to as *fertility awareness* or *periodic abstinence*. This method requires a woman to accurately predict when she is ovulating on

Vasectomy is a surgical method of contraception for men, where the vas deferens are cut, cauterized, and tied to block movement of sperm.

Tubal ligation is a surgical method of contraception for women, where the fallopian tubes are cut, cauterized, and tied to block movement of both sperm and ova.

Natural methods of birth control are methods that are designed to reinforce abstaining from sexual intercourse. They include fertility awareness, or determining the days a women is most fertile (i.e., releasing an egg) and, if pregnancy is not desired, abstaining from intercourse on these days. Another method is withdrawal, or removing the penis from the vagina just before orgasm.

the basis of body temperature and other signs and determine "safe" vs. "unsafe" days for intercourse. Accurately monitoring body temperature is key—body temperature drops slightly just before ovulation and rises slightly afterwards. A woman using the fertility awareness method takes her temperature with a special thermometer (called a *basal body temperature thermometer*) every morning before she gets out of bed. When her temperature drops and then rises, she can assume that ovulation is taking place. She abstains from intercourse on the 10–12 days per month she is fertile (from about seven days prior to ovulation to about three days after). Since so much effort is required and the margin for error is great, periodic abstinence has a failure rate of 14–47 percent.

Withdrawal is also considered a method of natural birth control. With this method, at the point of orgasm the penis is removed from the vagina so that ejaculation occurs outside the vagina. But withdrawal is very ineffective for two reasons: first, some sperm are in the pre-ejaculate fluid and second, withdrawal requires a significant amount of self-discipline.

What Is Your Risk? *Unintended Pregnancy*

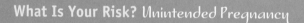

Approximately 50 percent of the pregnancies in the United States are unintended. According to the Centers for Disease Control, unintended pregnancy rates in the United States have been declining, and the rates are highest among women 20 years of age or younger (approximately one million teenage girls in the United States have an unintended pregnancy each year) and those 40 years of age and older. Unintended pregnancies are emotionally and financially costly.

The more frequently a woman has sexual intercourse with men, the more likely she is to become pregnant, even if she and her partners use contraception. Risk also goes up if directions are not correctly followed for the method of contraception employed.

In theory, most contraceptive methods should be close to 100 percent effective. The main reason they fail is human error. It is important not only to pick birth control methods that work well but also to use them according to their directions. Birth control methods can be combined—for instance, using spermicide with condoms or a diaphragm. This greatly improves effectiveness.

It is important to select birth control methods that fit well with your lifestyle and habits. For example, if you tend to be forgetful, a daily birth control pill may not the best choice for you, since if you forget to take doses in the correct time period, the pill will be ineffective. Likewise, if you aren't motivated to do the careful temperature monitoring required by many natural birth control methods, the chance of pregnancy also goes up.

EMERGENCY CONTRACEPTION

Emergency contraception can be used after unprotected sex or when contraception fails (such as a condom breaking). Emergency contraception usually consists of a "morning after" pill that contains enough hormones to cause a woman's period to come early. This "restarts" a woman's monthly fertility cycle, so that pregnancy does not occur.

Physicians used to prescribe certain birth control pills as emergency contraception, but recently the FDA approved an emergency contraceptive product called Plan B. It consists of two pills; the first is taken no more than 72 hours after unprotected intercourse, and the second, 12 hours after the first. It is available over the counter to women 18 years of age and older. Women under 18 need a prescription.

TERMINATION OF PREGNANCY

In everyday language the term **abortion** usually refers to ending a pregnancy by choice. But medically speaking, the word *abortion* is more generic, describing both "natural" losses, when the body rejects a developing embryo or fetus, as well as surgical or medical procedures that interrupt pregnancy. *Miscarriage* is the common term for a **spontaneous abortion** that occurs in the first half of a pregnancy. Death of a fetus after week 20 in a pregnancy is often referred to as *stillbirth*. And medically speaking, ending a pregnancy by choice is usually referred to as **artificial abortion**.

Pregnancies end via spontaneous abortion about 20 percent of the time, usually within the first 90 days of pregnancy. Many of these pregnancy losses are due to genetic problems in the developing fetus or from problems in the uterine environment. Often, levels of progesterone, which must be high the first 90 days of pregnancy until a placenta develops fully, decline suddenly and significantly. When levels get too low, the pituitary gland secretes a chemical called oxytocin, which causes the uterus to contract and expel the embryo or fetus.

Methods for terminating a pregnancy by choice differ based largely on the stage of pregnancy during which they are performed. During the first trimester, a surgical procedure called dilation and curettage (D&C) may be used to remove the embryo from the uterus. The cervix is dilated and a suction curette, a hollow tube, is inserted into the uterus; the contents of the uterus are then suctioned out. Another surgical procedure

---

Abortion is the expulsion of an embryo or fetus from the uterus before it has fully developed. **Spontaneous abortion,** often called *miscarriage,* is the body's rejection of the embryo or fetus. **Artificial abortion** is a medical procedure that is used when a woman chooses to terminate her pregnancy.

used during the first trimester is manual vacuum aspiration. This method is similar to suction curettage but can be performed earlier in pregnancy. Both procedures are performed under local anesthetic at a clinic or medical facility.

Drugs called *abortifacients* may also be used during the first trimester. They cause a change in the balance of hormones in the body and lead to uterine bleeding and expulsion of the embryo. RU-486, consisting of the two drugs mifepristone and misoprostol, is an example of an abortifacient.

The most common second trimester abortion method is dilation and evacuation (D&E), a procedure somewhat similar to a D&C. Other options include labor and hysterotomy. In labor induction abortions, which are performed rarely, saline solution and prostaglandins are injected into the uterus, killing the fetus and inducing labor. The fetus is delivered two to four days after the procedure. Hysterotomy is a surgical procedure in which incisions are made in the lower abdomen and uterus and the fetus is surgically removed.

According to the Guttmacher Institute (2008), a prominent nonprofit organization that focuses on sexual health and public education, more than one million artificial abortions are performed in the United States each year. The typical profile of a woman who has an abortion is a never-married, white woman, under 25 years of age. Further, 89 percent of abortions are done during the first trimester and fewer than 1 percent are performed after the 20th week of pregnancy.

Although there can be physical complications with abortions, the risk is minimal, especially if done early in the pregnancy. Psychological and emotional consequences are difficult to measure because it is such a deeply personal issue and very much grounded in personal morality and religious beliefs. Long-term, scientifically sound studies, while difficult, should be conducted to determine psychological and emotional consequences of abortion.

THE ABORTION CONTROVERSY

Abortion has become one of the most highly charged issues of modern times in American politics and society. Opponents of abortion, the so-called pro-life camp, base their opposition on the belief that human life begins at the moment of conception. According to this view, ending that life at any time, for any reason, is morally wrong and ought to be illegal. On the other side, the so-called pro-choice camp believes that women should have the right to choose the circumstances under which they have children. According to this view, the decision regarding whether to continue a pregnancy or end it is a personal one that (within certain limits) should stay a private matter that is not interfered with by the government.

Fetal viability, or the age at which a fetus can survive outside the uterus, has become a key issue in the abortion debate. By 24 weeks gestation, there is a 40 percent chance for survival outside the uterus, whereas by week 28 in a pregnancy (near the beginning of the third trimester), the chance of survival is 90 percent. Many Americans who hold the pro-choice position are uncomfortable with late-term abortions of viable fetuses, according to public opinion polls. For example, in a July 2007 ABC News/Washington Post poll, 23 percent of respondents felt abortion should be legal in all cases, 34 percent felt it should be legal in most cases, and 42 percent desired it to be illegal in most or all cases. Further, a May 2007 Gallup Poll found 72 percent of respondents felt that a late-term abortion procedure called "partial birth abortion" should be illegal.

As the polls indicate, although some people are at the extreme ends of the spectrum regarding whether abortion should be legal, many Americans are in that "murky" middle ground. Most believe in the sanctity of life and feel uncomfortable about abortion and dislike the idea that so many occur, yet most are also uncomfortable outlawing it outright, especially in the first trimester.

LEGAL HISTORY OF ABORTION

Abortion was legalized in the United States in 1973 by the U.S. Supreme Court decision in *Roe v. Wade* on the basis of a constitutional right to privacy. The court ruled that during the first trimester of pregnancy, the states could not interfere with a woman's choice to terminate her pregnancy. Prior to this, many states had laws outlawing all abortions. During the second trimester, states could enact some regulations, especially those needed to protect the mother's health. During the third trimester, when the fetus is viable, states could restrict or prohibit abortions except those needed to protect the mother's health or life.

The right to abortion has been challenged frequently at the state level, and many of these cases have found their way to the Supreme Court. In listening to challenges, the Supreme Court has been especially sensitive to restrictions that impose an "undue burden" on a woman's right to the procedure, abortions performed on minors, and fetal viability. Since *Roe v. Wade*, Supreme Court rulings have included the following:

1. States cannot give a husband veto power when his pregnant wife decides to terminate her pregnancy.
2. States may require that a notice regarding abortion be given to both parents of an unmarried minor who is dependent on at least one of the parents or that consent be obtained. However, there is a provision for a judicial bypass (a judge may give permission for the abortion).
3. Medicaid funding cannot be used for abortion.
4. Late-term abortion called "partial birth abortion" is illegal as an elective procedure in all 50 states. The ban on the procedure was upheld in a recent Supreme Court decision (April 2007).

Health & the Media *Pregnancy Prevention*

Since 2000, the National Campaign to Prevent Teen Pregnancy has sponsored an annual contest with cash prizes for 13- to 21-year-olds to design a public service announcement (PSA). The assignment is to create a compelling magazine ad with a catchy slogan and image to spread the message of teen-pregnancy prevention. The top PSAs appear in magazines nationwide. This winning PSA reflects a realistic view of a teenager speaking to other teenagers. It suggests abstinence but also empha-sizes contraception for those who have sex. The message clearly communicates responsibility without being preachy. The National Campaign is working to build a more coordinated and effective grassroots movement and to influence cultural values by teaming with the entertainment media and other influential sectors in society.

just because you **can**

doesn't mean you **should!**

MAKE A DECISION

Four out of 10 girls get pregnant as a teen.
The only way to be sure you don't get pregnant —
or get someone pregnant — is don't have sex.
But if you do, use contraception. Every time.

The National Campaign to Prevent Teen Pregnancy
www.teenpregnancy.org

Source: **www.teenpregnancy.org**

✓ **NEED TO KNOW**

Pregnancy can be prevented. Knowing the options regarding contraceptive methods and how those methods work is important in making the best individual choice. Abstinence is the only 100-percent-effective method of contraception. Hormonal methods biologically simulate pregnancy through use of synthetic hormones, but they can have side effects. Barrier methods block movement of the sperm and prevent them from reaching the ovum. Surgical methods—vasectomy and tubal ligation—are invasive and should be considered permanent. The fertility awareness method requires careful body monitoring to determine the unsafe days for intercourse. When contraception fails, it is mostly due to human error. The choice to terminate a pregnancy through abortion is a hard one; the degree of invasiveness of the procedure is directly related to time in the pregnancy when the procedure is performed.

➤ Sexual Behavior

Hormones influence not only reproductive processes but also how people experience and express their sexuality. Humans have a biological urge for sexual activity known as the *sex drive* (or libido), driven primarily by testosterone. The sex drive also has cognitive and emotional components. For example, a person can become sexually aroused just by thinking or fantasizing about sex and sexual images.

The sex drive usually becomes intense in both boys and girls at puberty. The libido is highest for men in their late teens and early twenties and for women in their mid-twenties into their thirties.

The Centers for Disease Control and Prevention (CDC) has surveyed sexual behavior among Americans and has reported the following findings for adults aged 25–44 (Mosher et al., 2005):

- 97 percent of men and 98 percent of women have had vaginal intercourse.
- 90 percent of men and 88 percent of women have had oral sex with an opposite-sex partner.
- 40 percent of men and 35 percent of women have had anal sex with an opposite sex partner.
- 6.5 percent of men have had oral or anal sex with another man.
- 11 percent of women reported having had a sexual experience with another woman.

A CDC survey of people under age 30 also showed there is a high percentage of sexual activity in younger age groups. Roughly 40 percent of people report having sex for the first time between ages 15 and 17. Another 25–30 percent engage in sexual intercourse for the first time between ages 18 and 20.

FIGURE 5.6 HUMAN SEXUAL RESPONSE

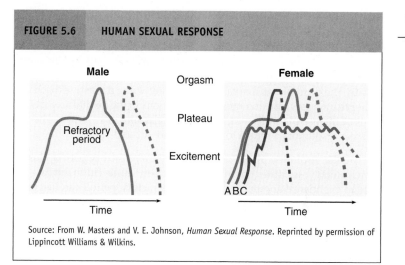

Source: From W. Masters and V. E. Johnson, *Human Sexual Response*. Reprinted by permission of Lippincott Williams & Wilkins.

Sexual behaviors are influenced by a variety of factors, including individual biology and personality, personal values and beliefs, family and cultural influences, and the media. People often wonder if they are "normal" in terms of what is sexually arousing to them, how frequently they engage in sexual activity, how they express themselves sexually (e.g., through masturbation, intercourse, etc.), and so on. For better or worse, there is no real answer to the question, What is normal sexual behavior? Sex drive and sexual behavior are deeply personal matters, and although there are some universals, there is also tremendous variation. Further, sex drive varies significantly over the course of the life span. To try to establish norms and benchmarks is misleading and ultimately meaningless.

THE HUMAN SEXUAL RESPONSE MODEL

Although scientists have long understood human reproduction, the physiology of the human sexual response was not well understood until the 1970s, when William Masters and Virginia Johnson conducted their ground-breaking clinical research on sexuality. Masters and Johnson studied the physiological changes that occur during sexual activity and identified four major stages in human sexual response: excitement, plateau, orgasm, and resolution. They also identified differences between the sexual response of men and women, adding to the body of knowledge about men's and women's sexual health.

According to the **human sexual response model** (Figure 5.6), the first phase is excitement, when both males and females become sexually

The **human sexual response model** is a four-stage model of the physiology of sexual response; the four stages are excitement, plateau, orgasm, and resolution.

aroused. Signs of arousal include erection of the penis in men and vaginal lubrication and swelling of the clitoris in women. Heart and breathing rates increase. As arousal intensifies, there is a transition to the plateau stage, a leveling off of sensation just before orgasm. Muscle tension increases, the penis increases in size, and the upper part of the vagina expands. The third phase is orgasm, a reflex involving a massive discharge of nerve impulses, causing muscle contractions in the genital area, sensations of intense pleasure, and, in men, the ejaculation of semen. The last phase is resolution, a return to a relaxed, pre-arousal state.

During the resolution phase, men experience a refractory period, during which blood vessels are constricted and the penis is flaccid so they are not able to experience another orgasm. The refractory period can last from minutes to hours. Women do not experience a refractory period.

As mentioned previously, women and men experience the sexual response differently. For example, the excitement and plateau phases tend to be longer for women then men—it generally takes women longer than men to become aroused. Another difference is that men experience one orgasm and women can experience multiple orgasms. These are normal differences between the sexes that may or may not make any difference in a relationship.

When a sexual problem does occur in a relationship, it may take the form of a man experiencing excitement, plateau, and orgasm while the woman is still experiencing excitement. As a result he is sexually satisfied while she is still only aroused. The solution generally recommended is that there be more foreplay to increase the woman's arousal level. It is more natural physiologically for men to extend the excitement and plateau phases than for women to try to shorten these phases. Issues involving the human sexual response are often issues affecting couples, and couples need to work together to deal with them. Good communication skills are essential to satisfying sexual relationships.

SEXUAL DYSFUNCTION

At some point in their lives, most people experience sexual problems or dysfunctions. **Sexual dysfunctions** are usually categorized as disorders of desire or arousal, orgasm disorders, and pain disorders.

Sexual desire disorders, or lack of interest in sex, can affect both men and women, as can sexual arousal disorders. Both disorders can be related to hormone levels, the ability to relax, and to a certain extent, wellness—that is, how well a person is functioning physically, mentally, and socially. Low levels of testosterone in men and estrogen in women can reduce

Sexual dysfunctions are common sexual disorders including sexual desire disorders, sexual arousal disorders, orgasm disorders, and sexual pain disorders.

desire and arousal, as can high levels of stress, emotional problems, worries and anxiety, and problems in the relationship. Certain medical conditions can also affect arousal, such as back pain, heart problems, endocrine disorders, or an enlarged prostate. Interventions for sexual desire and sexual arousal disorders include medications, relaxation techniques, and, if appropriate, counseling and education.

Sexual arousal disorder in men can result in erectile dysfunction (ED), also known as *impotence*. ED is the inability to achieve and/or maintain an erection long enough to have intercourse. ED is both a symptom of a condition and a condition itself. The causes of ED can range from low testosterone levels to depression and anxiety or vascular disease, including coronary artery disease. Sometimes medications that are used to treat a variety of conditions—including high blood pressure, diabetes, and depression and anxiety—can also cause ED as a side effect. The anxiety associated with ED can be emotionally damaging and can exacerbate the condition.

There are interventions that treat the symptom of erectile dysfunction and allow a man to achieve and maintain an erection long enough for intercourse without treating the underlying problem. Medications like Viagra act directly on the blood vessels that carry blood to the penis. When these blood vessels relax and dilate, they allow the erectile tissue in the penis to become engorged, producing an erection. Viagra allows a man to have an erection even in the midst of anxiety.

In women, sexual arousal disorders can result in the inability to relax vaginal muscles long enough to allow intercourse, to produce enough vaginal lubrication, or to attain orgasm. Intercourse can then be painful or undesirable. Unlike ED, sexual arousal disorders in women are not easy to treat with a drug. However, the symptoms can be treated with a lubricant to make vaginal penetration by a penis less painful and with muscle relaxants or minor tranquilizers to induce relaxation of vaginal muscles and allow orgasm to occur.

Both women and men can experience orgasm disorders, although such problems are more common in women. The chief symptom is delayed or absent orgasm. In many cases, lack of orgasm is due to timing differences between men and women, as described earlier, and the issue is more likely one of couple communication. Other causes of orgasm disorder include psychological or emotional problems, lack of knowledge, problems in the relationship, and the use of drugs or medications.

Sexual pain, or pain during or after intercourse, known as *dyspareunia*, is an unusual disorder that can affect both men and women. In women, dyspareunia may be caused by vaginismus, involuntary contractions of the vagina that make penetration painful, or by lack of vaginal lubrication. Vaginismus can have physical causes (e.g., pelvic inflammatory disease), which should be treated by a physician, or psychological causes, which may call for relaxation techniques or counseling. Lack of vaginal lubrication can be addressed with longer foreplay or with commercial lubrication products. In men, dyspareunia is generally related to infections of the urethra or inflammation of the urethra or foreskin, in some cases caused by a sexually transmitted infection. Men experiencing pain during or after intercourse should see their physician.

NEED TO KNOW

Human sexual response consists of excitement, plateau, orgasm, and resolution. This response is different for males and females. Males have shorter excitement and plateau phases, one orgasm, and resolution. Women experience longer excitement and plateau phases, can have multiple orgasms, and have a slower resolution. These natural biological differences can become problematic in a relationship, particularly for a woman, so good communication is needed to ensure mutual sexual satisfaction. Sexual dysfunctions can have physiological or psychological origins, and most are a combination of both. Sexual arousal disorders, erectile dysfunction, orgasm disorders, and sexual pain are examples of sexual dysfunctions which most often require medical intervention, which can range from medication to counseling or be a combination of the two. The dysfunctions are common and treatable.

➤ Gender Identity and Sexual Orientation

Up to this point this chapter has focused on the anatomy and physiology of human sexuality. The second half of the equation is how people express their sexuality. As noted at the beginning of the chapter, biological sex is determined at the chromosomal level and physically manifested in the appearance of the external genitals. Gender, on the other hand, is a concept defined more by a particular culture. Gender consists of the traits that a culture ascribes to males and females, contributing to what are considered "masculine" and "feminine" attributes and behaviors. **Gender identity** is the sense a person has that he or she is male or female.

By 18–30 months of age, children have a clear sense of whether they are boys or girls. Between the ages of 5 and 7, children solidify their sense of gender identity and strive to be consistent with their identity by employing stereotypes as rules. Between the ages of 7 and 12, children achieve gender stability, which is the cognitive understanding that gender is permanent. Both gender identity and stability are normally well formed prior to puberty.

Gender identity is a person's sense of being male or female.

In rare instances and for mostly unknown reasons, some individuals experience a conflict between their biological sex and their gender identity. Boys or girls may feel they are "really" the opposite sex, rather than gender that their body has. Individuals who experience this sense of gender dysphoria may be considered to have gender identity disorder and may be referred to as *cross-gender identified* or *transgendered.* Gender identity is not the same as sexual orientation. In other words, a transgendered person may either be homosexual or heterosexual.

Sexual orientation is commonly defined as an enduring emotional, romantic, and sexual attraction to members of one's own sex or of the opposite sex. It is generally recognized that sexual orientation exists along a continuum, with interest in romantic relationships exclusively with members of the same sex at one end of the continuum (homosexuality) and interest in romantic relationships exclusively with members of the other sex on the other end of the continuum (heterosexuality). Being attracted to and interested in members of both sexes falls in the middle of the continuum (bisexuality).

People can fall anywhere along this continuum, although social pressures encourage most people to identify themselves as heterosexual. The National Center for Health Statistics (2005) reported that among men ages 18–44, about 90 percent think of themselves as heterosexual, 2.3 percent say they are homosexual (gay), 1.8 percent report being bisexual, 3.9 percent "something else," and 1.8 percent did not answer the question. Among females in the same age group, about 90 percent say they are heterosexual, slightly over 1 percent identify as homosexual (lesbian), and almost 3 percent say they are bisexual.

It is not clear what causes a person's sexual orientation, but it is most likely an interaction of environment and individual biology, including genetics and hormonal factors. People do not choose their sexual orientation, although they can choose to express it or conceal it. Gay men and lesbians are often the targets of homophobia (fear of homosexuality) and may experience prejudice, discrimination, and even violence. Sometimes people experience so much conflict about their sexual orientation that they conceal it from themselves, which can lead to depression and other psychological problems.

Homosexuality is not a mental illness. Rather, it is a normal variation in one aspect of human experience. Abundant research indicates that gay men and lesbians are as mentally healthy as their heterosexual counterparts and equally competent at citizenship, parenting, and relationships.

Sexual orientation is emotional, romantic, and sexual attraction to people of the same or the other sex.

NEED TO KNOW

Gender identity and sexual orientation are different. Gender identity is one's sense of being male or female. A person who experiences a conflict between his or her biological sex and gender identity may be said to have gender identity disorder. Sexual orientation is enduring emotional, romantic, and sexual attraction to members of one's own or the other sex. Sexual orientation exists along a continuum from exclusive heterosexuality through bisexuality to exclusive homosexuality. Sexual orientation is influenced by both biological (genetic, hormonal) factors and environmental (family, societal, cultural) factors. People do not choose their sexual orientation.

➤ Healthy Relationships

Sexuality is an integral part of adult intimate relationships, but it is just one facet of relationships. Healthy relationships meet many more human needs than the sexual one. In his hierarchy-of-needs model, Abraham Maslow identified love and belonging as basic human needs; these needs can be met only in relationships. Besides love and belonging, intimate relationships offer such comforts as emotional intimacy, affirmation and acceptance, companionship, connection to others, and security for the future. Healthy relationships are central to wellness.

COMMITTED RELATIONSHIPS AND MARRIAGE

Most Americans meet their emotional needs in committed partnerships, whether marriage or cohabiting relationship. As a highly sanctioned social institution, marriage offers a great number of benefits to people, including economic benefits. Approximately 74 percent of Americans marry at least once in their life, reflecting the importance placed on marriage by the majority of the population. Research studies indicate that marriage is also good for your health—married people live longer than unmarried people, score higher on assessments of mental health, have lower rates of certain illnesses, and report being happier. Strong and supportive relationships of all kinds can offer some of the same benefits.

It has been reported that about half of all couples marrying today in the United States will eventually divorce. This statistic can be misleading, however; a more realistic percentage may be 40 percent. According to a U.S. Census Bureau report, marriages "are most susceptible to divorce in the early years of marriage. After 5 years approximately ten percent of marriages are expected to end in divorce, and another ten percent divorce by the tenth anniversary" (Kreider and Fields, 1996). The remaining 20 percent of all divorces happen between the 11- and 50-year mark. This shows that after a couple's tenth anniversary, the likelihood of divorce greatly decreases.

The most important elements of a healthy relationship are respect, trust, support, honesty, accountability, and shared responsibility. Respect is expressed by not constantly negatively criticizing or judging your partner's beliefs and actions and by performing helping behaviors that make his or her life easier. Trust, honesty, and support involve sharing open communication, willingness to admit mistakes, and the ability to take responsibility for your behavior. Shared responsibility means that work in the relationship, both emotional work and physical work, is shared equally.

In an unhealthy relationship, on the other hand, power is often unequal and one partner tries to dominate or control the other. The Iowa Coalition Against Violence developed the following criteria to assess relationships. The following seven points summarize this criteria. In a healthy relationship, most answers will be yes.

1. I can explain what I like and admire about my partner.
2. My partner is glad I have other friends, and has other friends himself/herself.
3. My partner is happy about my interests, accomplishments, and ambitions.
4. My partner has interests, accomplishments, and ambitions outside of me.
5. My partner has a good relationship with his/her family.
6. My partner takes responsibility for his/her actions and doesn't blame others for failures.
7. My partner talks about feelings, listens to me, and respects my opinions.

To further assess your relationship, complete the Relationship Vulnerability Scale (Figure 5.7).

COMMUNICATION AND CONFLICT RESOLUTION SKILLS

One way to improve relationships is by developing better communication and conflict resolution skills. Communication is key in both avoiding and resolving conflict. Conflict is simply disagreement between two people. Clear, open, and honest communication between people can cut down on conflict in relationships. Although some conflict is inevitable because people think and feel differently about things, it is very important not to allow conflict to become a contest where one must win their point at all costs. Differences in opinions are not contests. There is not a winner and a loser.

All the approaches to resolving conflict are intended to have a win-win outcome. In resolving conflict, it is important to (1) make sure communication is not hostile; (2) try to keep your emotions in check so that they don't get in the way of hearing what the other person is saying; (3) accept differences in opinions and feelings; (4) learn that it is OK to disagree; (5) listen to what is being said—don't be too quick to defend yourself; and (6) communicate in such a way that both of you feel that you have resolved the disagreement—even if you are not necessarily in agreement.

FIGURE 5.7   RELATIONSHIP VULNERABILITY SCALE

People begin and continue relationships for a variety of reasons. Sometimes these motives are not mutual. A person can be taken advantage of and eventually be hurt in the process. Relationships can sometimes evolve into dominant and submissive roles, without either person realizing it. This inventory is designed to help you evaluate your relationship and determine, to some degree, your chances of being in a vulnerable situation.

DIRECTIONS

Read each question carefully while reflecting on your present or most recent relationship. Check Yes or No according to your situation.

QUESTION	YES	NO
1. Is your partner often unavailable for phone calls at home or work?	——	——
2. Does he/she ask about the amount of money you earn or try to get involved in your financial planning?	——	——
3. Does your partner ever belittle your efforts and/or ideas?	——	——
4. Has your partner ever disappeared for any length of time (overnight, several days, a week) and not informed you of his/her whereabouts?	——	——
5. Does he/she live with you and contribute little or nothing to household maintenance?	——	——
6. Does your partner borrow money and seldom bother to repay it, or frequently ask you to buy him/her things, or always use your car?	——	——
7. Has he/she had one or more tragic misfortune(s) that needed your financial assistance?	——	——
8. Has your partner told you early in your relationship that he/she would like to be married and described a life of love and luxury for both of you but made no definite steps in that direction?	——	——
9. Do you stop your present activity or postpone your plans when he/she calls you to do something on the spur of the moment?	——	——
10. Is he/she the only person in your life?	——	——

11. Do you allow your partner to take the "upper hand" in your affairs? ___ ___

12. Have you ever noticed any discrepancies concerning what your partner has told you in regards to his/her name, background, family, etc.? ___ ___

13. When you go out does your partner avoid socializing with his/her or your family and friends? ___ ___

14. Do you usually wait for others to introduce you to potential partners instead of taking the initiative to meet new people on your own? ___ ___

15. When your partner describes his/her future goals, does it seem unclear as to where you fit into the future? ___ ___

16. Do you feel that you should be married to be happy? ___ ___

SCORING

Give yourself one point for each "yes" response to the questions.

Your score: _____ points

13–16 You are very vulnerable to being in a lopsided relationship which may result in hurt feelings in the future. You should seriously examine the contour and direction of your relationship with your partner. For you to continue with your present situation is almost certain to be a waste of time and energy.

9–12 You are vulnerable to being taken advantage of. Stop and ask yourself if you are getting out of this relationship what you are putting into it.

5–8 You are somewhat vulnerable to being hurt. Your relationship probably has potential but needs to be evaluated. You and your partner should discuss your future to determine what type of lifestyle you both desire.

1–4 You do not seem vulnerable to being dominated in your relationship. Keep the statements to which you responded "yes" in mind, and openly discuss them with your partner.

Source: Robert F. Valois and Sandra K. Kammermann, "Relationship Vulnerability Scale," page 108–109, Wellness, R.S.V.P., third Edition, 1986, Benjamin/Cummings Publishing Company, Inc., Menlo Park, CA, Copyright 1992 by Valois, Kammermann & Associates and the authors. Used with permission of Valois, Kammermann & Associates and the authors.

Web Site Resources

Alan Guttmacher Institute
www.guttmacher.org
American Society for Reproductive Medicine
www.asrm.org
Centers for Disease Control and Prevention (CDC)
www.cdc.gov
CrisisPregnancy.com
www.crisispregnancy.com/
MSN Health Center
http://health.msn.com
National Men's Health Network
www.menshealthnetwork.org
National Women's Health Network
www.womenshealthnetwork.org
Planned Parenthood
www.plannedparenthood.org
Sexuality Information and Education Council of the United States
www.siecus.org
Web MD (Pregnancy)
www.webmd.com/baby/

Knowing the Language

Abortion
Amenorrhea
Artificial abortion
Birth control pill
Bulbourethral glands
Cervical cap
Cervix
Clitoris
Condoms
Contraceptive implants
Depo-Provera
Diaphragm
Dysmenorrhea
Ectopic pregnancy
Embryo
Estrogen
Fallopian tubes
Fetus
Gender identity
Glans penis
Hormonal contraceptives
Hormones
Human sexual response (model)

IUD
Menopause
Menorrhagia
Natural methods (of birth control)
Ovaries
Ovulation
Progesterone
Prostate gland
Scrotum
Seminal vesicles
Sexual dysfunction
Sexual orientation
Spermicides
Spontaneous abortion
Testes
Testosterone
Trimesters
Tubal ligation
Uterus
Vagina
Vas deferens
Vasectomy

1. Identify and briefly describe the structures in the male and female reproductive systems that have similar functions.
2. Discuss how each of the following methods of contraception work: hormonal, barrier, vasectomy and tubal ligation, and fertility awareness/periodic abstinence.
3. What is the difference between spontaneous abortion and artificial abortion? What are the major issues inherent in artificial abortion?
4. What are the implications of the phases of human sexual response for men and women?
5. Identify and briefly describe the major types of sexual dysfunction in both men and women.

Exploring Ideas

1. What is the relationship between physiology and sexuality? How can acknowledgement of this relationship help in making low-risk choices with respect to sexual issues?
2. What major issues should be considered in contraception?
3. Is it better to treat the symptoms of sexual dysfunction or to try to treat the causes of sexual dysfunction?

Selected References

Basson, R. Are our definitions of women's desire, arousal and sexual pain disorders too broad and our definition of orgasmic disorder too narrow? *Journal of Sex and Marital Therapy* 28 (4): 289–300, 2002.

Blum, D. *Sex on the Brain: The Biological Differences Between Men and Women.* New York: Viking Press, 1998.

Cooper M., Baker P. Sex: The sensual man: Chapter 4 in *The MANual: The Complete Man's Guide to Life.* London: Thorsons, 1996.

Guttmacher Institute (2008). Facts on Induced Abortions in the United States.
http://www.guttmacher.org/pubs/fb_induced_abortions.html

Kinsey A, Pomeroy W, Martin C. *Sexual Behavior in the Human Female.* Bloomington, IN: Indiana University Press, 1948.

Kinsey A, Pomeroy W, Martin C. *Sexual Behavior in the Human Male.* Bloomington, IN: Indiana University Press, 1948.

Kreider, RM, Fields, JM. Number, timing, and duration of marriages and divorces: 1996. *U.S. Census Bureau Current Population Reports,* February 2002.

Masters W, Johnson V. *Human Sexual Response.* Boston: Little, Brown, 1966.

Masters W, Johnson V. *On Sex and Human Loving,* Vol 1. Boston: Little, Brown, 1988.

National Center for Health Statistics. Sexual behavior and selected health measures: Men and women 15–44 years of age, United States, 2002. Bethesda, MD: National Center for Health Statistics, 2002.

Nelson A, Hatcher R, Zieman M, Watt A, Darney P, Creinin M. *A Pocket Guide to Managing Contraception.* Dawsonville, GA: Bridging the Gap Foundation, 2005.

Oriel J. Sexual pleasure as a human right: Harmful or helpful to women in the context of HIV/AIDS. *Women's Studies International Forum* 5 (28): 392–404, 2005.

Potts A, Gaven N, Grace V, Vares T. The downside of Viagra: Women's experiences and perspectives. *Sociology of Health and Illness* 25 (7): 697–719, 2003.

Savin-Williams RC. Who's gay? Does it matter? *Current Directions in Psychological Science* (15):1, 40–44.

Wincze J, Carey M. *Sexual Dysfunction* (2nd ed.). New York: Guilford, 2001.

Wolf N. *Promiscuities: A Secret History of Female Desire.* London: Chatto and Windus, 1997.

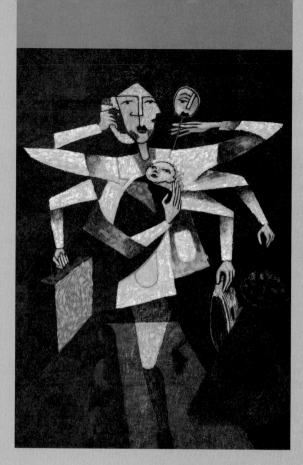

In the middle
of difficulty lies
opportunity.

— ALBERT EINSTEIN

Chapter 6

MANAGE STRESS

Stress is part of life. Too much can be harmful, yet too
little stress is unhealthy too. In this chapter, we focus on
understanding the concept of stress and how to recognize and
deal with excessive stress. We describe a variety of proven
stress management techniques and suggest new ways to think
about stress.

THE NATURE OF STRESS

DEFINING AND DESCRIBING STRESS

THE BIOLOGY OF STRESS: PHYSIOLOGICAL RESPONSES

THE PSYCHOLOGY OF STRESS: MENTAL AND EMOTIONAL RESPONSES

STRESS AND ILLNESS

SOURCES OF STRESS

SIGNS AND SYMPTOMS OF EXCESSIVE STRESS

CHRONIC STRESS AND HEALTH

STRESS—THE "BIG PICTURE"

MANAGING STRESS

TIME MANAGEMENT

KNOW THYSELF

STRESS MANAGEMENT TECHNIQUES

"THERE IS NEVER ENOUGH TIME, unless you're serving it," quipped Malcolm Forbes, the flamboyant business-magazine publisher. This quotation captures the modern view of stress in several ways. It reflects the sentiment that life is hectic and people continually rush about trying to do everything that needs to be done. It is also a joking reference to the difficulties of life behind bars should one end up in prison. This simple tongue-in-cheek comment shows how easily stress can be found in all aspects of life. For some people, common incidents like waiting in line or being stuck in traffic can be stressful. Yet, in the larger picture these are just minor inconveniences that pale in comparison with truly serious events such as those associated with extreme physical pain, mental anguish, or debilitating illness.

Stress is certainly part of our common conversational language. Hardly a day goes by when we don't hear someone say, "I'm under a lot of stress" or "I'm really stressed out." As college students, you can easily list your top stresses. They often arise from the challenge of balancing course work and financial pressures with social life and family relationships. Many students have jobs too, which adds another significant factor to the equation. Successfully coordinating all these activities requires self-management skills. As we found with eating and exercise, a proven approach for improving a desired lifestyle behavior is to learn the basic concepts, chart a plan, and then develop the necessary skills, and take action. In this case, the aim is to improve your ability to manage stress in a positive way.

Clearly, stress is part of living and varies widely across a continuum. Much of the time to a remarkable degree, we can control and manage the many demands and pressures in our lives. But it can be difficult. College students rank "dealing with stress" as a top concern. In this chapter, we examine the concept of stress through a broad, objective lens. You will find that stress can be a positive influence in your life, a force to be understood and reframed to your benefit, not simply something to be dreaded or avoided. We also review how to recognize excessive stress, and we present effective coping strategies.

➤ The Nature of Stress

The origin of the word *stress* can be traced to its use in physics, where it refers to the amount of force, pressure, or strain (load) put on an object to bend or break it. For example, when building a bridge or an airplane, engineers need to know the level of stress that component materials (woods, metals, plastics) can withstand before they break or fail. Decades ago, researchers in biology and medicine borrowed the term and applied it to the tensions and pressures that living organisms experience.

At the onset, let's define a few basic terms, because *stress* and related words have multiple meanings even across the biological and social sciences. **Stress** refers to the collective psychobiological responses that occur when a person's natural balance is disrupted. Throughout the animal kingdom, organisms inherently strive to maintain physiological balance, or homeostasis. Any factor or force that disrupts homeostasis is technically known as a stressor.

A **stressor** can be physical or psychological, and both types are wide-ranging. Imagine that you decide to go for a run on a cold day and inadvertently trip over a curb and land squarely on your knee. (It's easy to imagine the pain and see the bloody gash!) In this scenario, several physical stressors can be identified: the exertion of exercise, exposure to a low temperature, and the tissue damage from the impact of the fall. There is also the momentary psychological stressor of the fall itself when you know you can't catch yourself and you're going down.

Let's extend the story. Later that day you complete a difficult math assignment, participate in a group meeting that turns argumentative, and finally return to your dorm room for a quiet break—only to discover that your roommate has invited a few friends over. The psychological stressors include the mental challenge of the math assignment and the emotional frustrations that can arise when working or living with others. And, as in these examples, stressors are often multiple and overlapping, not just occasional, isolated events.

Stressors that deplete energy and cause a decline in performance or function lead to **distress,** or a negative stress condition. The word *stress* is typically used in this negative context, but technically, the correct term is *distress.* Conversely, stressors can also be positive. Stressors that motivate and result in improved performance or function lead to **eustress,** or a positive stress condition. Examples of eustress are a bonus for completing a specific project or the potential of exploring a new relationship with a person you find attractive. Knowing that stressors can lead to either distress or eustress, you can more easily see that stressors are not limited to threatening or unpleasant situations but also include those that are exciting or simply new.

Stress refers to a person's collective psychobiological responses to challenging situations, such as those which are tiring, threatening, exciting, or new. The situation, event, or factors that cause the stress response are known as **stressors.** Stressors disrupt a person's natural state of balance (homeostasis) and can be positive as well as negative.

Distress, or negative stress, is created by stressors that deplete energy and result in impaired performance.

Eustress, or positive stress, is created by stressors that motivate and result in improved performance.

Stress also can be categorized by its duration; we describe stress as acute, episodic, or chronic. Acute stress is brief but intense. Examples includes being called on unexpectedly in class by a professor or losing control of your car and narrowly avoiding an accident. Episodic stress is regular or predictable but intermittent. Final exams and class projects at the end of every semester or a difficult family situation that you have to deal with during visits home are examples of episodic stress. Lastly, chronic stress is prolonged and continuous. New military recruits experience this during boot camp, where they are challenged physically and mentally with no letup over several months of basic training. Another example is a job that is unpleasant or unfulfilling but necessary to make a living. A high-stress job is often one in which you have responsibility for outcomes but little or no control over them. Arguably the most difficult chronic stress situations are those in which people must deal with constant discomfort or pain due to a health condition. The degree of distress is magnified if no viable options are available.

Before we review techniques for balancing and managing the stressors in our lives, let's briefly consider the concept of stress from two viewpoints—one biological, the other psychological. This background material will allow us to better understand the basis and rationale for different stress management techniques.

THE BIOLOGY OF STRESS: PHYSIOLOGICAL RESPONSES

The biological perspective is based on the principle that our responses to stress are regulated by the brain, which controls all body functions. The urge to act when threatened is rooted in our neurological and endocrine systems, whose coordinated stress responses provide the extra strength and energy needed to cope. These collective physiological responses—including an increase in heart rate and breathing, a tensing of muscles, and a focusing of attention—are known as the *fight-or-flight response*. The fight-or-flight response evolved as a survival mechanism in the early development of our species. Let's take a closer look.

Hans Selye, M.D. (1907–1982), known as the father of stress research, developed a model called the **general adaptation syndrome** to describe how animals, including humans, respond to stress. He defined a stressor as anything that disrupts homeostasis (physiological balance). In turn, he described the stress response as the body's adaptations designed to reestablish homeostasis. As seen in Figure 6.1, the general adaptation syndrome depicts three predictable stages.

The **general adaptation syndrome** is a model that describes the body's physiological responses to stressors in three stages: alarm, resistance, and exhaustion.

FIGURE 6.1   GENERAL ADAPTATION SYNDROME

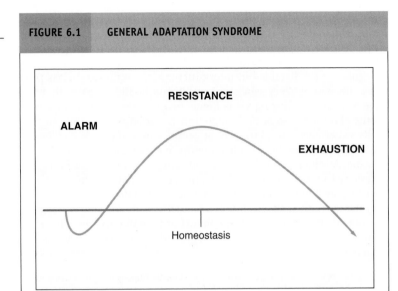

The general adaptation syndrome is shown as the time course of the body's resistance to a stressor (adaptive capacity). The baseline is the person's stable level of physiological balance (homeostasis). The three stages are *alarm* (this initial reaction to a stressor results in changes that briefly lower resistance), *resistance* (the body mobilizes to increase resistance to withstand the stressor), and *exhaustion* (extreme or prolonged stressors can override the body's ability to adapt, leading to illness and sometimes death).

This figure describes the complete general adaptation syndrome through the exhaustion stage. However, in most situations, our bodies successfully adapt to stressors and return to homeostasis at various points over time. The specific time course depends on the magnitude of the stressor and the individual's ability to adapt.

In the alarm stage, the brain's initial response to a stressor is to signal the **fight-or-flight response** throughout the systems of the body. This is achieved via the autonomic (involuntary) nervous system, the neuroendocrine system, and the voluntary nervous system. These complex systems can be thought of as a communication network that coordinates multiple physiological processes, some of which are activated while others are inhibited. For example, nutrients are released from energy stores to provide fuel for action, while blood vessels to the skin and digestive tract constrict to allow more blood to go to the muscles. Many of these changes

The **fight-or-flight response** is the acute stress response in which the autonomic nervous system triggers a set of physiological changes that ready the body for action. The fight-or-flight response corresponds to the alarm stage of the general adaptation syndrome.

are mediated through the release of chemical messengers (neurotransmitters) such as epinephrine (adrenaline) and cortisol. These chemical messengers are commonly referred to as *stress hormones*. All physiological changes heighten awareness and ready the body for action—fight or flight. Routine sensations and feelings such as hunger, comfort, joy, and sorrow are simply overridden. The effect is rapid and intense.

If the stressor continues, the body goes into the resistance stage and will continue to mobilize energy and biochemical resources (chemical messengers) as needed to withstand the threat. During this stage, the body's physiological processes are aimed at both adapting to the stressor and regaining homeostasis. If additional stressors occur during this phase, the body will likely not be able to meet the challenge because all resources are already being allocated to withstand the initial stressor. The cumulative stressors would overcome the body's capacity to adapt. In this sense, the body is particularly vulnerable during the resistance stage. If the body can successfully adapt to the stressor, there is a return to homeostasis. If, however, the stressor is too great or persists too long, the body moves into the exhaustion stage. In this stage, the stressor overcomes the body's capacity to adapt, with subsequent exhaustion, illness, and eventually death.

Visualize a lion stalking a gazelle and consider the biological alarm and cascade of effects that occur within the gazelle as it senses the presence of the lion (alarm stage). Due to a quick response and great speed, the gazelle may elude the lion. Alternatively, after a brief encounter, the gazelle may escape with wounds that will heal (resistance stage), or despite its best efforts to escape, the gazelle may in the end become exhausted and fall prey to the lion (exhaustion stage).

The fight-or-flight response (alarm stage of the general adaptation syndrome) is logical and purposeful as a means for dealing with short-term physical stress. Our ancestors regularly confronted wild animals. Just as with the gazelle, their ability to activate an innate emergency system was a key survival mechanism. Although this system has equipped humans for dealing with short-term physical stress, how well does it equip us for the stressors of modern life? How does it help us accommodate the mental or emotional stressors that are chronic or uniquely human?

THE PSYCHOLOGY OF STRESS: MENTAL AND EMOTIONAL RESPONSES

Psychologists point out that although a biological perspective of stress is critical to our understanding, it alone does not present the complete picture. A limitation of the biological model is that it does not explain the individual variability that we see in responses to stress. Research has shown that individuals do in fact respond differently to the same stressor because of differences in how they *perceive* and *interpret* the stressor.

Richard Lazarus, Ph.D. (1922–2002), a leading researcher on cognition and emotion, was among the first to propose that the interpretation of stressful events is more important than the events themselves. The ability of people to think about and assess future events—both the potential harms and challenges—makes them vulnerable in ways that other animals are not. Dr. Lazarus's research was primarily with humans, whereas Dr. Selye's work focused on laboratory animals. Research has confirmed that humans, due to their higher-level cognitive abilities, experience a wider range of mental and psychosocial stresses than do other animals.

Dr. Lazarus and his colleague Susan Folkman, Ph.D., defined stress as a particular relationship between the person and the environment that is appraised by the person as taxing or exceeding his or her resources and endangering his or her well-being. This definition is the basis of their **transactional model of stress and coping,** in which stressful experiences are seen as person-environment interactions (transactions). Two fundamental transactions are a person's judgment about the significance of the stressor and the person's self-appraisal of his or her ability to successfully cope with the stressor. This psychological perspective on stress allows opportunities for management at several points: during the initial appraisal of the stressor, during self-assessment of one's ability to control or cope, and during implementation of coping behaviors. We will discuss specific stress management approaches in the last section of this chapter.

These psychological concepts of stress were dramatically brought to life during the classic Stanford Prison Study, conducted by Stanford University researcher and social psychologist Philip Zimbardo and his colleagues in 1971. The intent of this experiment was to study the psychology of imprisonment by randomly assigning college men to roles as either prisoners or guards and then observing their interactions and behaviors for two weeks in a simulated prison environment. The unexpected occurred, conditions got out of control, and the study had to be shut down after only six days. Even though the college students knew they were subjects in a study, the "prisoners" soon lost the ability to cope, with some showing signs of depression and extreme stress. Some "guards" became ruthless in their positions of authority. These surprising and controversial findings highlighted the importance of perception, control, and coping and demonstrated that the interactions between the person and the environment are malleable and dynamic. (For complete documentation on this classic study, go to **www.prisonexp.org**).

The **transactional model of stress and coping** views stress as a transactional (person-environment) phenomenon dependent on the meaning of the stressor to the perceiver. The impact of the external stressor is first mediated by the person's appraisal of the stressor and then by the social and cultural resources at his or her disposal.

✓ **NEED TO KNOW**

The nature of stress is highly variable. Stressors can be physical or psychological, and they can occur acutely, episodically, or chronically. Dr. Hans Selye, a pioneer in stress research, used animal studies to develop the general adaptation syndrome, a model depicting the biological effects of stress. His basic concepts are still used today to understand the broad array of stress-related disorders. Dr. Richard Lazarus, a leading psychologist of the 20th century, conducted complementary research with humans, examining the role of cognition and emotion on the experience of stress. He and other psychologists have shown that individual responses to stressful events not only are highly variable but also depend on one's perceptions both of the stressors and of one's ability to cope. Integrating biological and psychological perspectives provides a holistic view of the complex relationships among stress, behavior, and health.

➤ Stress and Illness

The role of stress, particularly chronic stress, in causing or contributing to illness and disease is one of the most studied topics in medical science. Although parts of the puzzle remain unsolved, fundamental knowledge about the sources of stress and resulting signs and symptoms of excessive stress are well established. An update on type A behavior as a risk factor for heart disease, the potential link of stress to obesity, and recent insights on the connection between socioeconomic level and well-being are highlighted to show the varied pathways in which stress may influence our health.

SOURCES OF STRESS

The main sources of stress in America today are associated with changes in personal relationships and occupation. (Of course, as a student your "job" is to make progress in school and eventually earn your degree.) Some changes in life are traumatic, such as failing in school, the break-up of a close personal relationship, experiencing a major injury or illness, losing a job, or the death of a family member. As we now know, positive changes can also be stress-filled, such as graduating, getting married, having a child, or getting a job promotion.

In an effort to quantify the amount of stress a person is experiencing and the corresponding increased risk for stress-related illness, psychologists Thomas Holmes and R. H. Rahe developed their now-well-known Social Readjustment Rating Scale. Using a statistical analysis of responses from a large, diverse group of adults, they were able to assign values to a variety of events based on their perceived stressfulness. The resulting values indicate the relative impact of stressful events on health and give a sense of the wide range of stressors in our lives. In Table 6.1,

TABLE 6.1	EXAMPLES OF STRESSFUL EVENTS

Life Event	Point Value
Death of a spouse	119
Divorce	96
Fired from work	79
Major injury or illness	74
Pregnancy	67
Birth of a child	66
Parents' divorce	59
Marriage	50
Change residence to different city or state	47
Break-up of close personal relationship	47
Beginning or ending college	38
Making a major purchase	37
General work troubles	28
Change in personal habits	26
Vacation	24

Source: Miller MA, Rahe RH. Life changes scaling for the 1990s. *Journal of Psychosomatic Research* 43 (3): 279–292, 1997.

a few different events are listed to illustrate their findings. The events listed are representative. You could add items, many of them likely to carry high values.

Our environment also encompasses multiple sources of stress, many of which are seemingly omnipresent. Most Americans are city dwellers and encounter crowding, pollution, and noise in their daily lives. Separately, and even more so in combination, these stressors have been shown to harm health, particularly mental health. Collectively referred to as *urban press,* such negative environmental stressors are often beyond personal control. Conversely, positive environmental stressors can be found in the community via the arts, sports, museums, and parks. These can be sought out for excitement and enjoyment by individuals and groups.

SIGNS AND SYMPTOMS OF EXCESSIVE STRESS

Recognizing major life-changing events, such as those at the top of the stress scales, is not a problem. However, recognizing our *responses* to these events is not always so straightforward. Identifying the more subtle combination or accumulation of less dramatic daily or episodic stressors and our responses to them can require a focused of awareness and analysis. There are clues, though, and we should be alert to them. The following 10 questions capture common signs and symptoms of excessive stress.

- Have you become anxious and easily depressed?
- Have you become indecisive and generally apathetic?
- Have you become irritable and easily angered?
- Have your memory and concentration deteriorated?
- Have you experienced an increase in headaches or digestive problems?
- Has your blood pressure become elevated?
- Has your sleep pattern changed (insomnia/excessive sleep)?
- Have your eating habits changed (appetite loss/binge eating)?
- Have you increased your use of alcohol or drugs?
- Have you developed any nervous habits or phobias?

If you answered yes to one or more of these questions, reassess the stressors in your life. First, can you identify them? Is it likely that they are causing the signs and symptoms? And if so, are you taking the time and making the effort to address both the stressors and your responses to them? (See the Breaking It Down box "Sleep: An Update on a Primal Need.") A discussion of stress management, including practical strategies and techniques, is provided later in this chapter.

If you are currently facing demanding or distressing situations that are taxing your ability to make it through the day, or if you are showing signs of stress that are not subsiding, see a counselor or health specialist at your counseling center or student health center. These professionals are there to assist you, so don't hesitate to make an appointment and meet with them.

Breaking It Down Sleep: An Update on a Primal Need

The need for sleep is as fundamental to life as the need for food and water. We literally cannot live without sleep. In fact, forced sleep deprivation is used as a means to break down prisoners during interrogation. Despite extensive research, scientists have yet to understand why sleep is so vital—this essential question remains a mystery. However, they do know a great deal about the characteristics of sleep; for example, the types (shallow vs. deep sleep) and structure (sequence, organization) of sleep and how these aspects change from infancy to old age. Of particular interest is how normal sleep patterns are affected by sleep disturbances such as insomnia, sleep apnea (breathing interruptions during sleep), and narcolepsy (daytime "sleep attacks"). Sleep-related problems affect about one out of five Americans of all ages, races, and socioeconomic classes. More and more physicians are being trained in sleep medicine, a specialization offered through the American Boards of Internal Medicine, Pediatrics, Otolaryngology (ear, nose, throat), and Psychiatry and

(Continued)

Neurology. Patients with sleep problems can see a specialist at over 1,000 accredited sleep centers spread throughout the United States.

Both science and personal experience tell us that the relationship between sleep and stress is reciprocal. Stressors can definitely disrupt sleep—we've all had nights when emotional turmoil or a major deadline has kept us up. And, conversely, not getting enough sleep is also a stressor, so the potential for a vicious cycle exists. For college students, the effects of inadequate sleep on learning are especially relevant. The evidence shows that sleep loss results in impairment in learning capacity, that is, in higher cognitive functions such as attention, memory, and problem solving. Studies in which sleep was actively restricted or optimized showed a corresponding worsening or improvement in learning and academic performance. Establishing a healthy sleep routine is often a matter of recognizing and then eliminating or minimizing sleep disrupters:

Caffeine consumption—avoid coffee, sodas, pills, and, yes, chocolate too within a few hours of bedtime.

Exercise—by all means engage in regular exercise, but complete your workout a few hours before bedtime.

Indigestion—avoid problem foods and have antacids on hand just in case.

Reaction to medicines—be aware of active ingredients that may interfere with sleep, and find substitutes.

Other sleep disrupters, such as pain, emotional upset, or illness, can be more difficult to deal with but are still generally manageable, and in most cases these are short-lived. If you have recurring or chronic sleep problems, see a health care professional at your student health or counseling center. Depending on your specific situation, you may be referred to a sleep medicine specialist for a complete sleep-disorder evaluation. Even though today's high-tech world seemingly runs 24/7, humans are still subject to the biological control of circadian (daily) rhythms that dictate our need for regular restful sleep. Sleep deprivation interferes with our ability to learn and function, and in that sense it becomes an added stressor that further hinders our ability to cope. The opposite is true as well: maintaining healthy sleep habits goes a long way in helping us deal with stressors that are beyond our control. For more information about the science and medicine of sleep and tips for getting restful sleep, go to

National Sleep Foundation
www.sleepfoundation.org

American Academy of Sleep Medicine
www.sleepeducation.com

CHRONIC STRESS AND HEALTH

As we now know, the body's response to stress can be both helpful and harmful. From an evolutionary perspective, it equips us for survival—to face emergencies with speed and strength. But in the 21st century, the stressors we face are more often psychosocial than physical, and more typically chronic than acute. Long-term activation of the stress response resulting from the interplay between the nervous system and stress hormones can have detrimental effects on the body's major systems. When anxiety and worry about work and relationships don't let up, stress hormones continue to circulate throughout the body in high levels, never leaving the blood and tissues.

Simply put, persistent stress can damage the same physiological systems activated or affected by the stress response in the first place. At the head of the list are the nervous, endocrine, cardiorespiratory, metabolic, immune, and gastrointestinal systems. Over time, unrelenting stress and the accompanying biochemical turmoil translates into an increased risk for a vast array of disorders and diseases. Stress can both cause diseases and worsen existing ones. Heart disease, obesity, and depression are three of the most common stress-related conditions. Stress has also been shown to accelerate the aging process. This can be seen in photos of American presidents taken before and after their terms. For example, in Figure 6.2 the impact of the presidency is captured in the face of Bill Clinton who served two terms (1993–2001). Moreover, in 2004 at age 58, President Clinton was diagnosed with heart disease (significant blockage in the coronary arteries) and subsequently had bypass surgery.

| FIGURE 6.2 | THE PRESIDENCY AND PREMATURE AGING: BILL CLINTON IN 1992 AND 2003 (AT AGES 45 AND 56) |

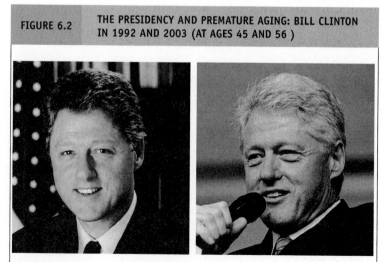

Sources: The photo from 1992 is an official White House photo. The photo from 2003 was taken during a 2003 Kennedy Library Forum.

Nearly 50 years ago, two cardiologists, Meyer Friedman and R. H. Rosenman, developed the concept of **type A** personality and identified it as a psychological risk factor for heart disease. They found that people with classic type A personality continually put themselves in stressful situations, which over time resulted in far more heart attacks than happened to people who were not type A. Today we are all familiar with type A behavior and easily recognize it in others. Type A individuals are competitive, aggressive, and time-driven; they never seem to miss a step. In contrast, type B individuals are methodical, move at a slower pace, and are generally easygoing. In reality, most of us fall somewhere in between the classic type A (driving, impatient) and type B (unhurried, calm) dispositions.

Further research on type A behavior and heart disease has yielded additional important findings. It turns out that type A behavior can be broken down into three components—excessive competitiveness, time-urgency, and **hostility**—and the hostility component is the primary culprit behind the continual activation of the stress pathways that lead to disease. Hostility—a combination of anger, aggression, and cynicism—may be a better predictor of heart disease than traditional risk factors like cigarette smoking, hypertension, and high cholesterol. See the "What Is Your Risk?" feature and take the 10-question hostility screener.

> **Type A behavior** is characterized by excessive competitiveness, time-urgency, and hostility. People with this profile tend to engage their stress response systems on a chronic basis. The **hostility** component has been identified as the primary trait that puts people at risk for the development of heart disease and other stress-related medical conditions.

What Is Your Risk? Screening for Hostility

Persons who exhibit high levels of hostility are endangering their health. Hostility has three aspects: anger, which is an emotional response to other people's "unacceptable" behavior; aggression, which refers to behaviors in response to negative emotions such as anger and irritation; and cynicism, which is a mistrusting attitude toward the motives of others. The 10 questions below attempt to get at these underlying aspects of hostility. (Remember though—as with any short assessment—this survey is only a screener.) Check any of the following statements that are true for you. Be as honest and objective as possible.

_____ 1. I often get annoyed at checkout cashiers or the people in front of me when I'm waiting in line.

_____ 2. I usually keep an eye on the people I work or live with to make sure they do what they should.

_____ 3. I often wonder how homeless people can have so little respect for themselves.

_____ 4. I believe that most people will take advantage of you if you let them.

_____ 5. The habits of friends or family members often annoy me.

_____ 6. When I'm stuck in traffic, I often start breathing faster and my heart pounds.

_____ 7. When I'm annoyed with people, I really want to let them know it.

_____ 8. If someone does me wrong, I want to get even.

_____ 9. I'd like to have the last word in any argument.

_____10. At least once a week, I have the urge to yell at or even hit someone.

The higher the number of "true" statements, the higher the estimate of one's hostility level. Five or more "true" statements suggest that you are excessively hostile. If you were unsure of many answers, consider asking someone close to you—a friend whose judgment you trust or a spouse—to profile you with the same 10 questions. Instruct this person to answer each question as he or she believes you would answer. If the score from this person's rating of you is similar to yours, then it's likely that your self-rating is accurate.

If your score indicates excessive hostility, take steps to address it. For example, discuss the results with a clinical psychologist at the campus counseling center. Also, an excellent book with practical information on developing behavioral skills to reduce anger is *In Control* by Redford and Virginia Williams.

Source: Williams V, Williams R. *Lifeskills*. New York: Times Books, 1997. Used with permission of the authors.

Stress and Obesity

Connections between chronic stress and seemingly unrelated conditions continue to be uncovered. The role of chronic stress in the current obesity epidemic is one example. As researchers continue to unravel how the body's stress response system is regulated, the details of the actions and interplay between the brain and multiple chemical messengers are becoming clearer. It is now known that caloric input, energy stores, and body weight are intertwined with the chronic stress response network.

The details of these interactions are exceedingly complex and require specialized training to fully understand. However, the essence is that problematic eating behaviors, including the overconsumption of so-called comfort foods (pleasing foods typically high in carbohydrates and fat), may be stimulated by elevated levels of stress hormones. At the metabolic level, these surplus calories tend to be stored in the abdominal area and over time result in abdominal obesity, which is strongly related to type 2 diabetes, heart disease, and stroke. In other words, stress can make us put on fat more easily, especially if we seek consolation in snack foods. This chronic stress–obesity connection offers another example of the dynamic interactions among physiological systems, emotions, and coping methods.

Social Standing and Health Status

It's no surprise that the most disadvantaged in society face more stress-related illness due to the continual struggle for life's necessities (food, clothing, housing). Discrimination and limited access to health care compound the difficulty of their situation. Governmental and private-sector agencies work diligently to reduce these inequities.

Recent research in public health has produced a related new finding with wide-reaching implications. It appears that certain psychosocial factors are at work not just among the poor but across the entire socioeconomic spectrum. Based on longitudinal analysis of demographic, psychological, and health variables in large population studies, a British research team led by Michael Marmot, M.D., professor of public health at University College, London found that it's not socioeconomic level that determines health (quality of life, longevity) but the underlying and related factors of individual autonomy and social participation.

Dr. Marmot labels this the **status syndrome.** Higher status usually affords more opportunities for individual control and meaningful relationships. Lower status means that external forces are more likely to determine one's fate. In other words, a person's health appears to be tied to his or her place in the social gradient above and beyond income, level of education, health behaviors, and genetic predisposition. Evidence from psychosocial research also supports the central proposition that explains the status syndrome: individual control and opportunities for social engagement are critical for lessening the risk of stress-related disorders and maximizing well-being and longevity.

STRESS—THE "BIG PICTURE"

This is an opportune time to step back and reconsider the "big picture" about stress and disease. As alluded to earlier, there are two complementary

---

The **status syndrome,** a recent concept in public health, refers to the effect of social position on a person's quality of life and longevity beyond that accounted for by education and income; it appears that risk for stress-related health problems are mediated through the opportunity for, or lack of, individual autonomy and social participation.

views on this issue. The first is the mainstream medical view rooted in biology: stress triggers specific physiological changes that make us more vulnerable to illness and disease via molecular, cellular, and genetic mechanisms. The second is anchored in a mind-body view, in which the excessive stress-poor health connection is due to psychosocial factors such as stress perception, coping abilities, individual autonomy, social support, and modern-day environmental stressors. Each view is incomplete without the other. A recent finding illustrates the convergence of the biological and psychological viewpoints.

In the year 2000, researchers reported that women appear to display an alternative stress response which they dubbed the **tend-and-befriend response.** It turns out that the classic fight-or-flight stress response was based largely on studies of male laboratory animals. When similar studies were conducted with female animals, their stress responses—which are in part mediated by sex-specific hormones—were, not surprisingly, somewhat different from the stress responses of males. Females demonstrated an added dimension of protecting offspring and preferring the companionship of others. When stressed, females—both lab animals and humans—exhibit nurturing-of-children behavior and seek companionship, especially from other females. Indeed, clinical and social psychologists know that women are more likely than men to seek out and provide social support when facing difficult situations. Researchers are careful to note that the tend-and-befriend response is not a universal female phenomenon but rather is a general gender-related behavioral tendency. The tend-and-befriend finding is another step forward in understanding variability in how we respond to stressors. Moreover, it illustrates the power of understanding stress from a holistic perspective that unifies biological and psychosocial knowledge.

Finally, let's not forget the essential role of stress in living a full life. Because uncontrolled chronic stress is clearly linked to a variety of health problems, it's easy to forget that stress is primarily a positive force in our lives. Think of stress in the context of excitement, challenges, and new experiences. Stress is not just good or bad but an undulating blend of positive and negative stressors. This motley assortment of forces and events that we dub stress is not optional. Rather it's an unavoidable part of living and personal growth. In times of high stress, we often say we long for a stress-free life, when in fact we actually mean a life with a manageable level of stress. Certainly, after a prolonged period of hard work or difficulty, a few days of carefree living are welcomed and can be restful and restorative—but then it's back to a routine with roles, responsibilities, and expectations. In a matter of days or weeks, a truly stress-free life

The **tend-and-befriend response** to stressful events is females' protective and caring behavior of offspring and preference for companionship. This type of stress response behavior appears to have both biological and psychological underpinnings.

would become boring, as many people discover when they retire. As long as our lives focus on goals and challenges, a healthy level of stress will be part of the equation. The key is to recognize stress and manage it to our benefit when we can. In many situations, we can use stress to reach our goals, whether at school or work or with family or friends.

✓ **NEED TO KNOW**

Excessive stress can cause or worsen a wide range of illnesses. The primary sources of stress include significant changes in personal relationships, responsibilities, or daily routine. Excessive stress often produces signs and symptoms which should alert you to assess your situation and take action. Recent research findings about type A behavior and hostility, stress and obesity, and social standing and health status illustrate the diverse ways in which stress can impact our health. Yet, not all stress is negative. Stress is a varied blend of positive and negative stressors that enriches life and helps define who we are.

➤ Managing Stress

Many adults are quick to tell college students to enjoy themselves; they often add that their college years were the best times of their lives. Whether this is selective memory or wistful longing for a time with fewer responsibilities is open to speculation. What we do know is that for increasing numbers of students today, the college years are not carefree, joyful times but rather full of anxiety and stress.

Along with many positive societal changes in recent decades, there have been negative trends too. Mass media and particularly television continually bring news of violence, illness, death, wars, and natural disasters into our daily lives. At the same time, we have become more separated from families and neighbors who might be able to help if these events were to actually directly impact us. For many college students, family support systems are unstable (more parents are separated, divorced, and remarried), financial worries are commonplace (college costs and student loans are mounting, more students are working to help pay for school), and the employment situation after graduation is bleak for many majors. Add these to the traditional sources of student distress—homesickness, difficulty making friends, poor grades, broken romances, easy access to drugs and alcohol, and sleep deprivation—and you have a situation that can be challenging to even the most resilient students.

Despite these challenges, colleges are still filled with opportunities. With planning, exploration, and follow-through, you can find your place, succeed in college, and have fun along the way.

Now that you have some background on the biology and psychology of stress, as well as the signs and symptoms of chronic stress, let's consider how you can manage the stress in your life. There are three key aspects to successful stress management. The first relates to the importance of using time management to reach your goals and avoid unnecessary stress. The second aspect focuses on understanding your own personality and temperament and how you perceive and respond to stress. And the third deals with identifying healthy coping strategies—including specific stress management techniques—that meet your needs.

TIME MANAGEMENT

The transition from high school to college presents many challenges. For many students, the greatest challenge is learning to manage their time effectively. Going to college means greater personal independence and less parental oversight of day-to-day activities. With increased freedom comes more responsibility for routine tasks previously handled by parents, such as meal planning and cooking, keeping the home organized and clean, and scheduling appointments. When these new duties are suddenly added to a student's normal college activities—attending classes and labs, completing assignments, studying for tests, making new friends, and participating in extracurricular activities—it's easy to become overwhelmed. Commuting and part-time jobs are often part of the mix as well. Even for the best prepared, the transition to college life requires adjustment and flexibility. Given these factors, it should come as no surprise that poor time management is a root cause of many stressors college students face.

Time management simply means the planned efficient use of one's time. It is the prioritization, scheduling, and execution of responsibilities to one's personal satisfaction. Because everyone has the same amount of time, it's up to each of us to make the best use of it. We certainly don't want to squander time, the very currency of life. The good news is that time management does not have to be complicated. It can be boiled down to three steps: perform a time audit, prioritize activities, and develop an action plan.

Perform a Time Audit

Analyze how you use your time. Write down all your activities on several representative days and make a chart showing the time allocation over the 24-hour periods. Next, categorize your activities into committed time (e.g., classes, work, family), maintenance time (e.g., personal hygiene, eating, exercising, necessary chores, sleeping), and discretionary time, which is free time to use as you wish. Identify blocks of time that could be better used. For example, are small blocks of time being lost that could be re-arranged to be used more efficiently?

Time management is the prioritization, scheduling, and execution of responsibilities to one's personal satisfaction.

Prioritize Your Activities

First things first. Organize your activities by importance and urgency into four categories: 1) urgent and important, 2) not urgent but important, 3) urgent but not important, and 4) not urgent or important. For example, studying for an exam may be both urgent and important, whereas spending time with family and friends is not urgent but important. Attending a sale may be urgent but not important, while watching TV soap operas is not urgent and not important. Prioritizing is not always straightforward, but it is critical. It is time well spent. Not prioritizing leads to many stressful situations because the most important activities are not given the special consideration they deserve.

Develop an Action Plan

Create a plan and execute. Based on your time audit and prioritization of activities, you can develop a schedule and to-do list. Many students use appointment calendars/planners; others prefer to use electronic PDAs (personal digital assistants). Both are fine because they both allow you to translate the first two steps into action by having a planned schedule and a timeline for tasks and projects. Execution is the final phase—the act of carrying out or completing the tasks you set out to accomplish. All the analysis and planning is for nil if you don't roll your sleeves up and actually do the work. A large part of time management is the drive to get tasks done and do them well. When you reach this point, your system for time management is in place. With time and practice, the steps will eventually become second nature.

Few of us learn time management as part of our formal education yet it is fundamental to being productive and preventing negative stressors. Colleges now recognize the importance of time management to student success and routinely cover this topic in freshman seminars. Other noncredit, short courses are often offered periodically through Student Services. If you feel your time management skills need sharpening, investigate what's offered on campus and get a refresher course. An online resource is the University of Chicago's Student Counseling & Resource Service's Virtual Pamphlet Collection with links to time management information used at colleges and universities across the country **(http://counseling .uchicago.edu/resources/virtualpamphlets/time_management.shtml).**

KNOW THYSELF

How we view our level of personal control in the world can have a major bearing on our response to stress. To better understand this personal control–human behavior connection, clinical psychologist Julian Rotter, Ph.D., developed the concept of **locus of control** and devised a scale to

Locus of control is a psychological concept referring to a person's beliefs about the underlying causes of events in his or her life.

measure it. Locus of control is simply a set of beliefs about the relationship between behavior and subsequent outcomes. These beliefs are described in one of two ways—an **internal control** orientation or an **external control** orientation. For most people, one orientation dominates their view and approach to living. Take a short (only 20 questions) locus-of-control survey online to see how you rate **(www.dushkin.com/connectext/psy/ch11/survey11.mhtml).**

Those with an internal control orientation believe that outcomes of their actions depend on what they do. These "internalizers" presume that they chart their own course and control their destiny. They believe that they are autonomous and, as masters of their fates, also bear responsibility for what happens to them. In contrast, those with an external control orientation believe that outcomes are based on events outside their personal control and that they have little influence. That is, outcomes are determined by powerful others, by luck or fate, or are simply unpredictable. These "externalizers" believe they are subject to external forces, and their actions often show that they feel little or no responsibility for what happens to them.

A major difference between these attribution styles is that people with an internal locus of personal control know how to act to get their desired outcomes, whereas people with an external locus of personal control seem not to have this knowledge. Rather, externalizers tend to wait passively for whatever comes their way. Yet, we should be mindful that various factors may shape our sense of autonomy—it's not simply a matter of choice. For example, those who face discrimination—because of poverty, lack of education, race, religion, gender, age, or other factors—may have learned from experience that what they do doesn't have much effect.

Locus of personal control plays a major role in our motivation, expectations, self-esteem, and risk-taking behavior, and it even plays a role in the outcome of our actions. Consequently, how we view the world and our effect on it has a major influence on how we perceive and cope with stressors. Clearly, an internal locus of control is important for behavior change including stress management.

Like hostility, locus of control is unequivocally linked to the stress-health relationship. Knowledge about these dimensions of our personality can be revealing and instructive. Our responses to stress and our coping methods are shaped by many factors, including personal experience, family background, social and societal influences, and the specific situational context. Some factors are within our control and others are beyond our control.

People with an **internal control** orientation believes that outcomes are contingent on their actions; people with an **external control** orientation believes that outcomes are determined by events or forces outside their personal control.

As suggested earlier, if you are concerned about a personality score or characteristic, or if the level of stress in your life is causing you problems with getting through the day, make an appointment with a counselor at the campus counseling center or student health center. You will find professionals whose job it is to help you cope with your experiences. They will be glad to talk with you and can provide guidance and resources.

STRESS MANAGEMENT TECHNIQUES

Stress management is mostly about techniques to assist us in dealing with challenges that are surmountable. These approaches are effective *within limits*. The challenges faced by a refugee, a homeless person, a terminally ill person, or the victim of a violent crime are in a different realm from the more routine stressors that most people face in their everyday lives. Standard stress management techniques will not solve truly dire situations, nor were they developed with that in mind. Disastrous circumstances and traumatic experiences require different approaches, resources, and expertise. As a side note, a sincere effort to consider our personal crises in light of those faced by people who lack the most fundamental needs can add perspective. A further step would be to assist those with greater needs. Whether it's volunteering at a homeless shelter or aiding an elderly neighbor with a project, a simple act of service and kindness to others can provide a restorative break from our own personal struggles.

Most of us can benefit from stress management. As referred to earlier when discussing Lazarus and Folkman's transactional model of stress and coping, accurate appraisal of the stressor followed by effective coping is central to successful stress management. Initially, we make a judgment about the stressfulness of an event. How stressful is it? Is it manageable, positive, or irrelevant? Next is an appraisal of our coping options and resources. What options are available to me? Can I successfully apply the necessary steps to manage the stressor? Clearly, coping with modern day stressors is not automatic. Fight-or-flight is rarely the appropriate response. Indeed, coping is a process that's always changing. It's a learned pattern that requires effort. And remember that coping is an effort to *manage* the situation—complete control and mastery are not necessary (or possible) in most cases. Successful coping is dependent on your overall health and energy, a positive belief, problem solving skills, and social support.

To reinforce and complement the stress-management suggestions from psychologists Lazarus and Folkman, we provide the following strategies from neuroscientist Robert Sapolsky, Ph.D.:

- *Learn to accurately recognize signs of stress.* This is the important first step. We must learn to recognize the signs and to identify the circumstances most responsible for the stress response. As noted earlier, it's important to "know thyself."

- *Find an enjoyable outlet and practice it regularly.* Take part in an activity or hobby that helps you release frustrations, and set aside time to do it regularly. The kind of activity is not critical as long as it's one you enjoy and is not stressful to others.
- *Seek control in the face of stress, but be realistic.* A can-do outlook is important. We generally have options to control stressors in a positive manner. Gather information, make a plan, and take action, but be realistic. We cannot control events that have already occurred, nor should we try to control future events that are uncontrollable.
- *Develop social support through strong relationships.* Nurture your social network. We are social creatures and long to be part of something larger than ourselves, whether it's a family unit or some other kind of group. This is true even for the most independent and individualistic among us. Remember, though, that strong relationships work both ways—they are reciprocal and dynamic. To have a good friend, you must be a good friend.

In addition to these general strategies, specific stress management techniques are available. A few of the best known and accessible are described briefly below. The first four—deep breathing, progressive muscle relaxation, visualization, and meditation—are all based on inducing a relaxation response in which one consciously focuses on countering or reducing the natural physiological stress responses (e.g., increases in breathing rate and muscle tension). In contrast, physical activity dissipates stress by simulating the body's call to action inherent in the fight-or-flight response. All stress management techniques have been shown to be effective for some people, but no single technique works well for everyone. Consider these like choices on a menu. Depending on your personal characteristics, preferences, and experiences, some will appeal to you more than others. The key is to find an approach that meets your needs and fits your lifestyle.

The only way to find out which technique works for you is through trial and error. Nearly all college campuses provide a variety of courses and workshops on stress management techniques. Take a class. Experiment. Reading about the techniques is simply not enough. We learn by doing. Listen to your own reactions and trust your instincts. You will be able to tell which techniques really work for you.

Deep Breathing
Deep breathing is a simple technique that is easily mastered and takes only a few minutes. Sit or lie down in a comfortable position with a straight spine. Begin by breathing deeply, using the full capacity of the lungs. Expand the chest and abdomen with each deep inhalation and then empty the lungs with a complete exhalation. Don't strain; this should be done comfortably. Allow the chest to rise and fall with each breath. The breathing rate should be slower than normal. Attempt to balance the time of the inhalation (a few seconds) with that of the

Health & the Media Distress, Eustress, and Humor

When we think of stress, our images are nearly always negative—conflict, sickness, grief, or sadness—reflecting the turmoil and angst of the human condition. These negative aspects have been captured in art through the ages. Yet, we know stress also can be positive. In a modern view with a twist, both eustress and distress are captured in Gary Larson's *Far Side* cartoon. Chuckling at this cartoon should remind us that humor is a most useful stress buster. As Bob Newhart once said, "Laughter gives us distance. It allows us to step back from an event, deal with it and then move on." And Victor Borge noted, "Laughter is the closest distance between two people."

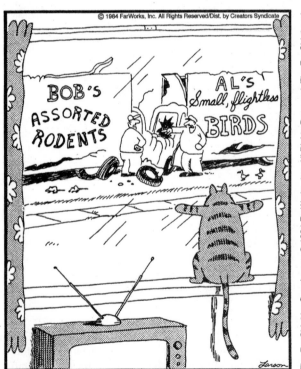

exhalation. Deep breathing is most effective if practiced daily for 5 to 10 minutes.

Progressive Muscle Relaxation

Progressive muscle relaxation is a technique in which one systematically contracts and relaxes different muscles in a sequential order coupled with deep breathing exercise. It can be performed in a seated or supine position. To try this technique, begin with the muscles of the right foot. Inhale deeply, contract the muscles, then exhale as you release the contraction and relax your foot completely. Notice how relaxation in this part of your body feels and enjoy the sensations. Next, go to the calf of your right leg, and proceed similarly through the major muscle groups in the rest of your body. The process takes only about 10 minutes and promotes relaxation by dissipating peripheral tension. Remain still and quietly enjoy the effects afterwards.

Visualization

Creative visualization, or the use of imagery, can be an effective stress reduction technique. This exercise is generally done in conjunction with deep breathing or progressive muscle relaxation, but it can be practiced by itself. Find a quiet place and make yourself comfortable—sit or lie down, with legs uncrossed and spine straight. Close your eyes and visualize a peaceful scene in nature—for example, a perfect, undisturbed place on a beach, an island, or a mountain or in a forest or a garden. It may be an actual place that you recall or a place that you are simply imagining. Immerse yourself in this beautiful and peaceful place by focusing on the details of the setting—see the colors and textures, hear the sounds, smell the fragrances, feel the breeze. With 5 to 10 minutes of visualization, you can create a mini-vacation and have a real break from the daily grind.

Meditation

Meditation is a technique that has been used for centuries in Asian cultures. In the 1970s, Harvard cardiologist Herbert Benson studied people who practiced Transcendental Meditation and noted their remarkable ability to reduce their blood pressure and heart rate. Dr. Benson became a leading proponent of mind-body medicine and helped make the meditation technique accessible to Americans through his book *The Relaxation Response*. He distilled meditation down to its essential techniques, removing them from their Eastern religious context.

There are many types of meditation, but most involve adopting a passive attitude toward one's thoughts as they come and go. To try meditation, find a quiet environment and sit comfortably with your eyes closed. Pay attention to your breathing, or silently repeat a word or phrase with each exhalation. As your mind wanders (and it will), simply notice it and bring your attention back to your breathing. Practice for 15 to 20 minutes every day or at least three or four days a week. Like deep breathing, progressive muscle relaxation, and visualization, meditation induces the relaxation response.

Physical Activity

Physical activity is one of the most natural ways to reduce stress, partly because it simulates the action of the classic fight-or-flight response. During exercise, we process (metabolize) stress chemicals and lessen the damaging effects associated with their accumulation. As discussed in Chapter 3 on fitness, regular physical activity imparts many health benefits, including an immediate reduction in tension and anxiety. Physical activity is convenient and readily available—when you are really stressed out, just put on your sneakers and go for a walk or a jog. You might be surprised by how effective 20 to 30 minutes of exercise can be in helping you deal with even the most difficult situations. The type of exercise is not critical. Nearly all types of activity reduce stress. The key is to find an activity that you enjoy, can maintain, and will engage in regularly.

In this section, we have provided both overall strategies and specific techniques to assist you in managing stress. A central theme woven throughout this chapter is the importance of balance. That is, to effectively deal with stress, we must strive to balance our lifestyle behaviors (nutrition, exercise, sleep) with work, family, and social responsibilities. Simply put, strong lifestyle behaviors better equip us to face stressors of all kinds, from the unexpected or uncontrollable to the minor annoyances in our daily routine. Moreover, self-knowledge, along with a

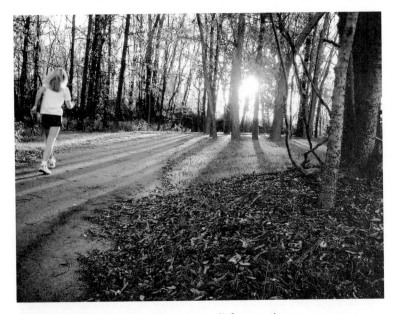

Regular exercise has many benefits—stress relief among them.

healthy lifestyle, provides the basis for the ongoing development of self-management skills that enable us to set and reach goals and overcome obstacles.

The college years are an opportune time to hone these life skills. Be pro-active, seek answers, and use campus resources. Stress is part of life, and to a great degree we have the ability to control stressors and our responses to them. Stress need not be dreaded—rather, it should be welcomed. Separate the wheat from the chaff—the daily hassles from more significant events—and realize that in most cases, stress can be a positive force in your life.

✓ NEED TO KNOW

The college years present different challenges for different people. For many, it's often a highly stressful time. To prevent unnecessary stress, use time management to reach goals. To manage excessive stress, understand how you perceive and respond to stress (locus of control). Based on self-knowledge and time-tested recommendations, develop a set of coping strategies. Find a stress management technique that works for you and practice it on a regular basis. Be aware that colleges provide many resources, from specific courses to professional counseling, to assist students in dealing with excessive stress. Be proactive—seek answers, use campus resources, and tailor your own approach to stress management.

Web Site Resources

American Academy of Sleep Medicine
http://www.sleepeducation.com
American Institute of Stress
http://www.stress.org
American Psychological Association (Stress)
http://www.apa.org/topics/topicstress.html
Medline Plus: Interactive Tutorial on Managing Stress
**http://www.nlm.nih.gov/medlineplus/tutorials/managingstress/
htm/index.htm**
National Institute of Mental Health
http://www.nimh.nih.gov
National Sleep Foundation
http://www.sleepfoundation.org
Stanford Prison Study
http://www.prisonexp.org
University of Chicago Student Counseling & Resource Service Virtual
Pamphlet Collection: Time Management
**http://counseling.uchicago.edu/resources/virtualpamphlets/time
_management.shtml**

Knowing the Language

distress
eustress
external control orientation
fight-or-flight response
general adaptation syndrome
hostility
internal control orientation
locus of control

status syndrome
stress
stressor
tend-and-befriend response
time management
transactional model of stress
and coping
Type A behavior

Understanding the Content

1. Define and provide examples of common physical and psychological stressors.
2. Discuss both the general adaptation syndrome model and the transactional model of stress and coping and then contrast.
3. Describe the signs and symptoms of excessive stress. What steps should a person take if they are experiencing these signs or symptoms?
4. Describe several stress management techniques and how they relieve stress.

1. How do modern day stressors differ from those of our ancestors who lived several thousand years ago? Consider how our society is organized differently today and the impact of technology on our daily lives.
2. The stress–illness relationship is reciprocal. Excessive stress can lead to or worsen disease, and, conversely, dealing with an illness can compound a person's level of distress. Have you experienced this firsthand with family or friends? Describe circumstances that show how stress can be both a cause and a consequence of illness.
3. Explain the concept of locus of control. Using yourself or someone you know well, describe and discuss how a person's locus of control positively or negatively impacts his or her ability to assess and cope with stress. How can one move along the locus-of-control continuum from more external to more internal control?

Selected References

Benson H. *The Relaxation Response*. New York: Morrow, 1975.

Colten HR, Altevogt BM (eds.). *Committee on Sleep Medicine and Research. Sleep Disorders and Sleep Deprivation: An Unmet Public Health Problem*. Washington, DC: The National Academies Press, 2006.

Covey SR. *The 7 Habits of Highly Effective People*. New York: Simon & Schuster, 1989.

Curio G, Ferrara M, DeGennaro L. Sleep loss, learning capacity and academic performance. *Sleep Medicine Reviews* 10: 323–337, 2006.

Dallman MF, Pecoraro N, Akana SF, et al. Chronic stress and obesity: A new view of "comfort food." *Proceedings of the National Academy of Sciences* 100 (20): 11696–11701, 2003.

Friedman M, Rosenman RH. *Type A Behavior and Your Heart*. New York: Knopf, 1974.

Holmes TH, Rahe RH. The social readjustment rating scale. *Journal of Psychosomatic Research* 11: 213–218, 1967.

Lazarus RS, Folkman S. *Stress, Appraisal and Coping*. New York: Springer, 1984.

Lovallo WR. *Stress and Health: Biological and Psychological Interactions* (2nd ed.). Thousand Oaks, CA: Sage, 2005.

Marmot M. *The Status Syndrome: How Social Standing Affects Our Health and Longevity*. New York: Henry Holt, 2004.

McEwen BS, Lasley EN. *The End of Stress as We Know It*. Washington, DC: Joseph Henry Press, 2002.

Miller MA, Rahe RH. Life changes scaling for the 1990s. *Journal of Psychosomatic Research* 43 (3): 279–292, 1997.

Rotter JB. Generalized expectancies for internal versus external control of reinforcement. *Psychological Monographs* 80 (whole no. 609), 1966.

Sapolsky RM. *Why Zebras Don't Get Ulcers* (3rd ed.). New York: Henry Holt, 2004.

Selye H. *The Stress of Life.* New York: McGraw Hill, 1956.

Selye H. *Stress in Health and Disease.* Boston: Butterworth, 1976.

Society for Neuroscience. *Brain Facts: A Primer on the Brain and Nervous System.* Washington, D.C.: Society for Neuroscience, 2006. **http://www.sfn.org/index.cfm?pagename5brainFacts**

Taylor SE, Klein LC, Lewis BP, et al. Biobehavioral responses to stress in females: Tend-and-befriend, not fight-or-flight. *Psychological Review* 107 (3): 411–429, 2000.

Wallis C. The new science of happiness. *Time* January 17, 2005.

Williams R, Williams V. *In Control: No More Snapping at Your Family, Sulking at Work, Steaming in the Grocery Line, Seething in Meetings, Stuffing Your Frustration.* New York: Rodale, 2006.

Williams V, Williams R. *Lifeskills: 8 Simple Ways to Build Stronger Relationships, Communicate More Clearly, and Improve Your Health.* New York: Times Books, 1997.

Zimbardo PG. Stanford Prison Study: A Simulation Study of the Psychology of Imprisonment Conducted at Stanford University, 1999–2008. **http://www.prisonexp.org**

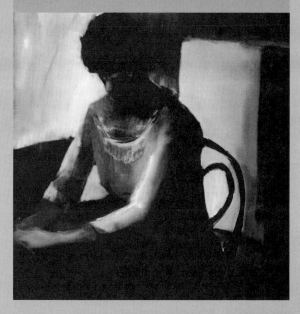

You can handle depression in much the same way you handle a tiger.... If depression is creeping up and must be faced, learn something about the nature of the beast. You may escape without a mauling.

— R. W. SHEPHERD

Chapter 7

MENTAL HEALTH AND DISORDERS

Until recently, mental illness was often kept secret. But today more people seek treatment openly, as anyone watching television will note upon seeing the frequent ads for anti-anxiety and anti-depression drugs such as Paxil and Zoloft. This openness is fortunate, given that mental illness is fairly common. Twenty percent of the U.S. population are affected by it, according to the Centers for Disease Control. Depression is the most common mental illness, and is also the leading cause of disability and suicide. In Chapter 7 we explore the concept and characteristics of mental health and common problems related to mental health; we then discuss mental illness and options for seeking help.

Mental Health

MIND, BODY, AND CULTURE

BASIC MENTAL HEALTH DEFINITIONS AND THEORIES

CHARACTERISTICS OF MENTAL HEALTH

Personal and Social Problems Related to Mental Health

SUICIDE

DRUG ABUSE

VIOLENCE

EATING DISORDERS

Mental and Personality Disorders

ANXIETY DISORDERS

MOOD DISORDERS: DEPRESSION AND MANIA

PERSONALITY DISORDERS

SCHIZOPHRENIA

Treatment

Theresa Foy diGeronimo state that over the previous 13 years, college campuses saw depression double, thoughts of suicide triple, and sexual assaults quadruple among students. He reports that 45 percent of college students say they are depressed, 10 percent claim they experience suicidal thoughts, and 44 percent report binge drinking. The behaviors associated with depression, suicide, and related alcohol abuse can greatly affect a student's academic and personal life.

Knowing the signs and symptoms of mental disorders, as well as the available treatments, is important for any student today. Most people will experience anxiety, depression, and difficulty adjusting to life's circumstances at some point. For some people these are short and self-correcting problems, but for others they can be long-term and significantly interfere with daily life.

Not that long ago there was little understanding of the physiology related to mental disorders, and there were not many treatments. But as the role of brain chemicals called *neurotransmitters* was unraveled, new drugs were developed in addition to the many counseling approaches already available. Further, since the underlying physical causes of disorders such as anxiety and depression are now better understood, people tend to view these illnesses as the physical diseases they are. The stigma of admitting to suffering from depression or anxiety has diminished greatly. There has never been more effective help available to those suffering with mental illness or disorders than there is today. Truly, there is no good reason for anyone to suffer in silence anymore.

➤ Mental Health

Maintaining good mental health is as important to good quality of life as maintaining good physical health is. We gauge **mental health** by assessing several factors, including how fulfilling people's relationships are, how well they adapt or cope with adversity, the level of their communication skills, their resilience, and their self-esteem.

MIND, BODY, AND CULTURE

The interdependence of the physical, mental, social, and spiritual dimensions of health are emphasized throughout the *Concise Guide*. This notion remains true in regard to mental health. The word **psychosomatic** refers to the mind's influence on the body. In Chapter 6 the body's physical

Mental health is the successful performance of mental functions resulting in productive activities.

Psychosomatic refers to the influence of the mind (*psyche*) on the way the body (*soma*) functions.

FIGURE 7.1   INTERACTION OF BODY, MIND, AND ENVIRONMENT

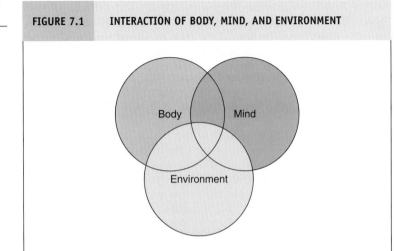

reaction to stress was discussed. Biology and emotions also influence each other, as shown in Figure 7.1.

When we are angry, our body responds by secreting certain types of chemical messengers called *hormones* which, in turn, influence neurotransmitters in the brain that relate to mood. When our body produces too little of certain neurotransmitters, depression can result. Just as the body has a fight-or-flight response to danger or stress (see Chapter 6), it also may respond to thoughts and feelings with back or chest pain, changes in appetite, constipation, high blood pressure, insomnia, upset stomach, weight loss, or weight gain.

Culture can also influence our mental health. When society emphasizes the importance of something an individual member of that culture can't attain, it causes conflict and potentially negative mind/body outcomes. Conversely, some institutions and organizations (such as religion or support groups) can greatly improve mental health and one's sense of well-being. This influence of culture is hard to measure but is nonetheless an important factor that individuals must include in making decisions regarding mental health.

BASIC MENTAL HEALTH DEFINITIONS AND THEORIES

When discussing mental health, there are a few basic terms you should know. *Behavior* is how someone acts. **Motivation** is something that causes a behavior. **Self-concept** is a set of core beliefs and values that

Motivation is the state of being energized to perform a task.

Self-concept is a stable set of beliefs about one's qualities and attributes.

FIGURE 7.2   MASLOW'S HIERARCHY OF NEEDS

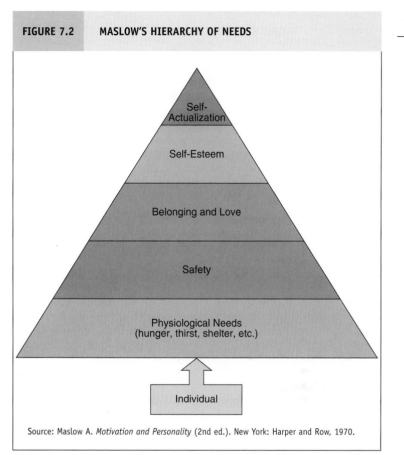

Source: Maslow A. *Motivation and Personality* (2nd ed.). New York: Harper and Row, 1970.

you feel describes yourself. **Self-esteem** is how you feel—either positively or negatively—about your core qualities and attributes. And finally, *assertiveness* is being very open and honest about declaring your rights, whereas *aggressiveness* is forceful behavior with the intent to dominate.

Maslow's Hierarchy of Needs

Abraham Maslow's (1970) hierarchy of needs is a model that describes the motivation for behavior. As shown in Figure 7.2, Maslow's contention is that people display behaviors in order to meet needs. Further, he describes five levels of needs. The first level is physiological needs—for food, water, and shelter.

Self-esteem is how one feels, good or bad, about one's qualities and attributes.

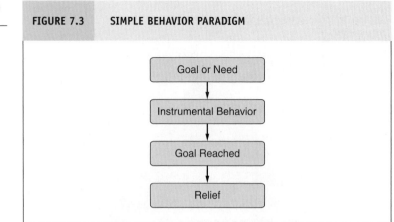

FIGURE 7.3   SIMPLE BEHAVIOR PARADIGM

Goal or Need

Instrumental Behavior

Goal Reached

Relief

Once our physiological needs are satisfied, the most basic psychological need is to feel safe and secure. If these two basic levels of needs are met, then people tend to be motivated by needs higher in Maslow's hierarchy, such as the desire for love and belonging or for self-esteem. Successful people who seem to be living life to its fullest might be seen as reaching the level of self-actualization, though some say this level is questionable, since we can never really know what our full potential is.

Simple Behavior Paradigm

Using Maslow's hierarchy of needs as a reference point, we can conclude that our behavior is either need-directed or goal-oriented. A simple paradigm to describe behavior is presented in Figure 7.3. The needs referred to in this figure can be the needs identified by Maslow (physiological needs, safety and security). Once the need is identified, people display an instrumental behavior to meet the need. If the behavior leads to achieving the goal, we get relief.

We discover early in life that the real world is rarely as simple as what Figure 7.3 describes. That is, our behaviors don't always result in a need being met. Often we display a behavior and the need is not met; the goal is not reached. The result of a need not being met is displayed in Figure 7.4. Basically, we experience tension, frustration, and conflict, and then we respond. For example, we often interpret family expectations and personal expectations for success as needs or goals. When the expectations are not met or the goal is not reached, how we respond can result in relief or in no relief, in which case the tension, frustration, and conflict can either increase or lessen.

Responding to Unmet Needs and Defense Mechanisms

When a need is not being met, the most simple response is anger. Another way to respond is to be assertive and challenge something (or someone)

FIGURE 7.4   **ALTERNATIVE BEHAVIOR PARADIGM**

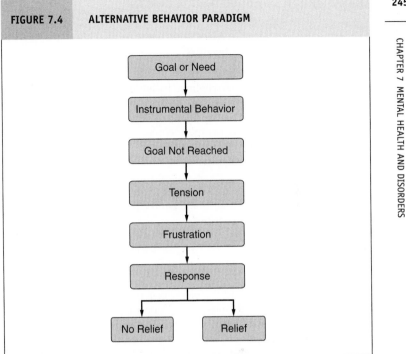

to try to get the need met. If anger and assertiveness do not work, then people often become aggressive, which involves either verbal or physical domination. It is not a good approach for resolving conflict and often is counterproductive, especially if the aggressiveness is extreme or violent.

Another common way we respond to unmet needs is to protect or defend our ego, our conscious state of how we perceive ourself; hence, these responses are called *defense mechanisms.* One such mechanism is rationalization, or making excuses for our need not being met. Another defense mechanism is denial, or simply not acknowledging that there is any frustration or conflict. Displacement is expressing our frustration by attacking another target—for example, a person may have a bad experience with a coworker but takes out her frustration on her spouse. Repression, or selective forgetting, is another defense mechanism—we refuse to think about the event that led to the frustration. Reaction formation is displaying behaviors that are the opposite of the ones that we are actually feeling. Finally, projection formation is accusing another person of the same unacceptable behaviors that we have displayed.

Use of defense mechanisms is normal. However, they can be harmful if they are overused to the point where the individual never deals directly with the problem.

The National Mental Health Association has identified ten characteristics of people who are mentally healthy:

1. They feel good about themselves.
2. They do not become overwhelmed by emotions such as fear, anger, love, jealousy, guilt, or anxiety.
3. They have lasting and satisfying personal relationships.
4. They feel comfortable with other people.
5. They can laugh at themselves with others.
6. They have respect for themselves and for others even if there are differences.
7. They are able to accept life's disappointments.
8. They can meet life's demands and handle problems when they arise.
9. They make their own decisions.
10. They shape their environment whenever possible and adjust to it when necessary.

These characteristics have some common themes that are related to Maslow's hierarchy of needs, the behavior paradigm, and the use of defense mechanisms. These themes include a positive self-image, good communication skills, a sense of humor, responding in a healthy way to unmet needs, and good problem-solving skills. It makes sense that people who display the characteristics of good mental health are well-balanced, good problem-solvers and accept personal responsibility for their behavior.

✓ NEED TO KNOW

Good mental health allows people to cope with the stresses and challenges of life. People's behaviors are motivated by their physical and emotional needs. According to Maslow's hierarchy, the most basic needs are the body's needs for food and shelter. Once those needs are met, people attempt to fill the most basic emotional needs, including a need for feeling safe and secure. When a need remains unmet, frustration results. Often people cope with unmet needs by using defense mechanisms such as denial, displacement, repression, reaction formation, and projection formation.

➤ Personal and Social Problems Related to Mental Health

Since mental health involves judgment, coping, communication, relationships, biology, and feelings, it is easy to see how most personal and societal problems are related to mental health. Some examples of social and personal problems related to mental health include suicide, drug abuse, violence, and eating disorders.

SUICIDE

Suicide is the eighth leading cause of death in the United States and the third leading cause of death among 15- to 24-year-olds. We know that depression is usually a precursor to suicide and that depression has a strong biological basis. So to say that suicide is "just" a mental health problem would be wrong.

Suicide can be examined in the context of the behavior paradigm discussed earlier. For example, when a need (food and shelter, safety and security, love and belonging, self-esteem) is not met, and tension, frustration, and conflict continues, then suicide can be the response. In the late 1800s sociologist Emile Durkheim identified three types of suicides (1951). An egoistic suicide is ending one's life as a response to not being able to assimilate into a group or society—for example, a student taking his life after having severe difficulty fitting into the college environment. By contrast, an altruistic suicide is taking one's life to advance a cause or an ideal. Lastly, anomic suicides occur when the person or group that provided a sense of security no longer exists. The loss of a social network can cause such persistent frustration, conflict, and depression that a person may choose suicide. An example of an anomic suicide would be an elderly man who kills himself after his wife dies.

Notice in all of these descriptions that the person chooses suicide. Life becomes so difficult that the person perceives suicide as the only remedy. Suicide as a choice represents the ultimate defeat.

Unfortunately, most suicides are preceded by warning signs that may go unnoticed. Such warning signs include feelings of hopelessness, withdrawing from family and friends, sleeping too much or too little, feeling tired most of the time, acting compulsively, losing interest in most activities, giving away prized possessions, social isolation, depression, acting irrationally, being preoccupied with death, behaving recklessly, abusing alcohol or drugs, and inability to concentrate. Many of the warning signs for suicide are also symptoms of depression, which is strongly related to suicide.

There are steps you can take to prevent suicide if you notice warning signs:

1. Always take suicidal comments seriously.
2. Try not to act shocked by what a suicidal person might say.
3. Do not handle the situation by yourself—get assistance from a health professional.
4. Listen attentively to everything that the person has to say.
5. Comfort the person with words of encouragement.
6. Let the person know that you are deeply concerned.

7. If you perceive the person is at high risk of suicide, do not leave him or her alone.
8. Talk openly about suicide.
9. If the person talks about committing suicide with a firearm that he or she owns, call the police so that they may remove the firearm.
10. Don't be judgmental.
11. Be careful about statements you make.
12. Listen; be gentle, kind, and understanding.
13. Let the person express emotion in the way that he or she wants.

It takes time and patience, but you must understand that the suicidal person is in pain and sees few other options. With medical intervention, the crisis can end, and through therapy the person can recover.

DRUG ABUSE

Much information regarding drug abuse is discussed in Chapter 4. Here it is important to note that attempting to modify one's mood can be a response to tension, frustration, and conflict. The extent to which one binge drinks can be directly related to coping problems. Also, stimulants, depressants, and hallucinogens can serve as chemical Band-Aids that exert a psychoactive effect to lessen the intensity of the response to tension, frustration, and conflict. However, this is a quick fix, and it is counterproductive to solving the problem, because of the potential for a new problem: drug dependence.

In some ways it is understandable that drug misuse and abuse is such a common problem related to mental health. The effects are immediate and can be powerful enough so that one's problems just don't seem as bad—that is, until the effects of the drug wear off. When that happens, the problems are still there, and some people respond immediately by modifying their mood to feel better once again. It's not long before using drugs as a coping mechanism creates compound problems—first, not only having to cope with the initial problem, but second, now having to deal with a drug problem.

VIOLENCE

According to a Centers for Disease Control study, the cost in the United States of medical care, rehabilitation, and loss of productivity due to violence is estimated at more than $224 billion a year. In 2003 the CDC reported that homicide claimed the lives of over 20,000 Americans, whereas suicide was responsible for the deaths of over 30,000 Americans. Homicide is the second leading cause of death for people between 15 and 34, and it is the leading cause of death for African Americans in this age group. There were nearly 30,000 firearm-related deaths in 2001, and more than 2 million nonfatal violence-related injuries occurred in the United States.

Violence is a serious mental health issue and is largely preventable. Violent behaviors and mental illness are not necessarily related—that is, only a small percentage of those who are diagnosed as mentally ill are violent. The causes of violence are related to larger social problems such as stress, dangerous environments, unemployment, drugs, and poverty. Like many other topics we will cover in this chapter, violence represents a choice, and this choice can be the response to frustration, tension, and conflict described in the earlier paradigm.

Breaking It Down Predicting Violent Behavior

In April 2007, Seung-Hui Cho, a senior at Virginia Polytechnic Institute and State University, shot to death two students near their campus dormitory rooms. A short time later Cho chained the doors of a classroom building and systematically murdered 30 additional students and faculty before committing suicide as police approached him. The so-called Virginia Tech Massacre is the most deadly school shooting in U.S. history.

The biggest question is what motivated Cho to murder so many? A Governor's Task Force report could not find definitive explanations for Cho's actions. However, it uncovered many warning signs that indicated Cho might be a threat either to himself or to those around him.

Cho appears to have been a lonely young man with poor social skills. Students taunted and bullied him in high school, most likely because he was Korean and had poor English language skills. Not being able to express himself well, he internalized this rejection and became an introvert with an undisciplined fantasy life. He fantasized about committing violent acts. Cho sent a video manifesto to NBC News the morning of his attack at Virginia Tech. These actions reflected a stoic, determined, irrational man who wanted to make people pay the ultimate price for his problems. His victims were simply in the wrong place at the wrong time.

In the years leading up to the massacre, some people noticed that Cho needed help. He was referred and evaluated for psychological care, but sadly, he was never made to continue with therapy. Cho's violent fantasies and sense of alienation from people around him worsened. That, combined with the easy ability to buy weapons, resulted in the massacre.

Several lessons can be learned from the Virginia Tech Massacre. A key point is that Cho fit the profile of a lonely, ostracized person who was capable of acting out violently. Unfortunately, the people around him were not networked in such a way that the full threat could become obvious before Cho acted out. When Cho was referred to counseling and didn't follow through, there was no mechanism to track what was happening with him. Strict privacy laws helped create a situation where Virginia Tech University staff and faculty had no comprehensive

(Continued)

record of the incidents that the faculty and staff at his high school had reported. If there had been such a record, perhaps when several female college students accused Cho of stalking them, charges might have been pressed and Cho might have been forced to get help. Instead, Cho's brushes with mental health authorities and the criminal justice system remained slight, so he wasn't flagged in the gun dealers' database as a person who should not be allowed to purchase firearms. Without guns, the scope of whatever Cho chose to do would have been greatly diminished.

It should be noted that most people with Cho's apparent history of mental disorders and social problems do not resort to lashing out at others. If they act out, usually they turn their anger inward and take their own life. However, suicide has great cost not only to the person but also to the person's family and friends. Although stopping people from taking violence out on innocent bystanders is extremely important, preventing suicides is also an important goal, and it can be achieved with the same steps that can minimize the chance of another school massacre.

The Virginia Tech Massacre shows that individuals, both teachers and other students, often have good instincts about pinpointing people who could benefit from counseling, psychiatric medications, and in some cases, hospitalization to prevent violent acts. The challenge is to track at-risk individuals so that they don't fall through the cracks like Cho did. With a good tracking system, easing of the privacy laws in situations like these, and the right people involved in discussions about the behaviors they are observing and the appropriate interventions, horrible incidents like this one can be prevented.

EATING DISORDERS

As discussed in Chapter 2, the eating disorders anorexia nervosa and bulimia nervosa cause people to starve themselves or engage in binge-and-purge eating behavior. Eating disorders can be a response to unmet needs relating to self-esteem or perception of body image. According to the National Eating Disorders Association, the causes of eating disorders are psychological, interpersonal, and social. Psychological factors include low self-esteem, feelings of inadequacy or lack of control in life, and depression, anxiety, anger, or loneliness. Interpersonal factors include troubled family and personal relationships, difficulty in expressing emotions and feelings, history of being teased or ridiculed based on size or weight, and history of physical or sexual abuse. Social factors include cultural preferences that glorify thinness and place value on obtaining the "perfect body," narrow definitions of beauty that include only specific body weights and shapes for women and men, and cultural norms that value people on the basis of physical appearance and not inner qualities and strengths. These psychological, social, and cultural factors are all related to the Maslow model and the behavior paradigm described earlier.

nervosa has the following symptoms:

- Fear of being fat when at or below normal weight;
- Restricting eating so weight falls more than 15 percent below what is considered healthy;
- Distorted body image that creates a sense of obesity even when overly thin; and
- In women, the absence of at least three consecutive menstrual cycles.

Bulimia nervosa according to the American Psychiatric Association, is characterized by binge eating and inappropriate compensatory methods to prevent weight gain, such as self-induced vomiting or misuse of laxatives and diuretics. Bulimia has the following symptoms:

- Recurrent episodes of binge eating (at least twice a week for three months);
- Complete loss of control during eating binges;
- Persistent overconcern with body shape and size;
- Regular self-induced vomiting or use of laxatives or diuretics to prevent weight gain; and
- Strict dieting, fasting, or exercise to prevent weight gain.

Binge eating disorder is a relatively new classification of eating disorders. It is characterized by overeating as a response to frustration and conflict. Unlike bulimia, binge eating disorder does not involve purging after overeating.

Eating disorders have serious physical consequences. Anorexia nervosa can result in low blood pressure, reduction of bone density, muscle loss and weakness, and kidney failure. Bulimia nervosa can result in gastric rupture, inflammation of the esophagus, tooth decay, peptic ulcers, and pancreatitis. Eating disorders when extreme can result in death. No one knows how many deaths each year are related to eating disorders, primarily because official statistics of cause of death, such as kidney failure or suicide, do not show whether there is a link to an eating disorder. However, studies of anorexic patients have reported death rates from 4 to 25 percent (University of Maryland Medical Center, 2002).

✓ NEED TO KNOW

Many personal and social problems are related to mental health, including violence against others, suicide, binge drinking, drug use, and eating disorders. While each of these problems may have a biological component as a cause, they all also relate to the psychological, social, and cultural factors described by both the Maslow hierarchy of needs and the behavior paradigm model.

Anorexia nervosa is an eating disorder characterized by self-starvation, excessive thinness, and a distorted body image.

Bulimia nervosa is an eating disorder characterized by binge eating and compensatory methods to rid the body of food.

Binge eating disorder is characterized by excessive overeating.

➤ Mental and Personality Disorders

Mental disorders are perhaps the most misunderstood kind of illness. We often use terms like *schizophrenic, bipolar,* and *obsessive-compulsive* to describe people, but in reality these are clinical terms that are used to identify profound disorders. Medical and psychodynamic perspectives are used in discussing abnormal behavior. The medical perspective is grounded in the physiological reasons for a condition, and the psychodynamic perspective contends that these disorders are a result of psychological conflicts and represent a means of coping with these conflicts. There is ample evidence supporting each perspective as well as a combination of perspectives—that is, both medical and psychodynamic factors interact—and the consequence is a condition that can be diagnosed.

ANXIETY DISORDERS

Anxiety is excessive worry and concern that is extremely unpleasant and involves apprehension, fear, and panic. Symptoms of anxiety disorders include trembling, jumpiness, inability to relax, racing heart, irritability, hyperactivity, insomnia, and apprehension. There are several classifications of anxiety problems. **Generalized Anxiety Disorder** is constant and uncontrollable worry and concern about everything. When anxiety comes on after a traumatic event—anything from a violent attack to an accident or the sudden death of a loved one—**Post-traumatic Stress Disorder** (PTSD), where persistent frightening thoughts, feelings and memories interfere with one's life, may result. **Panic disorders** are sudden, overwhelming attacks of fear. Usually the attacks are short but frequent. A person experiencing a panic attack has uncontrolled thoughts of impending doom for themselves or someone else, experiences intense anxiety symptoms, and may even pass out.

Phobias are fears of specific events, objects, or situations. There are many different kinds of phobias. Example are autophobia (fear of being alone), pharmacophobia (fear of taking medicine), musophobia (fear of mice), microphobia (fear of microbes), hydrophobia (fear of water), acrophobia (fear of heights), and claustrophobia (fear of being in closed spaces). The number of potential phobias is infinite. The response to a phobia can be

Anxiety is excessive worry and concern.

Generalized Anxiety Disorder (GAD) is constant and uncontrollable worry or concern about everything.

Post-traumatic Stress Disorder (PTSD) is an anxiety disorder that can occur after experiencing a frightening event in which physical harm may have occurred.

Panic disorders are sudden, overwhelming attacks of fear.

Phobias are fears of specific objects or events.

intense anxiety symptoms like those in panic attacks. People who have claustrophobia and find themselves in an enclosed area such as an elevator or closet may experience panic attack symptoms.

Finally, **Obsessive-Compulsive Disorder** (OCD) is a condition characterized by repetition of the same act over and over again (compulsion) as a response to persistent unwanted thoughts or images (obsession). The behavior is acted out in a ritualistic manner. Examples of OCD symptoms include constantly checking a door to make sure it is locked or constantly washing one's hands.

MOOD DISORDERS: DEPRESSION AND MANIA

Mood disorders are serious and disabling instabilities in emotions. The extremes of mood disorders are depression and mania.

Depression is feelings of worthlessness, indecisiveness, guilt, sadness, and apprehension. We wouldn't be human if we didn't experience depression at points in our lives because of deaths, disappointments, and conflicts. Usually, however, the intensity of these feelings wanes and the depression naturally lifts. But sometimes depression is a long-lasting state rather than a passing mood. In this case, depression can cause many personal, professional, and relationship problems for the person. **Mania** is characterized by an elevated mood in which the person appears extremely excitable and hyperactive, makes grandiose and incomprehensible statements, and has rambling thoughts.

There are three types of depressive illness: major depression, dysthymia, and bipolar illness. According to the National Institute of Mental Health, symptoms of major depression include

- sadness, irritability, excessive crying, anxiety, or hopeless feelings;
- decreased energy and feelings of fatigue;
- loss of interest or pleasure in usual activities;
- appetite and weight changes;
- sleep disturbances;
- thoughts of death or suicide attempts;
- difficulty concentrating, making decisions, remembering; and
- chronic aches and pains not explained by any other physical condition.

Obsessive-Compulsive Disorder (OCD) is repetition of an act over and over again as a response to unwanted thoughts.

Depression is characterized by feelings of worthlessness, indecisiveness, guilt, sadness, and apprehension.

Mania is characterized by an extremely elevated mood and subsequent hyperactive behaviors.

Dysthymia is a form of depression which is long-term and less severe than major depression, but it still impairs functioning to some degree. **Bipolar disorder,** which sometimes is referred to as *manic-depressive illness,* includes two states: extreme elation (mania) followed by the extreme low of depression. If the symptoms of depression are experienced only during a specific season, such as winter, when the days are short, the diagnosis may be **Seasonal Affective Disorder** (SAD).

Depression is a serious college health issue and certainly an impediment to academic success. It is important for anyone who experiences five or more of the symptoms of depression for two weeks or longer to seek some help from a health professional.

> **Dysthymia** is a form of depression which has long-term but less severe effects than major depression.
>
> **Bipolar disorder** (sometimes referred to as *manic-depressive illness*) involves swings between mania (extreme elation) and depression.
>
> **Seasonal Affective Disorder** (SAD) is symptoms of depression experienced during a specific season of the year.

What Is Your Risk? What Is Your Risk for Clinical Depression?

Depression is a common mood disorder. It is estimated that 16 percent of Americans experience a major depressive episode over the course of their lifetime and 13–14 million Americans experience major depression each year. Many factors can predispose people to becoming clinically depressed. Some of the more common factors include gender, age, social status, family history, personal loss, medical disorders, and medications.

A greater percentage of women report being depressed than men. The reasons are not clear but they may be related to hormones, differences in expressing emotions, and differences in problem-solving behaviors. Levels of estrogen can influence emotions, and if there are problems with estrogen levels, certainly depression can result. Women tend to be less inhibited than men in expressing their emotions, so symptoms of depression are often more noticeable both to them personally and to others. Men who are experiencing depression commonly mask the depression through use of alcohol or other drugs. This results in fewer reported diagnoses of depression among men.

As people gets older, the more likely they are to experience depression. It has been estimated that one-third of people over 65 experience depression. The many reasons for this include changes in biology related to age and life events that are difficult to adjust to—personal or family illness and life stressors associated with age, such as financial problems. Generally speaking, the challenges that come with being poor can be so overwhelming that depression can result.

Medical disorders also put people at higher risk of depression for a number of reasons, regardless of age. The biology associated with the medical disorder can affect certain hormones, which can cause depression. Also, a very serious disorder can cause one to feel despair and thus to be depressed.

Personal loss is a normal precursor to depression. We all have or will experience personal loss, and depression is an expected response. However, if depression remains the only way the person is "coping" or "responding," then it can become problematic and interfere with life.

Certain medications can affect neurotransmitters and cause depression; these include thyroid medications, birth control pills, and pain medications. Although these types of drugs have therapeutic value, they can change the biology enough in some individuals to cause depression.

For more specific application of risk factors associated with depression, complete the Depression Screening Questionnaire in Figure 7.5.

A person in a manic episode is hyperactive, believes he or she can do anything, and often talks in a rambling, incoherent manner. Although elation can be a symptom some people actually enjoy, a manic episode can make people delusional and their actions can badly disrupt their life and relationships. Symptoms of mania include repeatedly starting new tasks, outbursts of inappropriate anger, grandiose sense of knowing more than others, extravagant spending, and energetic exercise. Hospitalization may be required to stabilize the person's mood in severe cases.

PERSONALITY DISORDERS

Personality disorders are groups of persistent behaviors that impair social, academic, or professional functioning or cause personal distress. Common personality disorders include paranoid personality disorder, schizoid personality disorder, and schizotypal disorder.

A person suffering from **paranoid personality disorder** is excessively distrustful and suspicious of others, expects to be abused by others, doesn't confide in others, and may be extremely jealous. Schizoid personality disorder can result in extreme detachment from social situations and limited emotions in interpersonal relations. Finally, a person with a schizotypal disorder is usually socially isolated, exhibits bizarre behaviors and beliefs about the world, and is suspicious of others.

Paranoid personality disorder is characterized by excessive distrust and suspicion of others.

FIGURE 7.5   **DEPRESSION SCREENING QUESTIONNAIRE**

1. Falling Asleep:
❑ I never take longer than 30 minutes to fall asleep
❑ I take at least 30 minutes to fall asleep, less than half the time
❑ I take at least 30 minutes to fall asleep, more than half the time
❑ I take at least 60 minutes to fall asleep, more than half the time

2. Sleep During the Night:
❑ I do not wake up at night
❑ I have a restless, light sleep with a few brief awakenings each night
❑ I wake up at least once a night, but I go back to sleep easily
❑ I awaken more than once a night and stay awake for 20 minutes or more, more than half the time

3. Waking Up Too Early:
❑ Most of the time, I awaken no more than 30 minutes before I need to get up
❑ More than half the time, I awaken more than 30 minutes before I need to get up
❑ I almost always awaken at least one hour or so before I need to, but I go back to sleep eventually
❑ I awaken at least one hour before I need to, and can't go back to sleep

4. Sleeping Too Much:
❑ I sleep no longer than 7–8 hours/night, with out napping during the day
❑ I sleep no longer than 10 hours in a 24-hour period including naps
❑ I sleep no longer than 12 hours in a 24-hour period including naps
❑ I sleep longer than 12 hours in a 24-hour period including naps

5. Feeling Sad:
❑ I do not feel sad
❑ I feel sad less than half the time
❑ I feel sad more than half the time
❑ I feel sad nearly all the time

6. Decreased Appetite:
❑ My usual appetite has not decreased
❑ I eat somewhat less often or lesser amounts of food than usual
❑ I eat much less than usual and only with personal effort
❑ I rarely eat within a 24-hour period, and only with extreme personal effort or when others persuade me to eat

7. Increased Appetite:
❑ My usual appetite has not increased
❑ I feel a need to eat more frequently than usual
❑ I regularly eat more often and/or greater amounts of food than usual
❑ I feel driven to overeat both at mealtime and between meals

8. Decreased Weight (Within the Last Two Weeks):
❑ My weight has not decreased
❑ I feel as if I've had a slight weight loss
❑ I have lost 2 pounds or more
❑ I have lost 5 pounds or more

9. Increased Weight (Within the Last Two Weeks):
- ❏ My weight has not increased
- ❏ I feel as if I've had a slight weight gain
- ❏ I have gained 2 pounds or more
- ❏ I have gained 5 pounds or more

10. Concentration/Decision Making:
- ❏ There is no change in my usual capacity to concentrate or make decisions
- ❏ I occasionally feel indecisive or find that my attention wanders
- ❏ Most of the time, I struggle to focus my attention or to make decisions
- ❏ I cannot concentrate well enough to read or cannot make even minor decisions

11. View of Myself:
- ❏ I see myself as equally worthwhile and deserving as other people
- ❏ I am more self-blaming than usual
- ❏ I largely believe that I cause problems for others
- ❏ I think almost constantly about major and minor defects in myself

12. Thoughts of Death or Suicide:
- ❏ I do not think of suicide or death
- ❏ I feel that life is empty or wonder if it's worth living
- ❏ I think of suicide or death several times a week for several minutes
- ❏ I think or suicide or death several times a day in some detail, or have actually tried to take my life

13. General Interest:
- ❏ There is no change from usual in how interested I am in other people or activities
- ❏ I notice that I am less interested in people or activities
- ❏ I find I have interest in only one or two of my formerly pursued activities
- ❏ I have virtually no interest in formerly pursued activities

14. Energy Level:
- ❏ There is no change in my usual level of energy
- ❏ I get tired more easily than usual
- ❏ I have to make a big effort to start or finish my usual daily activities (for example, shopping, homework, cooking or going to work)
- ❏ I really cannot carry out most of my usual daily activities because I just don't have the energy

15. Feeling slowed down:
- ❏ I think, speak, and move at my usual rate of speed
- ❏ I find that my thinking is slowed down or my voice sounds dull or flat
- ❏ It takes me several seconds to respond to most questions and I'm sure my thinking is slowed
- ❏ I am often unable to respond to questions without extreme effort

16. Feeling Restless:
- ❏ I do not feel restless
- ❏ I'm often fidgety, wringing my hands, or need to shift how I am sitting
- ❏ I have impulses to move about and am quite restless
- ❏ At times, I am unable to stay seated and need to pace around

| FIGURE 7.5 | DEPRESSION SCREENING QUESTIONNAIRE *(Continued)* |

About Scoring This Psychological Questionnaire
Each of the four possible answers to each quiz is given an ascending numerical value from 0 to 3, and the total test score is the sum of the following:

- The highest number from questions 1–4
- The number from question 5
- The highest number from questions 6–9
- The total of each question from 10–14
- The highest number from questions 15–16

The quiz measures different criterion domains for depression. If you take the quiz online (http://counsellingresource.com/quizzes/qids-depression/ index. html), it will be scored electronically, and one of five different information pages will appear with a description of the results for scores in your range.

Test Score Key: 0–5 (None), 6–10 (Mild), 11–15 (Moderate), 16–30 (Severe), and 31 or more (Very Severe).

Source: This screening form was developed from the Quick Inventory of Depressive Symptomatology Self-Report (QIDS-SR).

SCHIZOPHRENIA

Schizophrenia is a severe personality disorder that involves distorted thoughts and perceptions, atypical communication, inappropriate emotion, abnormal motor behavior, and social withdrawal. There are five types of schizophrenia.

Paranoid schizophrenics experience delusions and auditory hallucinations. They trust no one and are constantly on guard because they are convinced that others are plotting against them. Catatonic schizophrenia is characterized by excessive inactivity. The person can retain the same posture for long periods of time and may alternate between violent behavior and being immobile and totally unresponsive to the outside world. Disorganized schizophrenics experience extreme delusions, hallucinations, and have inappropriate patterns of speech, mood, and movements. Extreme laughing and crying at unsuitable times are hallmark signs of disorganized schizophrenics.

A schizophrenic who experiences delusions, hallucinations, and disorganized behavior but lacks other specific symptoms is classified as an undifferentiated schizophrenic. Finally, residual schizophrenia is a condition in which at least one episode of schizophrenia has occurred but there are currently no prominent psychotic symptoms.

Schizophrenia is a severe mental disorder that involves distorted thoughts and perceptions, atypical communications, inappropriate emotion, and abnormal motor behavior. Forms of schizophrenia include paranoid, catatonic, disorganized, undifferentiated, and residual.

✓ **NEED TO KNOW**

Mental disorders are some of the most misunderstood illnesses. When people's behavior appears different, oftentimes it is incorrectly interpreted as a disorder. Mental disorders, like physical disorders, have common sets of symptoms that are characteristic of those having the disorder. The symptoms can range from mood disorders to severe disorders such as anxiety disorders, mania, and schizophrenia.

➤ Treatment

Psychotherapy and biomedical therapy are two approaches used to treat many of the disorders described in this chapter. In most instances a combination of both psychotherapy and biomedical therapy is used.

Psychotherapy is performed by a psychotherapist. A psychotherapist can be a psychologist, psychiatrist, a psychiatric nurse, or a counselor. In all instances there are licensure and certification requirements for people performing psychotherapy. (See Chapter 12 for a more detailed explanation of the educational backgrounds of various health professionals.)

The psychological techniques employed in psychotherapy include such approaches as psychodynamic, humanistic, person-centered, gestalt therapy, existential therapy, and behavior therapies, systematic desensitization, implosive therapy, flooding, biofeedback, aversive conditioning, token economy, cognitive therapy, rational-emotive therapy, feminist therapy, and group therapy. See Figure 7.6 for a roundup of the different techniques.

The biomedical approach involves the use of drug therapies to treat the disorder. In general the drugs used in treating these disorders include anti-anxiety drugs, anti-psychotic drugs, anti-depressant drugs, lithium, and electroconvulsive therapy. (Some of these drugs were discussed in Chapter 4.) Anti-anxiety drugs are minor tranquilizers such as Valium and Xanax. These drugs are designed to be used short-term. Anti-psychotic drugs are major tranquilizers that are used long-term and are capable of acting on the psychotic process itself. Anti-depressant drugs such as Prozac, Zoloft, and Paxil act on neurotransmitters and are helpful in controlling depression. Lithium is used to control the swings in bipolar mood disorders.

Electroconvulsive therapy (ECT) is a procedure in which electrodes administer shocks to the patient, who experiences a seizure and then lapses into unconsciousness. When conscious, the patient feels better because the ECT has affected nerve cells and the root physiological causes of depression. Exactly what happens neurologically after ECT is unclear, but it provides relief for some people. Because it has some serious risks, ECT is normally used only when all other treatments have failed. ECT can speed or slow the heartbeat and cause memory loss. When psychotherapy and biomedical therapy is not effective in keeping a person functional,

FIGURE 7.6   APPROACHES TO PSYCHOTHERAPY

Aversive conditioning: Client experiences unpleasant stimuli (shock, verbal insults) after behaving undesirably.

Behavior therapy: Uses principles of social learning to assist people in forming accurate perceptions of their feelings and themselves.

Biofeedback: Monitoring of body functioning to provide feedback to the client.

Cognitive therapy: Client is taught to understand the irrationality of their thoughts or behaviors.

Encounter groups: Confrontational strategies used to allow members to express true feelings.

Existential therapy: Emphasis is on free will and using the free will to develop insight and self-understanding.

Family therapy: A form of group therapy directed at families.

Feminist therapy: Focuses on role of society and the role of discrimination in daily life.

Flooding therapy: Client is placed in a real situation that they fear, normally accompanied by the therapist.

Gestalt therapy: An approach that employs role playing and confrontation.

Group therapy: Apply psychotherapeutic principles to group.

Humanistic therapies: The focus is on conscious thoughts and present times as opposed to psychodynamic (unconscious thoughts and past experiences).

Implosive therapy: Clients imagine and deal with their worst fears in a safe environment with a therapist.

Marital therapy: Husband and wives in therapy together to assist them in a more productive relationship.

Modeling: Client watches another person perform the feared behavior and with the help of the therapist copies that behavior.

Person-centered therapy: Creation of a warm, supportive environmen t where a person feels accepted and can reveal true feelings.

Psychodrama: Role-playing strategies used including role-reversal.

Psychodynamic therapies: Freudian "insight" therapies and involvesfree association and dream analysis and can be focused on the unconscious and past experiences.

Self-help groups: Support groups to assist people in displaying behaviors to reduce risk of recitivism to a previous problem behavior (alcohol dependence).

Sensitivity groups: Strategies used to promote self-awareness and trust of others.

Systematic desensitization: Uses principles of relaxation and visualization.

Token economy: Tokens are given as rewards for behavior in an effort to shape the behavior.

Health & the Media *Advertising Anti-depressants*

Zoloft is a selective serotonin reuptake inhibitor (SSRI), the most widely prescribed anti-depressant among that category of drugs. Drugs like Zoloft have made a positive difference in many people's lives. However, in 2004 Zoloft advertisements contained a cartoon character that asked, "Are you sad or anxious? Tired all of the time? Not sleeping well? Losing interest in things and people you love? Do these feelings stop you from enjoying life? These could be the signs of depression. When the cause is unknown, Zoloft can help." The ads were deemed misleading by the Federal Drug Administration (FDA) and pulled because the possible risks and side effects from taking Zoloft were not adequately described. The issue of whether drug companies should advertise to consumers directly—in effect, asking them to go to their doctor to get a specific drug, rather than going to the doctor with a problem and allowing the physician to evaluate prescription needs—remains very controversial today.

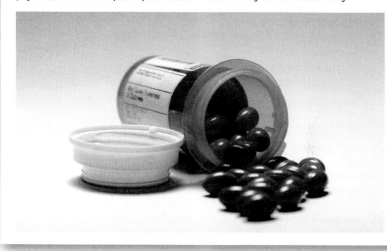

institutionalization may be the only remaining option, especially for people who may be dangerous to themselves or others.

✓ NEED TO KNOW

People who suffer from mental or emotional problems should be encouraged to know that interventions can help. After the condition is properly diagnosed, the appropriate treatment can be prescribed. Treatment can include counseling or medication or both. There have been tremendous advances in medications used to treat mental and emotional conditions. Medications such as anti-anxiety drugs and anti-depressants have made a positive difference in many lives. Even people with profound mental problems might not need to be institutionalized as they were years ago. There are many options both in medications and counseling.

Web Site Resources

Anxiety Disorders Association of America
www.adaa.org
Centers for Disease Control
www.cdc.gov
Freedom From Fear
www.freedomfromfear.com
Internet Mental Health
www.mentalhealth.com
Mental Health of America (formerly National Mental Health Association)
www.nmha.org
National Eating Disorders Association
www.nationaleatingdisorders.org
National Institute of Mental Health
www.nimh.nih.gov
Obsessive-Compulsive Foundation
www.ocfoundation.org
Substance Abuse and Mental Health Administration
www.samhsa.gov
Suicide.org: Suicide Awareness, Prevention, and Support
www.suicide.org/

Knowing the Language

Anorexia nervosa
Anxiety
Binge eating disorder
Bipolar disorder
Bulimia nervosa
Depression
Dysthymia
Generalized Anxiety Disorder
Mania
Mental health
Motivation

Obsessive-Compulsive Disorder
Panic disorders
Paranoid personality disorder
Phobias
Post-traumatic Stress Disorder
Psychosomatic
Schizophrenia
Seasonal Affective Disorder
Self-concept
Self-esteem

Understanding the Content

1. What is Maslow's hierarchy of needs and what does it have to do with mental health?
2. What can happen when needs are not met? What is the range of responses to tension, frustration, conflict?
3. What are the characteristics of good mental health?
4. What are the differences between mood disorders and personality disorders?
5. What are the common treatments used in treating mental disorders?

1. How does one know the difference between someone who is different and someone who is mentally ill?
2. How can a clear understanding of mental health lessen the personal and social problems related to mental health?
3. Why is it so hard for people to admit they are having mental health problems? What can be done to help create a better environment for people to seek help?

Selected References

American College Health Association. *National College Health Assessment: Reference Group Summary.* Baltimore, MD: American College Health Association, 2002.

American Psychiatric Association. *Diagnostic and Statistical Manual of Mental Disorders* (4th ed.). Washington, DC: American Psychiatric Association, 2000.

American Psychiatric Association. *Let's Talk Facts About Eating Disorders.* American Phychiatric Association, 2005.

Durkheim E. *Suicide: A Study in Sociology* (trans. Simpson G, Spaulding JA). New York: Free Press, 2000.

Glanze W. *Mosby's Medical and Nursing Dictionary* (5th ed.). St. Louis, MO: Mosby, 2002.

Kadison R, diGeronimo T. *College of the Overwhelmed.* San Francisco: Jossey-Bass, 2005.

Kitzrow M. The Mental health needs of today's college students: Challenges and recommendations. *NASPA Journal,* 41(1): 165–183, 2003.

Marano H. A nation of wimps. *Psychology Today* 40:25–32, 2004.

Maslow A. *Motivation and Personality* (2nd ed.). New York: Harper and Row, 1970.

Narrow WE, Rae DS, Robins LN, Regier DA. Revised prevalence estimates of mental disorders in the United States. *Archives of General Psychiatry* 59(2): 131–145, 2002.

National Institute of Mental Health. *Eating Disorders.* Bethesda, MD: National Institute of Mental Health, 2002.

National Institute of Mental Health. *Facts about Anxiety Disorders.* Bethesda, MD: National Institute of Mental Health, 2003.

Nordenberg L. Dealing with the depths of depression. *FDA Consumer* 32 (4) July–Aug. 1998.
www.fda.gov/fdac/features/1998/498.dep.html

Shortell S, Kaluzny A. *Health Care Management: Organizational Design and Behavior.* Albany, NY: Delmar, 2000.

Sontag D. Who was responsible for Elizabeth Shin? *New York Times,* April 28, 2002.

Steers RM, Porter LW. *Motivation and Work Behavior.* New York: McGraw-Hill, 1987.

Taylor S. *Health Psychology* (5th ed.). New York: McGraw-Hill, 2003.

U.S. Department of Health and Human Services. *Healthy People 2010.* Washington, DC: U.S. DHHS, 2000.

U.S. Public Health Service. *Mental Health: A Report of the Surgeon General.* Washington, DC: U.S. PHS, 2002.

Wrobel G. Accessing Medicaid Funding for School Based Mental Health Programs. Presented at the National Association of School Psychologists, Washington, DC, February 10–12, 2001.

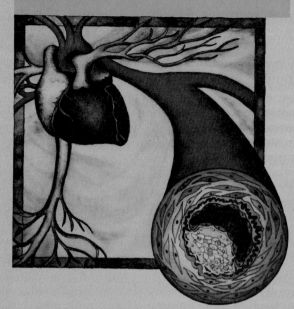

Cardiovascular disease is an equal opportunity affliction. In fact, more women than men die from heart disease, and the same is true for stroke.

— AMERICAN HEART ASSOCIATION

Chapter 8

CORONARY HEART DISEASE AND STROKE

In this chapter, we focus on understanding coronary heart disease (CHD) and stroke, the two most common types of cardiovascular disease. We discuss the underlying disease process of atherosclerosis and review the signs, risk factors, and treatments for CHD and stroke. Prevention measures to reduce risk of CHD and stroke are highlighted.

IN THE YEARS following World War II, America was buzzing. Families reunited, new families began, suburban communities around cities mushroomed, and the economy boomed. Life was upbeat. Americans were optimistic about their health, too. In contrast to the hard times of the Great Depression and World War II, people living in the postwar period benefited from major advances in health and medicine. For example, public health systems ensured cleaner water and sanitary-waste disposal, while the advent of antibiotics brought major killers like tuberculosis and pneumonia under control. Yet, these good times were overshadowed by the rise in death and disability due to cardiovascular disease.

Due to the growth in desk jobs and the popularity of labor-saving devices such as the washing machine and motorized lawn mower, people were getting much less physical activity than their parents had. In addition, the typical American diet changed to one where whole milk, butter, and red meats were commonplace rather than special occasion foods. Additionally, in 1950 the world was mostly unaware of the dangers of tobacco, which was especially unfortunate, given that about half of all American adults smoked.

Although heart disease rates in the United States had been increasing since the late 1930s, doctors had little advice for their patients on the control or prevention of heart conditions. Doctors thought that atherosclerosis was an inevitable part of the aging process and that blood pressure increased with age to enable the heart to pump blood through an older person's narrowed arteries. Similarly, the causal connections linking smoking, high-fat diet, and sedentary living to heart disease were not yet established. Doctors had scant evidence that modifying certain behaviors could help their patients prevent serious heart and vascular conditions. The standard treatment for people who survived a heart attack was four to six weeks of strict bed rest. Today people are encouraged to get up and walk as soon as they are medically stable, often within the first day following a heart attack or associated surgery.

In the 1950s, researchers began to investigate the potential roles of a high-fat diet and physical inactivity on the increased rates of cardiovascular disease. By the 1970s a growing body of scientific studies provided strong evidence that both of those lifestyle habits contributed to the rise in cardiovascular disease. Today complex surgeries and powerful drugs are available to treat the many forms of cardiovascular disease. But an advancement at least as important as those sophisticated medical treatments is our understanding that cardiovascular disease can often be prevented. Staying active, not smoking, and making good dietary choices throughout life greatly reduces our risk of what remains the number-one cause of death in the United States.

This chapter focuses on understanding the two most common types of cardiovascular disease: coronary heart disease (CHD) and stroke. The underlying disease process of atherosclerosis is reviewed, followed by a synopsis of CHD and stroke, including their signs, risk factors, and treatments. The cardiovascular risk factors that are modifiable, along with preventive lifestyle behaviors, are emphasized throughout.

➤ Cardiovascular Disease

Cardiovascular disease is a general term that encompasses a broad array of diseases of the heart (*cardio-*) and blood vessels (*-vascular*). Cardiovascular disease has been the number-one killer in the United States for many decades. In recent years, four of every ten deaths among Americans are due to cardiovascular disease. Coronary heart disease (CHD) and stroke are the two most common types, together accounting for about 70 percent of all cardiovascular deaths. Other cardiovascular deaths are attributable primarily to congestive heart failure, a decline in the heart's pumping capacity (7 percent); high blood pressure, or hypertension (6 percent); and peripheral arterial disease (4 percent). The final 13 percent of cardiovascular deaths are caused by a variety of other less common heart and blood vessel disorders. Less than 1 percent of deaths are due to congenital cardiovascular defects or rheumatic heart disease.

A disease process called **atherosclerosis** causes both CHD and stroke. The term derives from the Greek words *athero,* meaning "gruel" or "paste," and *sclerosis,* meaning "hardness." Atherosclerosis involves a buildup of patchy deposits—primarily fatty substances, cholesterol, cellular waste products, and calcium—inside the arteries. These deposits are collectively referred to as *plaque.* As the plaque accumulates, the arteries thicken and harden, becoming less elastic.

The process of plaque deposition is not uniform or equally distributed within an artery, but rather it is irregular and scattered. As plaque accumulates within an artery, blood flow is increasingly restricted as the inner diameter of the vessel becomes rougher and smaller. The combination of less elasticity of vessel walls and increased pressure within vessels weakens arteries and makes them vulnerable to rupture. As atherosclerosis develops, susceptibility for a blood clot to form and block a narrowed artery increases. A clot can form within a narrowed artery (thrombus), or a clot can form in another part of the body and migrate to a narrowed artery (embolus). Complete obstruction of an artery or, less frequently, the bursting of an arterial wall can occur. If this occurs in the heart, we call it a *heart attack.* If it occurs in the brain, we call it a *stroke.*

Atherosclerosis is the process in which the inner layers of arteries become irregular and thick due to accumulation of plaque (fatty deposits); over time, this process can lead to obstructive buildup within the arteries and weakening of the arterial walls.

Atherosclerosis may also occur in arteries far from the heart or brain—in the legs, pelvis, or arms, for example. This condition is known as *peripheral arterial disease.* It is much less common than heart attack or stroke as a cause of death, but it can be painful and limit one's activities. Cramping and fatigue in the legs during walking are early symptoms.

Atherosclerosis is a process that occurs throughout the body, although it may progress at different rates from one site to another. With that in mind, it's clear that a person at risk for any one of these three conditions—heart attack, stroke, or peripheral vascular disease—is also at risk for the other two. Moreover, atherosclerosis is often an underlying or contributing factor to hypertension and congestive heart failure.

Until the 1990s, atherosclerosis was chiefly considered a disease of middle age. It was viewed as a disease that could start in childhood but usually developed during mid-life and beyond. New studies have significantly shifted this view. We now know that atherosclerosis can progress more rapidly and earlier in life, even in people in their 20s. At the other end of the age range, older people who have tightly controlled their cardiovascular risk factors have relatively low rates of heart disease and stroke. Such evidence indicates that age by itself is not as strong a determinant of atherosclerosis as was once believed; this evidence provides a powerful incentive to reduce one's risk factors regardless of age.

Atherosclerosis is initiated by inflammation with subsequent scarring and calcification of the innermost layer of the artery (endothelium). Substantial evidence demonstrates that premature onset or accelerated atherosclerosis is caused by tobacco smoke, high blood pressure, high cholesterol, physical inactivity, obesity, and diabetes—all of which are largely modifiable. These and other risk factors are discussed later in this chapter. In the next two sections, we will present the key terms and concepts about heart disease and stroke, respectively.

CORONARY HEART DISEASE

Do you wonder what it feels like to have a heart attack? In the opening paragraphs of her book *Heartsounds,* Martha Weinman Lear tells the true story of her physician husband having a heart attack and the string of events that followed it:

> He awoke at 7 A.M. with pain in his chest. The sort of pain that might cause panic if one were not a doctor, as he was, and did not know, as he knew, that it was heartburn.
>
> He went into the kitchen to get some Coke, whose secret syrups often relieve heartburn. The refrigerator door seemed heavy, and he noted that he was having trouble unscrewing the bottle cap. Finally he wrenched it off, cursing the defective cap. He poured some liquid, took a sip. The pain did not go away. Another sip; still no relief.

Now he grew more attentive. He stood motionless, observing symptoms. His breath was coming hard. He felt faint. He was sweating, though the August morning was still cool. He put fingers to his pulse. It was rapid and weak. A powerful burning sensation was beginning to spread through his chest, radiating upward into his throat. Into his arm? No. But the pain was growing worse. Now it was crushing—"crushing," just as it is always described. And worse even than the pain was the sensation of losing all power, a terrifying seepage of strength.

On some level he stood aside and observed all this with a certain clinical detachment. Here, the preposterous spectacle of this naked man holding a tumbler of Coke and waiting to die in an orange Formica kitchen on a sunny summer morning in the 53rd year of his life.

I'll be dammed, he thought. I can't believe it.

Coronary heart disease (CHD)—also referred to as *coronary artery disease*—is a condition in which the blood supply to the heart muscle (myocardium) is partially or completely blocked due to atherosclerotic narrowing of one or more coronary arteries. CHD causes about one out of every five deaths in the United States. CHD was once widely thought to be a disease of men, and even today many people still believe this to be the case. But the statistics consistently show this to be false. CHD is the single largest killer of American males *and* females, with the total number of deaths (over 600,000 deaths in 2004) about evenly split between the genders (51 percent are women).

On average, men develop CHD about 10 years earlier than women because until menopause, women are somewhat protected from the disease by their high levels of estrogen. Among women, heart disease is often perceived as an "older woman's disease," and it is the leading cause of death among women aged 65 years and older. However, heart disease is also the third leading cause of death among women aged 25–44 years and the second leading cause of death among women aged 45–64 years. With regard to race/ethnicity, the prevalence of CHD for people age 18 and older is similar for whites (12 percent) and blacks (10 percent) and lower for Hispanics (6 percent) and Asians (5 percent).

CHD is a chronic, progressive condition. As the plaque builds up in the coronary arteries, the blood flow channels become more and more restricted, with a likely outcome being chest pain or **heart attack** if the

Coronary heart disease (CHD) is a condition in which the coronary arteries are narrowed or blocked, usually because of atherosclerosis.

Heart attack is tissue death (infarction) to part of the heart muscle (myocardium) due to an insufficient blood supply when a coronary artery becomes blocked. The medical term for heart attack is *myocardial infarction*.

artery becomes completely blocked. The medical term for chest pain is *angina pectoris,* or more commonly just **angina.** Typical angina is uncomfortable pressure, squeezing, or pain in the chest and it can vary widely in intensity. Angina often occurs when the heart needs more blood during physical exertion such as climbing a flight of stairs or running for a few seconds. Angina may also occur when experiencing strong emotions. Some people may have unstable angina in which chest pain occurs unexpectedly at rest. Nitroglycerin is the drug most often used to treat angina. This drug is a coronary vasodilator. It causes the blood vessels to relax and thus allows the channels inside the vessels to open up and improve blood flow.

A heart attack, or myocardial infarction, occurs when one or more of the coronary arteries are blocked. This can happen when a plaque tears or ruptures, creating a snag where a blood clot forms and completely blocks the artery. If the blood supply is cut off for more than a few minutes, the cardiac muscle cells suffer permanent damage and die. Depending upon the severity of the heart damage, the consequences can vary widely from a minor heart attack to sudden death. Fifty percent of men and 64 percent of women who died suddenly of CHD had *no previous symptoms* of the disease. This is a sobering statistic. Many of you may know of a person who died this way.

STROKE

Stroke is a disorder in which an artery to the brain becomes blocked or ruptures, resulting in death of brain tissue. When counted separately from other cardiovascular diseases, stroke ranks third among all causes of death behind diseases of the heart and cancer. Strokes accounted for about 1 out of every 16 deaths in the United States (over 150,000 deaths) in 2004. More women than men die from stroke (about 91,000 vs. 59,000). Strokes are also the second most common cause of disabling neurologic damage after Alzheimer's disease. Of those who survive a stroke, 15–30 percent suffer long-term disabilities. Over two-thirds of all strokes occur in people older than 65. In adults over 55, the lifetime risk for stroke is greater than one in six. Women have a higher risk than men, perhaps due to their longer life span. With regard to race/ethnicity, blacks are more likely than whites, Asians, or Hispanics to have a stroke and die from it. Although strokes are much more common in older people than in younger

Angina, or angina pectoris, is the medical term for chest pain or discomfort caused by a restricted blood supply to the heart.

A **stroke** is brain-cell injury caused by a blockage or rupture of a blood vessel in the brain. Stroke is characterized by loss of muscle control, mental function, vision, sensation, and/or speech and other symptoms that vary with the extent and severity of brain damage. The medical term for stroke is *cerebrovascular accident.*

adults, they do sometimes occur in younger individuals, especially if there is uncontrolled high blood pressure.

Most strokes are due to atherosclerosis, the same underlying disease process that leads to heart attacks. In a stroke, the arteries supplying blood to the brain are affected. For this reason, strokes are sometimes referred to as "brain attacks." The medical term for stroke is *cerebrovascular accident,* so called because the disorder affects the blood vessels (*-vascular*) to the brain (*cerebro-*). There are two types of stroke: ischemic and hemorrhagic. The term *ischemic* refers to decreased blood flow due to constriction or obstruction of an artery. Most strokes (about 87 percent) are ischemic. In these cases, an artery to the brain has become blocked or occluded. Deprived of their blood supply and thus oxygen and nutrients, the affected brain cells can be permanently damaged.

A transient ischemic attack, sometimes called a *mini-stroke,* is a less serious variation of the ischemic stroke. In a transient ischemic attack, blood supply to part of the brain is compromised but only for a brief time. In this case, normal blood flow re-establishes quickly and brain tissue does not die. However, a transient ischemic attack is a warning sign of an impending ischemic stroke.

Hemorrhagic strokes are less common (about 13 percent of all strokes) but are more dangerous than ischemic strokes. In this type of stroke, a blood vessel ruptures where the arterial wall has weakened. This not only prevents normal blood flow but also results in blood leaking into or around brain tissue, which in turn leads to life-threatening complications. Hemorrhagic strokes are more lethal than ischemic strokes.

When a stroke occurs, the resulting brain injury causes a loss of muscle control, mental function, vision, sensation, or speech, or a combination of these functions. Strokes usually damage only one side of the brain. Because nerves cross in the brain, symptoms appear on the side of the body opposite the injured side of the brain. Strokes affect people in different ways, depending on the type of stroke (ischemic vs. hemorrhagic), the specific area of the brain, and the extent of the brain injury.

✓ NEED TO KNOW

Cardiovascular disease includes all diseases of the heart and circulatory system. Coronary heart disease (CHD) and stroke are the two major types of cardiovascular disease and are the first and third leading causes of death in America, respectively. Atherosclerosis, a chronic progressive process of obstructive plaque buildup and weakening of the arterial walls, is the underlying cause of both CHD and stroke.

Every adult in America should be able to recognize the symptoms of heart attacks and strokes and know the steps to take to activate the emergency medical system. Onset of symptoms should trigger an immediate response. You may be the only person available to provide assistance. Remember that emergency therapy for heart attack and stroke is critical for saving lives and reducing disabilities. The cardinal signs of a heart attack and of a stroke and the appropriate actions to take are presented in the next sections.

HEART ATTACK ALERT—KNOW THE SIGNS

In the opening to this chapter's section on CHD, Dr. Lear struggles with disbelief and pain as he experiences a heart attack (described in the excerpt from *Heartsounds*). As a doctor, he knows the signs, yet he is trying to deny them. The thought that it must be something else—it *cannot* be a heart attack—is a typical initial response for many knowledgeable adults. Many people experiencing a heart attack are not sure what's wrong and wait too long before getting help. Know the signs of a heart attack, not only for your own sake but for the sake of others who may be indecisive about getting emergency care.

What are the classical signs of a heart attack? Many think a heart attack is sudden and intense, like the Hollywood portrayal where the character suddenly clutches his chest in anguish and falls over dead after an intense physical effort or emotionally charged event. A heart attack can occur this way, but the truth is that two out of three people who have heart attacks experience warning signs a few days or weeks beforehand. A person may notice only mild pain or discomfort from time to time. Or chest discomfort (angina) may become more frequent and occur with less and less physical exertion. Even those who have had a heart attack may not recognize their symptoms, because the next heart attack can have entirely different ones.

The most recognizable symptom of a heart attack is chest pain that may spread to the back, neck, jaw, left arm, both arms, or abdomen. The pain can range from slight discomfort or pressure to an unbearable squeezing or crushing sensation. It may persist or go away and return. The location of the pain can vary—it may occur in one or more of these sites and not in the chest at all. People who have a heart attack without chest pain are more likely to be over 75, have diabetes or heart failure, or have had a stroke. The chest pain of a heart attack is similar to the pain of angina but is generally more severe, lasts longer, and is not relieved by rest or nitroglycerin. Pain in the abdomen is sometimes mistaken for indigestion. Shortness of breath often accompanies chest discomfort, but it also can occur before chest discomfort. Other symptoms may include breaking out in a cold sweat, nausea, or light-headedness.

To summarize, *heart attack warning signs* are

- chest discomfort or pain;
- discomfort in one or both arms, back, neck, jaw or stomach;
- shortness of breath; and
- cold sweat, nausea, or light-headedness.

It's worth repeating that women are as vulnerable to a heart attack as men. Heart disease is the number-one killer of both women and men, and women account for just over half of all heart attack deaths. There is an average age difference, with women being about 10 years older than men when they have a heart attack. Please note that women are less likely than men to believe they're having a heart attack and more likely to delay seeking emergency treatment. As with men, women's most common heart attack symptom is chest pain or discomfort. But women are more likely than men to experience some of the other symptoms, particularly shortness of breath, nausea/vomiting, and back or jaw pain.

STROKE ALERT—KNOW THE SIGNS

Strokes are most common in older people, but they are not rare among young adults. A stroke can occur even in a young fit person if known risk factors are not being controlled. It's important to be alert to the signs of both heart attack and stroke across the adult age range.

Unlike those of a heart attack, the signs of stroke are not widely recognized by the public. In a recent study by the Centers for Disease Control and Prevention, only 17 percent of American adults recognized the major warning signs. Admittedly, symptoms of a stroke can vary widely depending on the exact location of the blockage or bleeding in the brain. Each area of the brain is supplied by specific arteries. For example, if an artery supplying the area of the brain that controls the movement of the right arm is blocked, then the right arm becomes weak or paralyzed. Similarly, a loss of vision, sensation, speech, movement, or mental function can be the sign of a stroke, depending on the specific area of the brain affected.

The most common early symptoms of an ischemic stroke are sudden numbness, weakness, or paralysis of the face, arm, or leg on one side of the body; sudden confusion with difficulty speaking or understanding speech; sudden dimness or loss of vision, particularly in one eye; loss of balance or coordination, leading to falls; and sudden, severe headache. Symptoms of a transient ischemic stroke are the same but usually disappear within minutes. Symptoms of a hemorrhagic stroke are also largely the same as those of an ischemic stroke, but sudden severe headache may be more common along with nausea and vomiting, temporary or persistent loss of consciousness, and very high blood pressure.

- sudden numbness or weakness of face, arm, or leg, especially on one side of the body;
- sudden confusion and trouble speaking or understanding;
- sudden trouble seeing in one or both eyes;
- sudden trouble walking, dizziness, loss of balance or coordination; and
- sudden severe headache with no known cause.

A person does not have to experience multiple symptoms to be having a stroke. Even if only one symptom is present, seek medical attention right away. Some people decide to ignore symptoms if they last only a few minutes. Yet, such a decision is a high-risk gamble with much to lose. Transient ischemic attacks often signal that a major stroke is on the way. People who have a transient ischemic attack should see a doctor immediately.

ACT IN AN EMERGENCY

Starting medical treatment as soon as possible is critical when a person is experiencing a heart attack or stroke. The sooner emergency care is begun, the lower the risk of death or disability. There are clot-dissolving drugs and procedures that can open blocked arteries, but they must be delivered quickly—within the first one to three hours—to be effective.

It's critical to take action. Nearly everywhere throughout the country, a call to 9-1-1 will activate emergency medical service and ensure quick arrival by trained paramedics. Be sure to note as much of the following information as you can for the paramedics and emergency room team:

- What are the symptoms?
- What time did the symptoms begin?
- Does the person have any medical conditions?
- What drugs, if any, does the person take?

The paramedics will be able to start medical treatment, monitor the patient on the way to the hospital, call ahead to prepare the emergency team, and provide the quickest possible transport.

In the unusual instance where 9-1-1 is not available, drive the person to the nearest hospital emergency room. Call ahead if possible and alert them that you are coming. People who may have had a heart attack or stroke should not attempt to drive themselves, because an impaired driver is a hazard to everyone on the road.

Be aware that you may face obstacles in taking the appropriate action—primarily from the person you are trying to assist! Many reasons can surface to delay calling 9-1-1. People can't believe a heart attack or stroke is happening to them. Symptoms are not what they expected. People wait to see if the symptoms go away. They want to try and treat the symptoms themselves. They call a family member for advice. They call the doctor and wait for a return call. They try to make arrangements for children or other dependent family members before seeking emergency care. They fear large medical bills. Although these are rational reasons, none of them are good enough to postpone *emergency* treatment. Although it may be tempting to wait, a delay in calling 9-1-1 can result in death or life-long disability.

If the symptoms turn out to be related to some less serious problem, consider that as good news. The paramedics and emergency room team will not fault you for your quick and decisive actions to the known signs of a heart attack or stroke. Unfortunately, their dilemma is often just the opposite. They are sometimes unable to effectively treat people who waited too long before coming. In some cases, the time-sensitive window for using the most successful treatments may have closed.

Breaking It Down Defibrillators—From the Emergency Room to the Shopping Mall

Automatic External Defibrillators (AEDs)—you may have seen them conspicuously mounted in shopping malls, airports, fitness centers, and sports arenas. In the years ahead, you'll be seeing more of them—from work sites and churches to country clubs and casinos. They save lives. But how did the defibrillator come from the emergency room to the shopping mall?

We've seen the scene depicted on TV many times. The patient suddenly loses consciousness and has no pulse. It's a case of cardiac arrest and a "Code Blue" is called for immediate response by a trained team of nurses and doctors. The resuscitating team continues advanced cardiac life support until the patient recovers or dies. The good news—on TV and in real life—is that cardiac arrest is often reversed by the electric discharge of a defibrillator.

Nearly a quarter of all deaths in the United States are attributed to sudden cardiac arrest, which results from disturbances in the electrical activity of the heart—most commonly, ventricular fibrillation. During this abnormal heart rhythm, the ventricles begin to quiver—visualize a bowl of writhing worms—rather than contracting in unison. This causes a sudden cessation of normal circulation of the blood due to failure of the heart's ventricles to contract effectively. Cerebral hypoxia, or lack of oxygen supply to the brain, causes victims to immediately lose consciousness and stop breathing. If left untreated, cardiac arrest invariably leads to death within minutes.

Most of these deaths are due to underlying CHD and are associated with a heart attack. Sudden cardiac arrest occurs primarily in the middle-aged and elderly. Though the average age is about 65, some people are in their 30s or 40s. For many, there is no previous history of heart problems.

Sudden cardiac arrest is often the first symptom and it can occur any time, anywhere. By its very nature, sudden cardiac arrest is unpredictable.

The good news is that with the growing availability of AEDs in public places, successful treatment for cardiac arrest is much more likely. During ventricular fibrillation, electrical energy is present in the heart, but it is chaotic. If the heart can be shocked—called *defibrillation*—a normal heart rhythm may be restored. Due to advances in computer technology, AEDs are smart devices that "automatically" diagnose the abnormal heart rhythm and provide the necessary shock as appropriate. Learning to use an AED is highly intuitive and surprisingly simple. Many report that it's easier than learning CPR. AED courses last about three or four hours and include hands-on practice. AED training and related resources are offered through several organizations, including the American Heart Association and the American Red Cross.

The key to successful treatment is to be quick. The shorter the time from collapse to defibrillation, the better the chances of survival. If defibrillation is delayed for more than 10 minutes, survival rates drop to less than 5 percent. The challenge is to respond to every victim of sudden cardiac arrest within minutes. If the time from the 9-1-1 call to defibrillation is seven minutes or less, as many as one-third to one-half of sudden cardiac arrest victims found in ventricular fibrillation can be resuscitated.

Summary of the "Chain of Survival" for Sudden Cardiac Arrest

First person at the scene of the collapse: early access

- Recognize the emergency
- Decide to help
- Establish unresponsiveness
- Call 9-1-1 or local emergency number

Trained citizen: early CPR

- Provide rescue breathing
- Provide chest compressions if pulse is absent and AED is not yet available

Trained and authorized responder: early defibrillation

- Attempt to defibrillate as soon as AED is available

Professional medical personnel: early advanced care

- Give advanced medical care, including airway and breathing support and medications

Learn or maintain CPR and AED skills. If we needed help, we would hope that a bystander would know what to do. It may well be that we will be the bystander, not the victim. We need to be ready.

✓ **NEED TO KNOW**

You should know the warning signs of a heart attack and those of a stroke and how to activate the emergency medical system in your area. Time is of the essence. The sooner emergency care is begun, the lower the risk of death or disability. Learning CPR (cardiopulmonary resuscitation), knowing how to use an AED (automatic external defibrillator), and keeping your certifications current are excellent ways to keep up to date and maintain practical—and potentially life-saving—skills.

➤ Risk Factors

Since the 1970s, risk factors for heart disease and stroke have been described as one of two types: nonmodifiable or modifiable. Risk factors that *cannot* be modified or changed are age, gender, and heredity. Increasing age is a risk factor. Men are at greater risk than women. And a family history of early heart disease, particularly in parents, grandparents, or siblings is a risk factor. Early or premature heart disease is usually defined as occurring before age 65.

Risk factors that *can* be modified, treated, or controlled include six major factors and several other contributing factors. Three of the classic risk factors are smoking, high blood pressure, and elevated blood cholesterol. In the next few pages, we'll take a closer look at each of the major modifiable risk factors as these are the ones under our control. Dr. Paul Dudley White, the father of modern cardiology, once wrote that heart disease before age 80 is our fault, not God's or nature's will. That is, atherosclerosis is a largely preventable disease.

CIGARETTE SMOKING

A smoker's risk is directly related to the number of cigarettes smoked daily. The nicotine and carbon monoxide in tobacco smoke reduce the amount of oxygen carried in the blood. These and other substances in tobacco smoke reduce HDL ("good") cholesterol, damage blood vessel walls causing plaque to build-up, and may trigger the formation of blood clots. In addition to increasing one's chances of having a heart attack or stroke, smoking causes cancer and lung disease, is the strongest risk factor for peripheral arterial disease and sudden cardiac death, and harms the fetus during pregnancy. Moreover, constant exposure to the tobacco smoke of others (secondhand smoke) can be as harmful as smoking.

Cigarette smoking is the single most preventable cause of disease and death in the United States. Despite the multiple harmful effects of tobacco and large-scale efforts to curb its use, tens of thousands of Americans still smoke. The latest figures indicate nearly one in four Americans over the age of 16 smokes. On average, smokers have twice the risk of heart attack and stroke that nonsmokers have. Yet, remarkably, a large portion of a smoker's risk disappears two years after stopping; by 10 years, a former smoker's risk is similar to a nonsmoker's. If you smoke, the single best thing you can do for your health is to stop. All physicians agree on this point. Also, think of family and friends who smoke and what you can do to help them quit. (For suggestions, see You Can Quit Smoking Now! at **www.smokefree.gov)**

HIGH BLOOD PRESSURE

High blood pressure, or **hypertension,** is a condition in which blood pressure is consistently elevated over repeated readings on different days. Blood pressure is the force with which the blood pushes against the walls of the arteries. If blood pressure is continuously high, the heart is working harder than it should and over time this will damage both the heart and the blood vessels.

When blood pressure is measured, two values are recorded. The higher value, or systolic pressure, reflects the highest pressure in the arteries when the heart contracts. The lower value, or diastolic pressure, reflects the lowest pressure in the arteries during the relaxation phase following a contraction. Blood pressure is written as systolic pressure/diastolic pressure; for example, 120/80 mm Hg (millimeters of mercury). This reading is referred to as "120 over 80."

Blood pressure is measured with a sphygmomanometer—a soft rubber cuff connected to a rubber bulb that inflates the cuff and a meter that registers the pressure of the cuff. Listening with a stethoscope placed over the artery below the cuff, a health professional inflates the cuff until it compresses the artery tightly enough to temporarily stop blood flow. Then the cuff is gradually deflated. When the pressure in the cuff equals the maximum pressure in the artery, the artery opens and the sound of the blood rushing through the artery is amplified by the stethoscope. This is the systolic pressure. As the cuff pressure is reduced further, the sound suddenly becomes faint. This is the diastolic pressure—the pressure exerted when the heart relaxes between beats.

Hypertension is defined as a systolic pressure at rest that averages 140 mm Hg or higher, a diastolic pressure at rest that averages 90 mm Hg or higher, or both. As shown in Table 8.1, the higher the blood pressure, the greater the risks. In most people with hypertension, both systolic and diastolic pressures are high. Although hypertension can be successfully

---

High blood pressure or **hypertension** is a chronic elevation of blood pressure, defined as a systolic pressure of 140 mm Hg or higher and/or a diastolic pressure of 90 mm Hg or higher.

TABLE 8.1   CLASSIFICATION OF BLOOD PRESSURE

CATEGORY	SYSTOLIC (mm Hg)		DIASTOLIC (mm Hg)
Normal	<120	and	<80
Prehypertension	120–139	or	80–89
Hypertension Stage 1	140–159	or	90–99
Hypertension Stage 2	≥160	or	≥100

Note: High blood pressure is not diagnosed based on a single reading. If an initial reading is high, a second reading should be taken a few minutes later. Elevated readings should then be confirmed in the other arm.

Source: *Seventh Report of the Joint National Committee on Prevention, Detection, Evaluation and Treatment of High Blood Pressure*, 2003. **www.nhlbi.nih.gov/guidelines/hypertension**

controlled, in most cases (over 90 percent of the time) its actual cause remains a medical mystery. This condition is formally known as *essential* or *primary hypertension.*

Hypertension is widespread in the U.S. population, affecting nearly one in three adults. Of those with hypertension, about 30 percent don't know that they have it. There is a popular myth that persons can "sense or feel" when their blood pressure is high. This is a false belief. Some folks think that if they don't feel ill, they must be OK. The truth is that hypertension typically has no symptoms for many years. This is why hypertension is known as "the silent killer."

Compared to people with normal blood pressure, those with uncontrolled hypertension have a two- to three-fold greater risk of heart attack and a three- to four-fold greater risk of stroke. Other prominent risks include kidney damage and heart failure. Hypertension is significantly more common in blacks, adults over age 75, and the obese.

If you don't already know your blood pressure or if it's been more than a year since you had it checked, get a reading and record it. Everyone should know their blood pressure. If you have hypertension, work out a plan with your doctor to control it. There are a variety of approaches using combinations of weight reduction, dietary changes, aerobic exercise, stress management, and drug therapy.

HIGH BLOOD CHOLESTEROL

A **high blood cholesterol** level, technically known as *hypercholesterolemia,* is another important modifiable risk factor. A total cholesterol value equal

High blood cholesterol, or hypercholesterolemia, is an abnormally elevated total cholesterol level as measured from a blood sample.

to or greater than 240 mg/dL (milligrams per deciliter of blood) is defined as high, putting a person at increased risk of atherosclerosis and thus heart attack, stroke, and peripheral arterial disease. Elevated cholesterol values can be due to many factors: a diet high in saturated fats, smoking, obesity, physical inactivity, and diabetes. Like hypertension, high cholesterol has no symptoms, and many people are unaware that they have the risk factor. About one of five American adults has high blood cholesterol.

The National Institute of Health recommends that everyone age 20 and older should have their cholesterol levels measured. The preferred blood test is a fasting lipoprotein profile which measures not only total blood cholesterol but also its components: low-density lipoprotein (LDL) cholesterol, high-density lipoprotein (HDL) cholesterol, and triglycerides.

Cholesterol is transported throughout the circulatory system by combining with lipoprotein carriers that vary in size and weight (e.g., LDL, HDL). The LDL-cholesterol combination is readily deposited on arterial walls and is a major constituent of plaque. LDL cholesterol—a.k.a. the "bad" cholesterol—is the largest component of total cholesterol and the primary target for cholesterol-lowering treatment. Conversely, the HDL-cholesterol combination functions in just the opposite manner and prevents plaque build up in the arteries. Thus, HDL cholesterol is dubbed the "good" cholesterol. It is the only blood lipid in which higher levels are better.

The classification system for total, LDL, and HDL cholesterol is presented in Table 8.2. Notice the target values: total cholesterol under 200 mg/dL, LDL cholesterol under 100, and HDL cholesterol equal to or greater than 60. An overall index of CHD risk is determined from the ratio of total cholesterol to HDL cholesterol. Ratios range from 3 or less (e.g., 180/60) which would be low risk and highly desirable to 10 or higher (e.g., 250/25) which would be high risk and require medical follow-up. An ideal target is to keep the total cholesterol well below 200, with the HDL cholesterol accounting for 30 percent or more.

Average ratios (total cholesterol/HDL cholesterol) are 3.3 to 3.8 for young adult men and 3.0 to 3.5 for young adult women. The more favorable ratio in women is due to their higher levels of HDL cholesterol, which is associated with the female hormone estrogen. This is one reason why women are at lower risk for CHD and stroke through midlife. After menopause (as estrogen levels diminish), women lose this HDL cholesterol advantage, and the incidence of atherosclerotic diseases increases. For both genders, total cholesterol and thus LDL cholesterol levels increase with age.

How do we decrease LDL cholesterol and increase HDL cholesterol? For most people with borderline values, a prudent low fat diet and aerobic exercise, respectively, are effective approaches to improving the blood lipid profile. If your LDL level is high, it's important to meet with your doctor. Effective cholesterol-lowering (LDL) drug therapy is available as an additional treatment if needed.

TABLE 8.2   CLASSIFICATION OF BLOOD LIPIDS

TOTAL CHOLESTEROL (mg/dL)

<200	Desirable
200–239	Borderline high
≥240	High

LDL CHOLESTEROL (mg/dL)—PRIMARY TARGET OF THERAPY

<100	Optimal
100–129	Near optimal
130–159	Borderline high
160–189	High
>190	Very high

HDL CHOLESTEROL (mg/dL)

<40	Low
≥60	High

Note: Exclusive of the LDL cholesterol, a low HDL cholesterol (<40) is a major risk factor. Conversely, a high HDL cholesterol (≥60) is cardioprotective.

Source: *Third Report of the Expert Panel on Detection, Evaluation, and Treatment of High Blood Cholesterol in Adults,* 2004. **www.nhlbi.nih.gov/guidelines/cholesterol**

As you now see, understanding your lipid profile as a risk factor is not just a matter of knowing total cholesterol. Years ago, this was the case. But that was prior to the discovery of the lipid subcomponents and an understanding of their roles. Although the term *high blood cholesterol* (or hypercholesterolemia) continues to be widely used, it's now known to be an oversimplification. The more accurate term is **abnormal blood lipids** (or dyslipidemia, *dys-* means "abnormal"), which refers to elevations of total cholesterol, LDL cholesterol, and triglycerides and/or low HDL cholesterol. In the years ahead, the term *abnormal blood lipids* will eventually replace *high blood cholesterol.*

Everyone should know his or her blood lipid values. In a 2003 national survey by the CDC, only 60 percent of Americans aged 20 to 44 reported blood cholesterol screening during the preceding five years. If you have not had a lipoprotein profile performed within the past several years, get one. You should be as familiar with your cholesterol levels as you are with your height, weight, BMI, and blood pressure.

Abnormal blood lipids, or dyslipidemia, is elevated levels of total cholesterol, LDL cholesterol, and triglycerides and/or low HDL cholesterol as measured from a blood sample.

Health & the Media Health Messages That Strike a Chord

The American Heart Association (AHA) has long been a leader in communicating health messages to the public. In recent years, these messages have broadened from straightforward ads to raise awareness of risk factors and signs of a heart attack or stroke to more complex messages to motivate and enable behavior change. This new emphasis is captured in the "You're the Cure" campaign and encompasses not just individual behavior change but also advocacy for children, families, and communities. This print ad certainly strikes a chord. How can we not want to improve the health of children? It also makes us reflect on our responsibility as role models. The action points—advocating for daily PE and healthy food choices in school—clearly link the prevention of childhood obesity to reducing risk for heart disease and stroke. Highlighting the multiple benefits of healthy lifestyle behaviors is a key message that underlies chronic disease prevention. AHA is an excellent resource for up-to-date information on how to improve diet, exercise regularly, and manage risk factors.

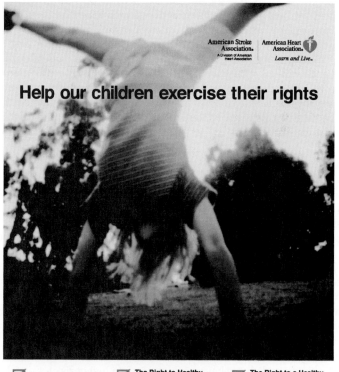

Until the 1990s, the American Heart Association identified only three *major* risk factors that could be changed: cigarette smoking, high blood pressure, and high blood cholesterol. Other modifiable risk factors, described as *secondary* or *contributing* risk factors, were associated with an increased risk for cardiovascular disease, but their significance and prevalence had not yet been precisely determined. However, as the research evidence continued to mount, it became clear that several of the secondary risk factors were of similar importance as the first three. Accordingly, physical inactivity in 1992 and then obesity and diabetes in 1998 were upgraded to *major* risk factors.

Physical Inactivity

Physical inactivity is an independent risk for heart attack and stroke. When inactivity is combined with overeating, obesity and diabetes can result. All contribute to the development of atherosclerosis. Conversely, regular moderate-to-vigorous exercise reduces the risk of heart and blood vessel diseases. Exercise can also favorably modify other risk factors by controlling blood cholesterol, obesity, and diabetes as well as lowering high blood pressure. Yet, only 3 in 10 adults are active enough to achieve these health benefits. Or put another way, 7 in 10 are not engaging in sufficient levels of physical activity. Although any increase in physical activity among the sedentary may impart some benefit, regularly engaging in moderate activities (e.g., 30 minutes of brisk walking five days a week) is known to improve cardiorespiratory function and lower the risk of cardiovascular disease. In general, physical activity follows a dose-response curve—the more active you are, the better. Refer to Chapter 3 for more information on physical activity and exercise guidelines.

Obesity

People with excess body fat—particularly if the fat is in the waist/trunk area (abdominal obesity)—are at higher risk of CHD. Obesity also contributes to the development of other risk factors for atherosclerosis: high blood pressure, high blood cholesterol, and diabetes. However, obesity puts people at higher risk of cardiovascular disease even if they don't have other risk factors. One in three American adults are obese (BMI of 30 or more; e.g., 5'5"/180 lb or 6'0"/221 lb = BMI of 30). Losing excess body fat reduces a person's risk for atherosclerosis as well as other associated disorders. In many cases, even modest weight loss (5 to 10 percent of body weight) can help significantly. Refer to the section on healthy weight in Chapter 2 for information on safe and effective weight loss and maintenance strategies.

Diabetes

People who have diabetes have a two- to six-fold higher risk for developing atherosclerosis than those without diabetes. Diabetes—defined as a high blood glucose level (fasting value of 126 mg/dL or higher)—is a disease in which the body does not produce or respond properly to insulin. The most common form of diabetes is type 2, which usually develops in adults during middle age. In recent years though, onset of diabetes is occurring at younger ages. Among Americans age 20 and older, 1 in every 11 persons has diabetes. Even when glucose levels are controlled, diabetics still have an increased risk of heart attack and stroke. Most diabetics die from cardiovascular disease. Diabetes damages the blood vessels and is linked with low HDL ("good") cholesterol, high triglycerides, and high blood pressure. Women who have diabetes are not protected from atherosclerosis before menopause. Also, physical inactivity and weight (fat) gain contribute to the development of diabetes. This dangerous combination of risk factors—elevated blood glucose, high blood fats, high blood pressure, and obesity—is called the metabolic syndrome (discussed in Chapter 10). For those with diabetes, regular medical checkups are essential. For everyone else, remember that diabetes is largely a preventable disease. Refer to Chapter 10 for an expanded discussion on diabetes.

What Is Your Risk? How the Framingham Heart Study Shaped Our Understanding of Risks

This chapter cites many statistics regarding risk factors and an individual's odds of developing cardiovascular disease. But how were those statistics arrived at? It may be surprising, but much of our information regarding heart disease risk factors comes from one massive study that began in the late 1940s.

During the first half of the 20th century, the rate of cardiovascular disease increased dramatically among Americans. The U.S. Public Health Service decided to undertake a large-scale study to investigate why. Researchers wanted to learn which biologic and environmental factors were contributing to the rapid rise in cardiovascular death and disability. They agreed on an epidemiological study, a new approach at the time, to learn how and why those who developed heart disease differed from those who remained disease-free.

In 1948, the town of Framingham, Massachusetts, located outside of Boston, was selected as the study site, and 5,209 healthy residents between 30 and 60 years of age, both men and women, were enrolled as the first study group. Each participant underwent a detailed medical history, a physical examination, and comprehensive laboratory tests. Every two years, participants returned for similar comprehensive medical examinations.

In 1971, 5,124 children (and their spouses) of the original participants were recruited for the "offspring study." Currently, the children of the offspring group, called "third generation" group, are being enrolled and will be studied to further understand how genetic factors relate to cardiovascular disease. The goal is to recruit 3,500 grandchildren of the original group. Over the decades, new diagnostic technologies have been added to the ongoing protocols.

(Continued)

The extensive longitudinal data from the Framingham Heart Study led to the identification of the major CHD risk factors. In fact, the Framingham researchers coined the term *risk factor* in 1961. Over the years, the researchers have examined key elements of American lifestyle and have found, for example, that a lifestyle typified by a poor diet, sedentary living, and/or excessive weight gain increased the risk factors. The Framingham study has played a central role in influencing health care professionals to place greater emphasis on prevention and on detecting and treating cardiovascular disease risk factors in their earliest stages. Results from Framingham also stimulated national awareness campaigns educating the American public to the risk factors for CHD and stroke, particularly tobacco use, high blood pressure, and high cholesterol levels.

Without question, the Framingham study has profoundly advanced our understanding of the major risk factors for cardiovascular disease. Over the past half-century, about 1,200 articles have been published in the leading medical journals. Most of what you read in this chapter is based on or confirmed by the Framingham Heart Study. In the years ahead, look for reports from the Framingham study as their researchers continue to update and expand our knowledge about the prevention and control of cardiovascular disease.

To estimate your risk for CHD and stroke, use the links below. Also, consider calculating the risk profile for one of your parents or grandparents. To get a sense of what your health status might be like in another 25 or 30 years, simply take a hard look at your parents. If you are concerned with what lies ahead, think about preventive approaches and be proactive. The Framingham study demonstrated that heart disease is largely a consequence of lifestyle and everyday choices.

Texas Heart Institute: How Healthy Is Your Heart?
http://hht.texasheartinstitute.org

Harvard School of Public Health: Disease Risk Index
www.diseaseriskindex.harvard.edu

OTHER RISK FACTORS

Although not considered major risk factors, other factors are known to contribute to heart disease and stroke risk. Some people have particularly intense cardiovascular responses (e.g., sharp spikes in heart rate and blood pressure) to stressful conditions. Under conditions of continual stress, this high physiological reactivity can contribute to the development of cardiovascular disease. People who score high on personality traits of anger and hostility are also at higher risk. Such individuals, primarily men, typically display an explosive temper or expect the worst from people. This is damaging to their own health as well as unpleasant for those around them. Third, drinking too much alcohol can raise blood pressure and triglycerides and cause other cardiac problems as well as contributing to obesity, alcoholism, suicide, and accidents. As a side note, moderate alcohol consumption has been shown to reduce CHD risk by elevating HDL cholesterol. However, the evidence is not strong enough to recommend that teetotalers should begin drinking to improve their cardiovascular health!

Always hunting for new clues that will lead to a more complete understanding of cardiovascular disease, scientists continue to search for additional risk factors. Examples include homocysteine, which is an amino acid that appears to be associated with atherosclerosis and clot formation; lipoprotein (a), which may be harmful due to its role in preventing the breakup of clots; and viruses and other infectious agents that may damage blood vessel walls and start the atherosclerotic process. As research progresses, specific biochemical markers for these and other risk factors may eventually lead to additional or better methods for predicting or diagnosing cardiovascular disease.

✓ **NEED TO KNOW**

Major risk factors for CHD and stroke are categorized as nonmodifiable and modifiable. The three nonmodifiable risk factors are increasing age, being male, and having a family history of CHD. The six modifiable risk factors are cigarette smoking, high blood pressure, abnormal blood lipids, physical inactivity, obesity, and diabetes. CHD and stroke are largely preventable diseases. Good nutrition, regular exercise, and maintaining a healthy weight are key elements to cardiovascular health.

➤ Interventions

The aim of this section is to provide a brief overview of the most common behavioral, pharmacological, and surgical approaches to reduce risk of heart attack and stroke and to treat atherosclerosis.

BEHAVIORAL APPROACH

If you have one or more of the six modifiable risk factors, the first step should be to consider lifestyle modification to reduce risk. Most primary care doctors will be glad to hear of your initiative to improve your health and help you develop an appropriate plan. Practical, science-based, online resources are cited throughout the *Concise Guide* to help you break the smoking habit, improve eating and exercise patterns, and reach and maintain a healthy weight. If you plan these risk-lowering behavior changes on your own, it would be smart to consult with your physician before starting. It is important to have your doctor's support. Depending on your overall health status and risk profile, your doctor may feel it necessary to prescribe medications immediately along with your steps to improve lifestyle behaviors.

Occasionally a doctor may not support a person's desire to improve health habits and recommend relying solely on medications to lower or control risk factors. This approach is not common, but it does occur. If the doctor's rationale is unclear, then get a second opinion. A time-honored principle in the practice of medicine is to do the patient no harm. This reminds us that—even in the 21st century, when drugs are available for nearly every known malady—medications should be used only as needed. If nondrug alternatives such as lifestyle changes are available and feasible, they should be tried first or at least in combination with medications.

PHARMACOLOGICAL APPROACH

This overview focuses on the use of medicines and the importance of patient-doctor communication to break tobacco dependence or treat and control high blood pressure and abnormal blood lipids. Dozens of other cardiovascular drugs are available to treat a multitude of related conditions. While discussion of these is beyond the scope of the *Concise Guide,* an excellent resource to learn about specific prescription and over-the-counter drugs is the *Physicians' Desktop Reference* Web site **(www.pdrhealth.com/drug_info/index.html).**

Nicotine replacement treatments via gum, inhaler, nasal spray, or patch are often prescribed for tobacco users who want to stop smoking, chewing, or dipping. Consult with your doctor about using nicotine or other drugs to help break the habit of tobacco dependence. He or she will gladly discuss drug treatment as well as counseling and behavioral options. Some doctors record history of tobacco use (i.e., current, former, never) as a vital sign along with their patients' pulse, blood pressure, temperature, and respiratory rate. If you use tobacco and value your health, talk to your doctor or other health care provider about stopping. Remember, it's never too late to stop!

Drugs to treat and control high blood pressure and high blood cholesterol are two of the most common types of drugs prescribed in the United States. There are a variety of both anti-hypertensive drugs and LDL-cholesterol-lowering drugs available. Doctors have many choices regarding specific drugs and dosages. Yet, a major challenge to doctors is noncompliance, or patients not taking their medications. During initial drug treatments, many people abruptly stop taking the medication due to unpleasant side effects and *do not follow up* with their doctor. It's critical for people to report side effects to their doctor so that adjustments can be made. Successful treatment depends on the patient and doctor working in partnership, with the patient taking an active role in his or her own health.

In a sense, noncompliance is a natural response. Most people with high blood pressure or high cholesterol feel fine; they don't have symptoms of sickness. Yet, they are told they have high blood pressure or abnormal blood lipids and it must be treated. In turn, the prescribed medicines may make them feel odd or ill or disrupt their normal patterns in some way— for example, they begin experiencing sluggishness, achiness, frequent trips to the toilet, difficulty sleeping, or a host of other side effects.

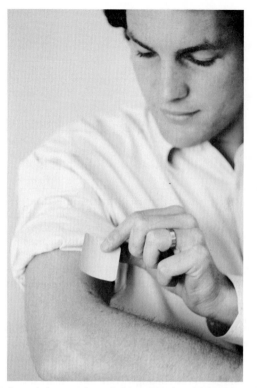

A nicotine patch can help a smoker quit by easing the withdrawal cravings the smoker experiences.

What is the solution? First, realize that high blood pressure and abnormal blood lipids need to be treated. The damage caused by either of these conditions is cumulative and permanent. If your doctor recommends drug therapy, side effects may occur. Be aware from the beginning that it may take several calls or office visits to find the right drug/dose combination. You need to be an active partner with your doctor to find a treatment that is satisfactory to both of you. Share this insight. If you know others who are having difficulty staying on their medicines, strongly encourage them to go back to their doctors.

SURGICAL APPROACH

Since the 1960s, coronary angiography, also known as *cardiac catherization*, has been the gold standard for determining the degree of blockage in the coronary arteries. After a series of initial diagnostic tests, angiography is typically performed when CHD is suspected. In this procedure, a tiny hollow tube or catheter is inserted into an artery in the arm or leg and guided to the heart, where a contrast dye is released and X-rays are taken. From the resulting images, the degree of atherosclerosis—the narrowing of the coronary arteries—can be measured. If severe blockage is present in one

FIGURE 8.1   CORONARY ANGIOPLASTY

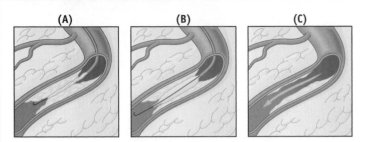

(A)   **(B)**   **(C)**

(A) From an artery in the leg or arm, a catheter (thin tube) is positioned in the narrow part of the coronary artery. A very thin wire tipped with an expandable balloon is threaded across the blocked area. (B) The balloon is inflated and deflated several times to compress the surrounding plaque and open the artery. The balloon is then deflated and the catheter removed. (C) The artery is now wider and blood can flow more easily.

Reprinted with permission **www.americanheart.org** © 2007, American Heart Association, Inc.

or more coronary arteries, the options are usually coronary angioplasty or coronary artery bypass surgery. Multiple factors are considered in determining whether a patient is a candidate for either surgical procedure.

Both types of surgery are amazingly common, remarkably safe, and in the vast majority of cases, successful in restoring functional capacity and relieving symptoms such as chest pain (angina). However, if patients don't follow prescribed lifestyle changes and drug treatments after surgery, the surgical benefits may be relatively short-term. Some people find themselves back on the operating table a few years later for a second surgery. Over 660,000 angioplasty procedures and nearly 430,000 bypass surgeries were performed in the United States in 2004. That's about 1,800 angioplasties and nearly 1,200 bypass surgeries per day every day throughout the year!

Coronary Angioplasty

Coronary angioplasty, or balloon angioplasty, is technically known as *percutaneous coronary intervention* (PCI) (*percutaneous* means "through the skin"). This catheter-based procedure is performed to open up a blocked coronary artery and restore blood flow to the heart muscle. Generally, coronary angioplasty is preferred to bypass surgery because it is less invasive and faster. During the procedure, the patient remains awake and

Coronary angioplasty is a surgical procedure in which a balloon-tipped catheter is inserted into a diseased narrowed coronary artery; inflation of balloon stretches the vessel opening, improving blood flow through it. Also called *balloon angioplasty,* and technically known as *percutaneous coronary intervention.*

FIGURE 8.2   CORONARY ARTERY BYPASS GRAFT

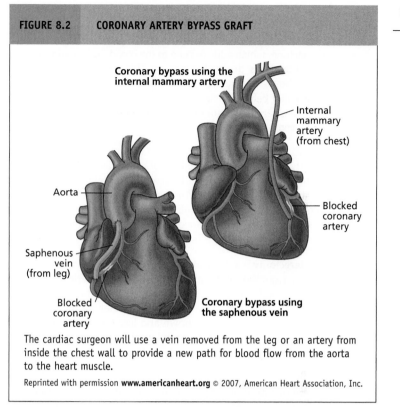

The cardiac surgeon will use a vein removed from the leg or an artery from inside the chest wall to provide a new path for blood flow from the aorta to the heart muscle.

Reprinted with permission **www.americanheart.org** © 2007, American Heart Association, Inc.

conscious. The procedure involves guiding a catheter (thin tube) through a large peripheral artery (usually the femoral artery) into the aorta and eventually into the narrowed artery. A small inflatable balloon at the end of a wire is then threaded into position and inflated. This compresses the plaque that narrows the artery. In most cases, a stent (a tiny wire mesh tube) is positioned in this newly opened artery and left permanently in place to help keep the artery open. After one or two days in the hospital, the patient usually returns home.

Coronary Artery Bypass Graft

Coronary artery bypass graft, commonly called *bypass surgery,* consists of grafting vessels taken from another part of the body (e.g., vein from leg, or artery from chest wall) to a coronary artery and the aorta. Blood flow is thus

Coronary artery bypass graft, or bypass surgery, creates a new route around a significantly narrowed coronary artery or multiple diseased arteries using a vein from the leg or an inner chest-wall artery, permitting increased blood flow to deliver oxygen and nutrients to the heart muscle. Bypass surgery is one of the most commonly performed major operations.

rerouted, skipping over (bypassing) the narrowed or blocked area. In the traditional surgery, an incision is made down the center of the chest from the neck to the top of the stomach, and the breastbone is parted. The patient is on a heart-lung machine, which adds oxygen to the blood and circulates blood to other parts of the body during the surgery. This open-heart surgery can take four to six hours depending on the number of blood vessels to be grafted. The modifier before *bypass*—for example, *triple* or *quadruple*—refers to the number of arteries that are bypassed. The hospital recovery stay is typically five to seven days.

Other surgical techniques and technologies are being used more frequently. One increasingly popular method, called *off-pump coronary artery bypass*, avoids use of the heart-lung machine. This operation allows the bypass to be created while the heart is still beating. Another less-invasive alternative is the use of smaller incisions that avoid splitting the breastbone. Lastly, some bypass procedures are being performed using surgeon-directed robotics.

Carotid Endarterectomy

Carotid endarterectomy is a surgical procedure done to prevent strokes by removing plaque from the carotid arteries. The carotid arteries are located on each side of the neck and extend from the aorta to the base of the skull. Narrowed carotid arteries are diagnosed using a variety of medical imaging techniques. Although less well known and less frequently performed than angioplasty or bypass surgery, carotid endarterectomy is a common operation (about 98,000 in 2004) and a safe and long-lasting treatment.

The patient may be given a general anesthesia or, alternately, only the neck area may be numbed to allow the patient to communicate with the surgeon during the operation. The surgery involves making an incision to expose the narrowed carotid artery. The artery is temporarily clamped or bypassed, and another incision is made directly into the blocked section of the artery. The surgeon removes the plaque deposits, stitches the artery, removes the clamps or the bypass, and closes the neck incision. The procedure lasts about two hours. Following surgery, the average hospital stay is one or two days.

Three of the most common cardiovascular surgeries have been reviewed. Surgical techniques are continually being modified and improved. Moreover, applications of new technologies are providing new options for removing arterial plaque—for example, miniaturized devices and tools using the latest laser, mechanical, and chemical technology.

All three cardiac procedures can be viewed in tutorials with animation graphics at **www.nlm.nih.gov/medlineplus/tutorial.html**

Heart Transplants

As an endnote to this section on surgical approaches, we'll take a look at the ultimate cardiovascular surgery—heart transplantation. For a few

---

Carotid endarterectomy is a surgical procedure in which a narrowed carotid artery is opened and the plaque is removed to restore adequate blood flow to the brain.

FIGURE 8.3   CAROTID ENDARTERECTOMY

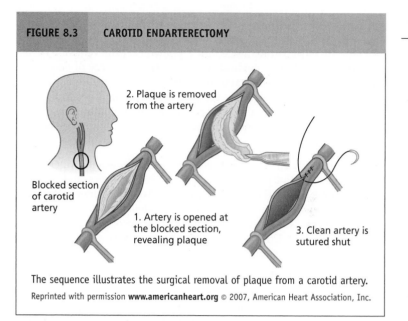

2. Plaque is removed from the artery

Blocked section of carotid artery

1. Artery is opened at the blocked section, revealing plaque

3. Clean artery is sutured shut

The sequence illustrates the surgical removal of plaque from a carotid artery.

Reprinted with permission **www.americanheart.org** © 2007, American Heart Association, Inc.

patients with advanced heart disease, it may represent the only option left. The first heart transplant was performed in 1967 in Groote Schuur Hospital, Cape Town, South Africa, by Professor Christiaan Barnard and his surgical team. It was a milestone in medicine. The patient only lived for 18 days, succumbing in the end to pneumonia. But his new heart beat strongly to the end. Dr. Barnard showed the world that a human heart transplant was possible. The science of organ transplantation is now highly refined and recipient outcomes are remarkably successful. Since 1990, there has been an average of over 2,000 heart transplants per year in the United States. Nationwide, over 180 medical centers perform heart transplants. Survival rates are about 85 percent for one year and nearly 70 percent for five years. As expected, the costs are enormous—surgery and treatments for the first year are estimated to be $400,000–500,000.

✓ NEED TO KNOW

Interventions to treat known risk factors for CHD and stroke can be categorized as behavioral, pharmacological, and surgical. Modifying lifestyle habits is a powerful approach to reducing risk factors. Motivation and perseverance are needed, but the cost and the side effects are minimal. Drugs are available to help people stop smoking and to control high blood pressure and abnormal blood lipids. Standard surgical procedures include angioplasty and bypass procedures to treat CHD, and carotid endarterectomy to prevent stroke. Effective interventions often use combinations of behavioral, pharmacological, and surgical approaches.

➤ Prevention

Humans are intrigued with scientific and medical achievements. We are particularly dazzled by medical advances. The discovery of new drugs and the refinement of surgical techniques to treat cardiovascular disease are shining examples. With the constant highlighting of medical breakthroughs, we tend to minimize or overlook the enormous human pain and financial costs that come with heart disease and stroke—that is, until it strikes close to home.

No one purposely chooses a path that leads to disease and surgery, with the emotional and physical toll of the incisions, the tubes, and the pills. But by default, this is the path many follow. And more often than not, it leads to a life with limitations and loss of independence. In retrospect, many heart disease survivors encourage young people to pay attention to their health *now*. Don't wait until you're 40 or have a heart attack before you take stock of your lifestyle.

To gain insight into the emotional dimension and impact on quality of life, you should discuss the process of heart surgery with someone who has gone through it. A family member or a neighbor may be willing to share a firsthand account of their disease progression, surgery, and rehabilitation. Surgical options can indeed be life-saving treatments. Yet, if one can prevent the need for surgery by following a healthy lifestyle, then the choice seems clear.

Over 90 percent of people who develop atherosclerosis or experience a heart attack or stroke have one or more of the major risk factors. Science-based guidelines are available for all six of the modifiable risk factors. To keep your risk low, don't smoke, eat a prudent diet, exercise regularly, and maintain a healthy weight. Monitor your blood pressure, blood lipid profile, and blood glucose level and intervene as necessary to keep them in a healthy range. The central message is simple: cardiovascular disease is largely preventable through our own actions. The lifestyle habits you establish now will have a bearing on whether or when you will face drug therapy and surgery in the years ahead.

If the public were to adopt preventive measures, premature death and disability across all ages would decline markedly. A few notable scientists assert that cardiovascular disease need not influence one's quality of life until the age of 80 or later. Esteemed cardiologist Dr. Paul Dudley White stated that "a high, even 100 percent, mortality from cardiovascular disease nor sudden death itself are to be regretted, provided they take place at an advanced age after a healthy, happy, and useful life right up to the last minute."

Specific Topics

American Red Cross—Health & Safety Services
   www.redcross.org/services/hss
Disease Risk Index (Harvard School of Public Health)
   www.diseaseriskindex.harvard.edu
How Healthy Is Your Heart? (Texas Heart Institute)
   http://hht.texasheartinstitute.org
National Cholesterol Education Program
   www.nhlbi.nih.gov/about/ncep/index.htm
National Heart Attack Alert Program
   www.nhlbi.nih.gov/about/nhaap
National High Blood Pressure Education Program
   www.nhlbi.nih.gov/about/nhbpep/index.htm
Sudden Cardiac Arrest Association
   www.suddencardiacarrest.org
Tobacco Cessation Guidelines
   www.surgeongeneral.gov/tobacco
You Can Quit Smoking Now!
   www.smokefree.gov

General

American Heart Association (AHA)
   www.americanheart.org
American Stroke Association (a division of AHA)
   www.strokeassociation.org
CDC's Division for Heart Disease & Stroke Prevention
   www.cdc.gov/dhdsp
MedlinePlus Tutorials on Diagnostic and Surgical Procedures
   www.nlm.nih.gov/medlineplus/tutorial.html
Physicians' Desktop Reference
   www.pdrhealth.com/drugs/drugs-index.aspx

Knowing the Language

abnormal blood lipids
angina
atherosclerosis
carotid endarterectomy
coronary angioplasty
coronary artery bypass graft

coronary heart disease
heart attack
high blood cholesterol
high blood pressure
   (hypertension)
stroke

Understanding the Content

1. Define atherosclerosis, coronary heart disease, and stroke.
2. How do the signs of a heart attack differ from those of a stroke?
3. What is the difference between a modifiable and a nonmodifiable risk factor? Provide examples of each.
4. Give an example of a behavioral, a pharmacological, and a surgical intervention to reduce risk for cardiovascular disease.

Exploring Ideas

1. Assume you are walking across campus early one morning and you see a person lying on the ground who appears to have passed out. What would you do?
2. Prescription drugs are available to control high blood pressure and abnormal blood lipids, yet many people stop taking their medicines. What are possible explanations for this situation? What are possible solutions?
3. What lifestyle behaviors will lower the likelihood that we develop atherosclerosis? Within the context of the modifiable risk factors, describe the key cardioprotective behaviors.

Selected References

American Heart Association (AHA). What Is Carotid Endarterectomy? www.americanheart.org/downloadable/heart/110065676921546%20WhatIsCarotidEndarterect.pdf

AHA. What Is Coronary Angioplasty? www.americanheart.org/downloadable/heart/110072340569149%20WhatIsCoronaryAngioplast.pdf

AHA. What Is Coronary Bypass Surgery? www.americanheart.org/downloadable/heart/110072228916148%20WhatIsCornryBypsSrgry.pdf

AHA. Heart Attack, Stroke and Cardiac Arrest Warning Signs. www.americanheart.org/presenter.jhtml?identifier=3053

AHA. *Heart Disease and Stroke Statistics: 2007 Update At-a-Glance.* Dallas: American Heart Association, 2007. www.americanheart.org/downloadable/heart/1166712318459HS_StatsInsideText.pdf

AHA. Heart disease and stroke statistics—2007 update: A report from the American Heart Association Statistics Committee and Stroke Statistics Subcommittee. *Circulation* 115: e69–e171, 2007. http://circ.ahajournals.org/cgi/content/full/115/5/e69

American Red Cross. Saving a Life is as Easy as A-E-D. www.redcross.org/services/hss/courses/aed.html

Centers for Disease Control and Prevention (CDC), Division for Heart Disease & Stroke Prevention. Men and Heart Disease Fact Sheet.
www.cdc.gov/DHDSP/library/fs_men_heart.htm

CDC, Division for Heart Disease & Stroke Prevention. Women and Heart Disease Fact Sheet.
www.cdc.gov/DHDSP/library/fs_women_heart.htm

CDC. Trends in cholesterol screening and awareness of high blood cholesterol—United States, 1991–2003. *MMWR* 54 (35): 865-870, 2005.
www.cdc.gov/mmwr/preview/mmwrhtml/mm5435a2.htm

Framingham Heart Study: A Project of the National Heart, Lung and Blood Institute and Boston University
www.framinghamheartstudy.org

Hurst JW. Meaningful quotations from Paul Dudley White. *Clinical Cardiology* 21: 617–618, 1998.

Lear MW. *Heartsounds.* Pp. 11–12. New York: Simon and Schuster, 1980.

National Heart, Lung, and Blood Institute (NHLBI), NIH. Heart and Vascular Diseases.
www.nhlbi.nih.gov/health/public/heart/index.htm

NHLBI, NIH. Seventh Report of the Joint National Committee on Prevention, Detection, Evaluation and Treatment of High Blood Pressure, 2003.
www.nhlbi.nih.gov/guidelines/hypertension

NHLBI, NIH. Third Report of the Expert Panel on Detection, Evaluation, and Treatment of High Blood Cholesterol in Adults, 2004.
www.nhlbi.nih.gov/guidelines/cholesterol

Piscatella JC, Franklin BA. *Take a Load Off Your Heart: 109 Things You Can Actually Do to Prevent, Halt, and Reverse Heart Disease.* New York: Workman Publishing, 2003.

U.S. Department of Health and Human Services (DHHS). Health Consequences of Smoking: A Report of the Surgeon General. 2004.
www.cdc.gov/tobacco/sgr/sgr_2004/index.htm

U.S. DHHS. Tobacco Cessation Guidelines.
www.surgeongeneral.gov/tobacco

World Health Organization (WHO) and CDC. *The Atlas of Heart Disease and Stroke.*
www.who.int/cardiovascular_diseases/resources/atlas/en/

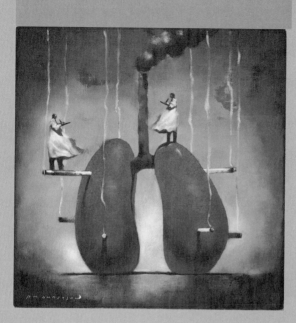

The truth is, if you asked me to choose between winning the Tour de France and cancer, I would choose cancer. Odd as it sounds, I would rather have the title of cancer survivor than winner of the Tour, because of what it has done for me as a human being, a man, a husband, a son and a father.

— LANCE ARMSTRONG

Chapter 9

CANCERS

In Chapter 9 we try to defuse the perception that cancer is synonymous with death. While people do die from cancer, there have been phenomenal advances in diagnosis and treatment. There is now hope where there was once none. This chapter discusses the basic disease process of cancer and also explains risks, prevention-oriented behaviors, early detection strategies, and treatment options.

ABC NEWS ANCHOR Peter Jennings and Dana Reeve, actress and wife of actor Christopher Reeve, have something in common: both died from lung cancer. Peter Jennings smoked heavily for many years and was diagnosed and died from cancer at age 67. Dana Reeve never smoked and was diagnosed and died from lung cancer at age 44. Jennings and Reeve are examples of what we do and don't know about cancer these days. One might expect Peter Jennings would eventually have a day of reckoning because of his risky lifestyle choice of smoking. But for Dana Reeve, what caused her cancer at such a relatively young age remains a mystery.

Reducing the impact of cancer is difficult because it requires proactive efforts on two fronts. People need to engage in healthy diet and behaviors throughout life to limit risk of developing cancer in the first place. Additionally, people should have regular screenings so in the event cancer does occur, it can be detected early and treated effectively. There are still many unknowns about why cancer strikes certain people and not others, and why some people respond better to treatment than others. But science continues to unravel these puzzles over time. Although the disease in both Reeve and Jennings followed the "traditional" pattern of late detection and a subsequently quick death, the good news is that more and more people are diagnosed with cancer early and respond favorably to treatments. Many become cancer-free after initial therapies and stay that way for the rest of their lives. And for others, cancer is not cured outright but is managed like a chronic disease, so that many people with cancer continue living productive lives despite being ill.

➤ Cancer

This year approximately 1,400,000 new cases of cancer will be diagnosed and over 550,000 Americans will die from the disease. One in four deaths in the United States is attributable to cancer. The good news is that, according to the American Cancer Society, the five-year survival rate for all cancers increased from 50 percent in 1974–76 to 65 percent in 2005. More people are surviving cancer because of education, early detection methods, and sophisticated treatment.

WHAT IS CANCER?

Cancer is a broad term that refers to the growth and spread of abnormal cells in the body. The cell is the basic unit of life. Cells that are alike group together and form tissue. Tissue makes organs, and organs make up body systems. There are nine major body systems: cardiovascular, respiratory, digestive, endocrine, skeletal, muscular, nervous, reproductive, and excretory. Figure 9.1 is a diagrammatic representation of the progression of cells to body systems.

Cancer is the growth and spread of abnormal cells.

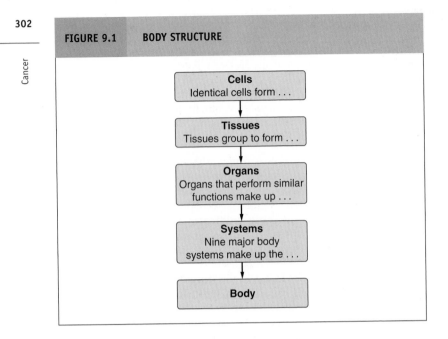

FIGURE 9.1 **BODY STRUCTURE**

Human cells have two major characteristics. They "survive" by dividing into new cells, and each type of cell has a specific function. For example, cells in the digestive system may secrete digestive enzymes, while those on the tongue may allow you to taste.

Normally cells divide and create the same types of tissues that they came from. But sometimes, something goes wrong in the division process. Two unhealthy cells derive from a normal one, and then those two cells continue creating more abnormal cells. The abnormal tissue created can make an organ unhealthy. Unhealthy organs will make a body system malfunction. If the process goes on unchecked, death will result.

CANCER TERMINOLOGY

A multitude of terms describe cancer and the disease process. The most basic ones are fairly simple. When a healthy cell becomes abnormal, it is said to mutate. Some **mutations** lead to cancers, but not all do. An abnormal cell that is not cancerous is referred to as **dysplasia.**

Chemicals from outside the body that influence cells to grow in abnormal ways are known as *carcinogens.* On the other hand, within the body, some

---

Mutation is the process by which a normal cell becomes abnormal.

Dysplasia is an abnormal cell that is not cancer.

FIGURE 9.2   LOSS OF CONTROL OF NORMAL CELL GROWTH

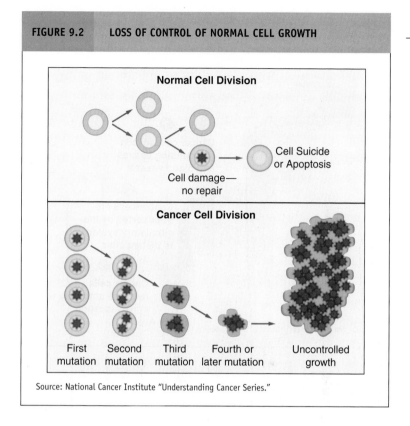

Source: National Cancer Institute "Understanding Cancer Series."

people have genes in their DNA that are known to be correlated with increased chance for certain types of cancers. These are referred to as **oncogenes.**

Finally, when cancer spreads from its point of origin to another area, the process is known as **metastasis.** For example, one might hear that the cancer has metastasized from the lungs to the bone, meaning that the cancer has spread from the lungs to the skeleton. Figures 9.2 and 9.3 show diagrammatic representations of all of these terms.

When abnormal cells divide, they normally form a structure referred to as a *tumor.* A tumor is a stacking of cells, sometimes also called a *growth.* Tumors do not have to contain cancer cells—a benign tumor is a growth of normal cells, and a malignant tumor is a growth of cancer cells. It

Oncogene are genes that increase the risk of cancer in a person who carries them.

Metastasis is the spread of cancer from its place of origin to somewhere else in the body.

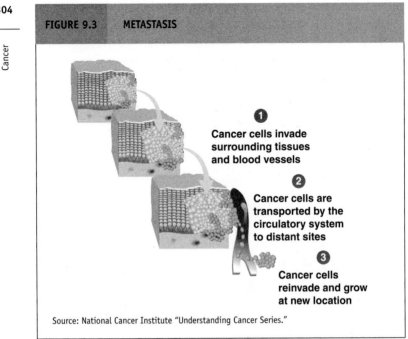

FIGURE 9.3   METASTASIS

1 Cancer cells invade surrounding tissues and blood vessels

2 Cancer cells are transported by the circulatory system to distant sites

3 Cancer cells reinvade and grow at new location

Source: National Cancer Institute "Understanding Cancer Series."

should be noted that just because something is referred to as *benign* doesn't necessarily mean it is not dangerous. Some benign tumors can significantly interfere with the function of an organ and body system and, as a result, can be life-threatening.

Often the terms *tumor* and *cyst* are used interchangeably, but this is incorrect. Cysts are a mass of cells with fluid in the center. Tumors have solid centers. Both, however, are growths. Another difference is that cysts are usually benign.

Tumors normally arise from certain types of body tissues and are named in a way that defines their origin. Tumor names also end with the suffix *-oma*. **Sarcomas** are tumors that arise from bone, cartilage, or muscle. **Lymphomas** originate in lymphatic tissue, and **carcinomas** arise from epithelial tissue, such as that in the skin, nose, and mouth. From a clinical perspective, the specific location of the tumor is often referred to when discussing the tumor. For example, the term *basal cell carcinoma* describes a tumor that is made up of basal cells found in skin.

Sarcomas are tumors that arise in bone, cartilage, or muscle.

Lymphomas are tumors that originate in lymphatic tissue.

Carcinomas are tumors that arise from epithelial tissue.

➤ Causes of Cancer

Many factors influence cellular change over time. Like many diseases, cancer generally has more than one cause.

HEREDITY

Deoxyribonucleic acid (**DNA**) is the cellular molecule containing the genetic code that organisms need to divide, grow, and function. There are 23 pairs of chromosomes in the nucleus of every cell in our body (except for red blood cells, sperm, and ova). Genes lie on the chromosomes and influence all sorts of body traits, from height and eye color to the propensity to develop certain types of cancers. If a person has a gene sequence that is linked with cancer, it usually means that at a certain point in a person's life, specific cells are more likely to grow abnormally than they would in a person without that oncogene.

In recent years health researchers have focused on decoding human DNA by mapping what different gene expressions do. Mapping the human genome is not a small task, because there are an estimated 20,000–25,000 genes in human DNA, with 3 billion chemical base pairs involved.

The alignment of the chemical base pairs spells out the genetic code, including disease. The Human Genome Project has estimated that there are about 1.4 million locations where single-base DNA differences occur in humans that seem to correlate with cancer and other diseases. The genetic sequences that are linked to a disease are sometimes referred to as "markers." In the case of cancer, having a marker does not mean the person will inevitably develop cancer. But it indicates that the person is at a much higher risk for developing a form of the disease if certain environmental variables are present. For example, people who have a marker for lung cancer but do not smoke have a low risk of lung cancer. If they do smoke, then their risk of lung cancer is very high—bigger than the risk of a smoker who doesn't have the lung cancer marker. Again, it is the marker combined with the unfavorable

DNA (deoxyribonucleic acid) is the genetic code inside nearly all cells that gives instructions on how the cell will divide, grow, and function.

environment (via smoking) that greatly increases the overall chance for cancer.

Although it sounds like science fiction, some day we may be able to alter a problematic line of code in a person's DNA and eradicate hereditary-linked cancers. Until then, the best way to deal with what we may be genetically predisposed to is to be aware of the kinds of cancer that run in our family, to try to live a healthy lifestyle, and to get early and regular screenings to minimize risks.

ENVIRONMENT

Some chemicals in our environment can cause cancer. These substances are called **carcinogens**. Some of the more common ones include sulfur dioxide, arsenic, asbestos, benzene, chromium, radon, soot, tar, vinyl chloride, wood dust, and ultraviolet light.

Sulfur dioxide is a product of combustion engines and is a component in air pollution. Exposure to sulfur dioxide over time can cause cell mutations that contribute to the development of lung cancer. Arsenic is found in pesticides and has been linked to lung, skin, and liver cancer. Asbestos, a risk factor for lung cancer, was once a key chemical in glues, home insulation, and tile products. As a result, many construction workers who worked before asbestos was outlawed in the late 20th century were put at risk for cancer. Similarly, petroleum workers are often exposed to benzene, which has been linked to leukemia, and metal workers must deal with exposure to chromium, a chemical that increases the risk of lung cancer.

Radon is an underground gas found in geological pockets in many parts of the United States. It can leak through the foundation of homes unnoticed because it has no odor. Prolonged exposure to radon can increase the risk of lung cancer. Excessive soot and tar exposure, such as that experienced by industrial workers, has been linked to lung, skin, and liver cancers. Frequent exposure to wood dust has been associated with nasal cancer. Finally, exposure to ultraviolet light from the sun is strongly related to the development of skin cancer.

Again, it is important to note that exposure doesn't automatically mean disease. But people who have high levels of exposure to carcinogens run greater than average risks for developing certain cancers, and the longer the duration of exposure, the higher the probability of getting cancer. Environmental health specialists are very skilled at implementing ways to reduce exposure, so although an occupation may be risky, certain precautions like protective masks, sunscreen, or special clothing can help minimize harmful exposures.

A **carcinogen** is a chemical or substance in the environment that can cause cancer in someone who is exposed to it.

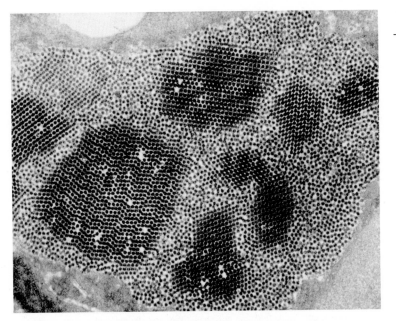

The Human Papilloma Virus (HPV) is a leading cause of cervical cancer in women. Pap Smear tests are important screening tools in finding abnormal cells early.

VIRUSES

Viruses are microorganisms that invade other organisms and use their cellular materials to replicate itself. (A more detailed explanation of viruses is in Chapter 11, "Infections.") Since cancer involves abnormal replication of body cells, it makes sense that if viruses are capable of disrupting the genetic mechanisms in cells, their process might be a contributing factor to cancer. Fortunately, only a few viruses are thought to actually cause cancer.

Herpes virus 2, the most common form of genital herpes, can affect cervical cells and increase a woman's risk of cervical cancer. The same holds true for women infected with human papillomavirus (HPV). Hepatitis B affects liver cells and may increase the risk of liver cancer. Epstein-Barr virus (EBV), the cause of mononucleosis, increases the risk of lymphoma, and human T-cell lymphotrophic virus is related to leukemia.

People who have been infected with cancer-linked viruses should be monitored more closely than those who have not. For example, a woman with a herpes 2 infection should have Pap smears to determine the health of the cervical cells on a more regular basis than a woman who isn't infected with herpes 2. Understanding the early signs of related cancers is important so people can seek medical help early, if necessary. A more thorough discussion about herpes and HPV, including the issues surrounding Gardasil, the vaccine for HPV, can be found in Chapter 11, "Infections."

As with so many diseases, the everyday choices we make can influence our risk for cancer. Lifestyles are a key factor in the etiology of many common cancers. Tobacco use is strongly implicated in the development of lung cancer. People who smoke 30 cigarettes or more each day have a 15 times greater risk of developing lung cancer than nonsmokers. Even smoke that non-smokers inhale—"second-hand smoke"—can increase the risk of lung cancer. Additionally, combining cigarettes and alcohol increases the risk of cancer of the esophagus. People who drink more than four drinks a day and smoke have a 40 times greater chance of developing cancer of the esophagus than people who don't combine heavy alcohol consumption with smoking.

Meat consumption and colon cancer are also related. The higher the consumption of red meat, the greater the risk of colon cancer. The population of the United States consumes large amounts of red meat and has one of the highest incidences of cancer of the colon. Specific information regarding reducing one's risk will be discussed later in the chapter.

✓ NEED TO KNOW

Cancer is multicausal. There are both hereditary and environmental components to cancer. Depending upon the type of cancer, the hereditary influence might be stronger that the environmental or vice versa. It is critical that people know the kinds of cancers that run in their families and learn which environmental variables are related to the development of the cancer so that they can limit their exposure to those variables. If a certain type of cancer is present in their family, people need to assume they have a genetic predisposition and limit their risk.

➤ Diagnosing Cancer

Diagnosing cancer requires an examination of cells to determine if they are normal or malignant (cancerous). The protocol for diagnosis involves the same steps used for identifying any disease. It begins when people explain their medical history, describe their symptoms, and are examined by a medical professional.

EXAMINATIONS AND BIOPSIES

When people have physical symptoms that are of concern, they usually visit a physician who asks about the severity of symptoms and the length of time they have been occurring. The physician performs physical examinations to determining health status, such as listening to the heart and lungs and measuring blood pressure. This examination may reveal suspicious findings that require further testing.

In the case of cancer, further testing can include examinations with imaging technologies such as X-rays, CT scans, or MRIs (see Chapter 12 for more explanation of some of these technologies). Some cancers leave traces in the blood, so tests may also be conducted on blood samples. For example, if a man has prostate cancer, his blood will show high levels of prostate specific antigen (PSA).

If something looks abnormal in blood work or a scan image, a biopsy is performed. A **biopsy** is the removal and examination of a segment of the abnormal tissue or tumor. The cells are examined in order to determine if they are benign or malignant. Biopsies can be performed in a range of ways. The least invasive type is with a needle inserted into the tumor which draws out cells for study. Other times, surgery may be needed to obtain a tissue sample. Most biopsies are uncomfortable but not highly painful.

STAGING OF CANCER

Once cells are determined to be malignant, the next step is to determine how serious and advanced the malignancy is. In other words, how deep is the cancer and has it metastasized? **Staging** is the term used to determine how invasive the cancer is. There are three types of staging: tumors (T), nodes (N), and metastasis (M). *T, N,* and *M* values are assigned after the diagnosis of cancer.

If a tumor cannot be measured or found, then it is called *TX*. When there is no evidence of a primary tumor, a *T0* is noted, which means that cancer has been diagnosed but the tumor has not been found. If the tumor has not started to grow into the surrounding tissues, then it is staged as *Tis*. Finally, *T1–T4* are used to describe the size and invasiveness of the tumor, with *T4* being the largest and most invasive.

N staging is also important because if the cancer has spread from the tumor to the lymph nodes, it very possibly has spread to other parts of the body, too. The notations in *N* staging include *NX, N0, N1, N2,* and *N3. NX* means that nearby lymph nodes cannot be measured. When the nearby lymph nodes don't contain cancer, an *N0* is assigned. *N1, N2,* and *N3* refer to the size, location, and number of lymph nodes involved. The higher the *N* value, the more lymph nodes involved and the more dangerous the cancer is.

M staging is used to describe the extent of metastasis of the cancer. Only three stages are used: *MX, M0,* and *M1. MX* means metastasis cannot be measured or found. *M0* means that there is no known distant metastases, and *M1* means metastases are present.

The evaluation of *TNM* will determine the course of treatment. As a general rule, the worse the *TNM* staging, the more intense the treatment. For

Biopsy is the removal and testing of a sample of cells or tissue to look for abnormalities.

Staging is a description of the size and spread of a cancer.

people who are diagnosed with cancer, the staging they want to hear or see on their medical chart is *TX, NX, MX.*

✓ **NEED TO KNOW**

Diagnosing cancer is a complex and sophisticated process. Depending on the type of suspected cancer, a diagnosis may involve physical exams, X-rays, blood evaluation, and biopsy. Cancer must be staged, or rated, for an effective treatment plan to be devised. Staging describes three factors: whether a tumor has been found, if the original cancer has been discovered in lymph nodes as well, and if metastasized cancer can be found outside the original cancer site. Cancer tumors that are small and have not spread are the easiest to treat successfully.

➤ Common Cancer Sites

Any cell in the body has the potential to become cancerous. Figures 9.4 and 9.5 show the estimated cancer incidences and deaths by gender for 2008. It will be quickly noticed that the more common sites for cancer to

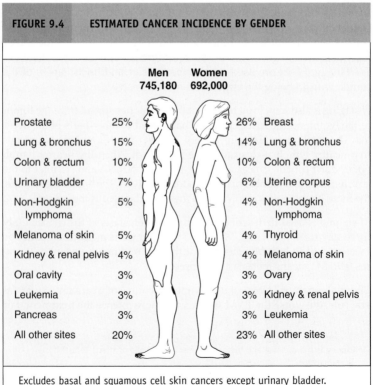

FIGURE 9.4   ESTIMATED CANCER INCIDENCE BY GENDER

	Men 745,180	Women 692,000	
Prostate	25%	26%	Breast
Lung & bronchus	15%	14%	Lung & bronchus
Colon & rectum	10%	10%	Colon & rectum
Urinary bladder	7%	6%	Uterine corpus
Non-Hodgkin lymphoma	5%	4%	Non-Hodgkin lymphoma
Melanoma of skin	5%	4%	Thyroid
Kidney & renal pelvis	4%	4%	Melanoma of skin
Oral cavity	3%	3%	Ovary
Leukemia	3%	3%	Kidney & renal pelvis
Pancreas	3%	3%	Leukemia
All other sites	20%	23%	All other sites

Excludes basal and squamous cell skin cancers except urinary bladder.

Source: Reprinted by the permission of the American Cancer Society, Inc. from www.cancer.org. All Rights Reserved.

FIGURE 9.5 ESTIMATED CANCER DEATHS BY GENDER

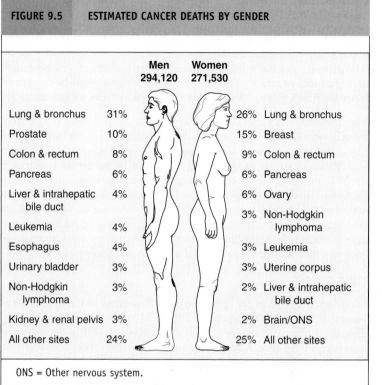

	Men 294,120	Women 271,530	
Lung & bronchus	31%	26%	Lung & bronchus
Prostate	10%	15%	Breast
Colon & rectum	8%	9%	Colon & rectum
Pancreas	6%	6%	Pancreas
Liver & intrahepatic bile duct	4%	6%	Ovary
		3%	Non-Hodgkin lymphoma
Leukemia	4%	3%	Leukemia
Esophagus	4%	3%	Uterine corpus
Urinary bladder	3%	2%	Liver & intrahepatic bile duct
Non-Hodgkin lymphoma	3%		
Kidney & renal pelvis	3%	2%	Brain/ONS
All other sites	24%	25%	All other sites

ONS = Other nervous system.

Source: Reprinted by the permission of the American Cancer Society, Inc. from www.cancer.org. All Rights Reserved.

develop include the breast, lung, colon, prostate, cervix, testicles, blood, and skin. We will examine these kinds of cancers with respect to signs and symptoms, risk factors, early detection, and treatment.

BREAST CANCER

Of the estimated 180,000 new cases of breast cancer each year, 99 percent are found in women and less than 1 percent are in men. Breast cancer is the most common form of cancer diagnosed among women and the second most common site for cancer deaths in women. The most common symptom of breast cancer is a lump in the breast or changes in the nipple. Although most lumps are benign, lumps still remain the most common symptom of breast cancer. Other symptoms include breast swelling, tenderness, nipple pain and/or dimpling, and nipple discharge. Any of these symptoms warrant immediate medical evaluation.

Like most cancers, the causes are unknown. Risk factors include a family history, a long menstrual history including periods that started early and ended late in life, obesity after menopause, postmenopausal hormone therapy, never bearing children, and having a first child after age 30. None of these events are strongly enough correlated with cancer to conclude cause and effect, but they are factors that increase one's relative risk.

Early detection of breast cancer is key to survival. The simplest early detection method is breast self-examination performed once a month. Women who properly practice self-examinations have a higher probability of identifying a lump or tumor so that less invasive procedures can be used to remove the lump. Figure 9.6 shows the proper procedures for examinations.

Mammography is a type of X-ray examination of the breast. If a lump or mass is seen in the X-ray image, it will be biopsied. Unless directed by a physician, the general medical consensus is that all women should begin yearly mammograms at age 40. The earlier the breast cancer is detected, the less intense the treatment. If the cancer hasn't invaded other tissue or the lymph nodes, then all that may be necessary is a lumpectomy (removal of the growth). If the cancer is more advanced, then removal of the affected breast, called *mastectomy,* might be necessary. In addition to surgery, there may be a need for follow-up chemotherapy and/or radiation, both of which will be discussed in the section on cancer treatment.

LUNG CANCER

Lung cancer accounts for approximately 15 percent of the new cases of cancer, or about 210,000 cases annually. It is the second most commonly diagnosed cancer among both men and women, and it is also the most common site for cancer deaths among both genders. The most common symptoms for lung cancer include persistent cough, sputum streaked with blood, chest pain, and recurring bouts with respiratory infections, such as pneumonia and bronchitis.

Lung cancer tumors can grow and spread without symptoms. Unfortunately, lung cancer has a lower rate of survival than other cancers, mostly because it is usually discovered late. By the time a tumor is visible on an X-ray, it is well advanced.

The most important risk factor for lung cancer is cigarette smoking. Other risk factors include exposure to secondhand smoke and to carcinogenic environmental chemicals. Although family history is always an important variable in the development of cancer, lung cancer is clearly more related to environmental exposure.

Chest X-rays, analysis of cells in sputum, and fiber-optic examination of the bronchial passages are detection methods. Unfortunately, they are not very effective for early detection. Treatment options include surgery, chemotherapy, and radiation.

COLON CANCER

Approximately 150,000 cases of colon cancer are diagnosed each year in the United States. It is the third most common cancer, in both incidence and mortality, for both men and women. The most common symptoms

FIGURE 9.6   BREAST SELF-EXAMINATION

BSE is a tool that may help you learn what is normal for you. BSE includes looking at and feeling your breasts. If you notice any changes in your breasts, see your health care provider right away.

Step 1: Lying Down

Feel for changes:

- Lie down on your back with a pillow under your right shoulder

- Use the pads of the three middle fingers on your left hand to check your right breast

- Press using light, medium and firm pressure in a circle without lifting your fingers off the skin

- Follow an up and down pattern

- Feel for changes in your breast, above and below your collarbone and in your armpit

- Repeat on your left breast using your right hand

These steps may be repeated while bathing or showering using soapy hands.

Step 2: In Front of the Mirror

Look for changes:

- Hold arms at your side

- Hold arms over your head

- Press your hands on your hips and tighten your chest muscles

- Bend forward with your hands on your hips

Studies have shown that BSE used alone does not decrease mortality rates.
Susan G. Komen for the Cure does not provide medical advice.
©2008 Susan G. Komen for the Cure® Item No. 806-301a-GA, General Audience 3/08

Monthly breast self-exams should always include visual inspection (with and without a mirror) to note changes in contour or texture and manual inspection in standing and reclining positions to note unusual lumps or thicknesses.

Source: Susan G. Komen for the Cure, 2008.

are rectal bleeding, blood in the stool, change in bowel habits, and cramping pain in the lower abdomen. Unfortunately, there are no early signs of the disease.

The major risk factors for colon cancer include family history, colon polyps, inflammatory bowel disease, low fiber diet, obesity, and a diet high in saturated fat and red meats.

Because there are no early signs of colon cancer, the emphasis is on early detection. Early detection can be done through a number of procedures. The simplest is a noninvasive procedure to determine if there is blood in the stool. Another procedure is an endoscopic exam called a *colonoscopy*; the person is given a sedative and a scope is inserted deep into the bowel so that the bowel wall can be examined for cancer. An endoscopic exam is recommended for all adults over 50 years of age.

Treatment for colon cancer can range from removal of the tumor to removal of sections of the colon. It depends on how advanced the cancer is. Follow-up with chemotherapy and radiation may also be necessary.

PROSTATE CANCER

Prostate cancer is the most commonly diagnosed cancer among men and typically affects men over 50 years of age. Many experts say that, like women's risk of breast cancer, if men live long enough, they will eventually develop prostate cancer. Approximately 220,000 new cases of prostate cancer are diagnosed each year.

Like many other of the cancers discussed, symptoms usually occur in the advanced stages. The common symptoms include weak or interrupted urine flow, inability to urinate, need to urinate frequently, blood in the urine, pain or burning with urination, and pain in the lower back, pelvis, or upper thighs. Symptoms usually mean the cancer has spread.

Risk factors for prostate cancer are age, ethnicity, and family history. The older a man is, the greater the risk. More than 70 percent of all prostate cancer cases are diagnosed in men older than 65. African American men have the highest prostate cancer rates in the United States.

Treatment options for prostate cancer usually include surgery, chemotherapy, and radiation. In early stage prostate cancer, radioactive seed implants can be inserted into the prostate to shrink the tumor. However, some prostate cancers are slow growing, and if a man is quite old, the cancer may be monitored and not removed because it might not present a threat to life and health.

CERVICAL CANCER

The cells of the cervix are susceptible to mutation especially with the presence of certain viruses such as HPV. Cervical cells can change and over time mutate into cancer cells without a woman experiencing other symptoms. Approximately 10,000 new cases of cervical cancer are diagnosed each year. Cervical cancer is the fourth most commonly diagnosed cancer in women and the eighth most deadly cancer for women.

Symptoms of cervical cancer don't usually occur until the abnormal cervical cells invade surrounding vaginal and cervical tissue. Then, the symptoms are usually abnormal vaginal bleeding and vaginal discharge. The main risk factor for cervical cancer is infection with HPV. Also, women who had sexual intercourse at an early age or who have had multiple partners are also at higher risk.

The Pap test is the most common early detection measure used to determine the health of the cervical cells and the first indication of cancer. A Pap test consists of a swab of cervical cells that are examined under a microscope. A trained lab technician can distinguish between healthy cells and cancer cells. Sometimes a Pap test will be reported as dysplasia. This term describes cells that aren't normal yet aren't cancer either. Women with dysplasia are monitored more closely and have Pap tests more often. If cervical cancer is diagnosed, then surgery, chemotherapy, and radiation are most likely to follow.

What Is Your Risk? Oral Sex, HPV, and Throat Cancer

Most young people think of oral sex as a low-risk behavior that prevents contraction of a sexually transmitted disease. Surveys have shown that approximately one in five ninth graders have reported engaging in oral sex.

It has been known for many years that sexually transmitted diseases can be spread through oral sex, despite its reputation for being safer than vaginal or anal intercourse. Recent studies also suggest that one type of STD, human papillomavirus (HPV) can cause throat cancer. Previously, HPV was thought to cause only genital warts and cervical cancer.

It is estimated that at any given time 20–40 million Americans are infected with HPV. Sixty percent of sexually active women will become infected, and HPV is one of the most common STDs diagnosed in student health centers. According to *New Scientist* magazine, people who have had more than five oral-sex partners in their lifetime are 250 percent more likely to have throat cancer than those who do not have oral sex.

Incidences of throat cancer are higher now than in years past, when it was thought to mostly be caused by environmental factors such as heavy smoking or heavy alcohol use. Given the high rate of both oral sex and HPV infection today, it seems that unprotected oral sex is not as safe as once thought.

TESTICULAR CANCER

Testicular cancer is called a "young man's cancer" because the majority of the almost 8,000 diagnosed cases each year occur in men 20–40 years of age. Like other cancers, testicular cancer in the early stages has no specific symptoms. A common symptom is a lump in the testicle. The lump may or may not be painful. Testicular swelling, hardness, and a feeling of heaviness or aching in the scrotum or lower abdomen are other possible symptoms of testicular cancer.

Risk factors for testicular cancer are not clearly understood. Undescended testicles are the major risk factor. In the absence of risk factor information, the key is early detection. The American Cancer Society recommends that men, especially between the ages of 20–40, practice testicular self-examination (TSE) once each month. Figure 9.7 highlights the simple TSE procedures.

Treatment for testicular cancer can range from chemotherapy to removal of the testicular lump to removal of the testicle or both testes.

LEUKEMIA

When blood cells mutate and become cancerous, leukemia can result. Approximately 45,000 new cases of acute and chronic leukemia are diagnosed each year, making it the fifth most common cancer diagnosed among males and females. Acute leukemia is the major form affecting children, and its symptoms appear quickly. Chronic leukemia is the major form affecting adults and is characterized by a slow progression of symptoms.

The major signs of leukemia are fatigue, paleness, weight loss, repeated infections, fever, bruising easily, nosebleeds, and other hemorrhages. Some of these symptoms are common to other conditions as well, making the diagnosing of leukemia difficult. The major risk factors for leukemia include exposure to environmental carcinogens, radiation, and specific types of viruses.

Other than paying close attention to ongoing fatigue, weight loss, and other symptoms with a follow-up diagnosis, there is no early detection method. Blood tests in suspect patients can indicate leukemia, and sometimes a bone marrow biopsy might be needed to examine bone marrow for cancer cells.

SKIN CANCER

Skin cancer is an epidemic. There are over a million cases of skin cancer diagnosed in the United States each year. The good news is that most skin cancer is curable if detected early. Symptoms of skin cancer are more ambiguous that other forms of cancer discussed because the symptoms are mostly changes on the skin so one has to notice those changes.

FIGURE 9.7   TESTICULAR SELF-EXAMINATION

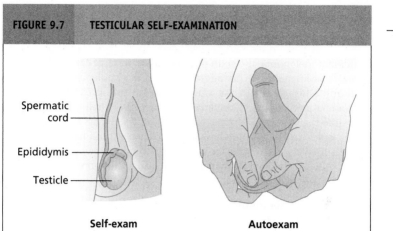

Spermatic cord

Epididymis

Testicle

Self-exam   **Autoexam**

Photo courtesy of TeensHealth.org

It's best to do a TSE during or right after a hot shower or bath. The scrotum (skin that covers the testicles) is most relaxed then, which makes it easier to examine the testicles.

1. Use both hands to gently roll each testicle (with slight pressure) between your fingers. Place your thumbs over the top of the testicle, with the index and middle fingers of each hand behind the testicle, and then roll it between your fingers.
2. You should be able to feel the epididymis (the sperm-carrying tube), which feels soft and ropelike, and is slightly tender to pressure; it is located at the top of the back part of each testicle. This is a normal lump.
3. Remember that one testicle (usually the right one) is slightly larger than the other for most men—this is also normal.
4. When examining each testicle, feel for any lumps or bumps along the front or sides. Lumps may be as small as a piece of rice or a pea.
5. If you notice any swelling, lumps, or changes in the size or color of a testicle, or if you have any pain or achy areas in your groin, let your doctor know right away.

Lumps or swelling may not be cancer, but they should be checked by your doctor as soon as possible. Testicular cancer is almost always curable if it is caught and treated early.

Source: This information was provided by KidsHealth, one of the largest resources online for medically reviewed health information written for parents, kids, and teens. For more articles like this one, visit www.KidsHealth.org or www.TeensHealth.org. Copyright: 1995-2008. The Nemours foundation.

There are three major types of skin cancer. **Basal cell carcinoma** usually appears as flat, firm, pale areas of the skin or as small, raised, pink or red shiny areas. **Squamous cell carcinoma** appears as growing

Basal cell carcinoma are flat, firm, pale areas of the skin or small, raised, pink or red shiny areas.

Squamous cell carcinoma appears as growing lumps with a rough surface or as flat, red patches that grow slowly.

lumps with a rough surface or as flat, red patches that grow slowly. **Malignant melanoma** is considered the most dangerous of the skin cancers.

Malignant melanoma, the sixth most common form of cancer diagnosed in males and females, is very aggressive, and the incidence is rising faster than any other cancer in the United States (Cottrell, 2005). Malignant melanoma appears as an unusual mole, and if untreated it will grow deep into the body and metastasize. Melanomas appear asymmetrical—that is, one side doesn't match the other. They also tend to have irregular borders and wide variation in colors including yellow, green, and red tinges. Finally, the size of melanomas tends to be more than 6mm, or about the size of a pencil eraser.

The chief risk factor for malignant melanoma is exposure to the sun. It is estimated that 65 percent of melanomas are related to ultraviolet (UV) exposure. There are three major forms of UV rays, called UV-A, UV-B, and UV-C. All forms of ultraviolet light are found in the sun's rays, and when the rays reach the skin, they traumatize the skin. The skin responds by secreting pigment, which is what causes a suntan. So a suntan is not a sign of health but rather a sign of the skin trying to protect itself from damage. Tanning booths are also a source of UV rays (see this chapter's Breaking It Down box, "Are Tanning Booths Safe?").

Early detection for malignant melanoma uses an A, B, C, and D screening. *A* stands for "asymmetrical." Symmetrical moles are usually not melanoma, which have irregular edges. Likewise, the borders (*B*) of the moles observed should be round, not irregular. The color (*C*) of a malignant melanoma is not brown, but might be brownish, red, yellow, or green. It does not look like a typical, common brown mole. Finally, a malignant melanoma will have a diameter (*D*) more than 6mm or the size of a pencil eraser. If any mole on the body has abnormal characteristics of A, B, C, and D, a follow-up evaluation is necessary. Figure 9.8 shows the A, B, C, D of identifying malignant melanoma.

Treatment for malignant melanoma is like that for other cancers: surgery, chemotherapy, and radiation. Generally speaking, the earlier a melanoma is diagnosed, the better the outcome. If found in the early stages, then all that may be necessary for treatment is the removal of the mole.

How much at risk are you of developing malignant melanoma? Complete the inventory in Figure 9.9 to assess your behaviors and relative risk for skin cancer.

Malignant melanoma is the most dangerous form of skin cancer because it is fast growing and can metastasize quickly.

FIGURE 9.8 IDENTIFYING MALIGNANT MELANOMA

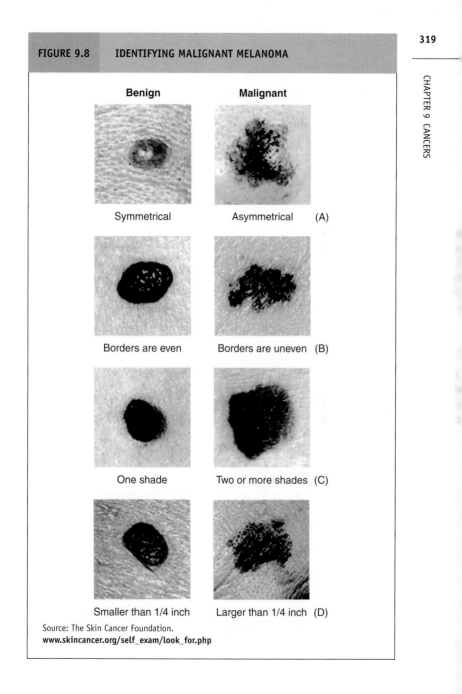

Source: The Skin Cancer Foundation.
www.skincancer.org/self_exam/look_for.php

FIGURE 9.9   ARE YOU AT HIGH RISK FOR MELANOMA?

Directions: If you are curious as to your risk for developing Melanoma, answer the following questions.

1. Do you have 50 or more moles on your body?
    ❑ YES   ❑ NO

2. Do you have one atypical mole?
    ❑ YES   ❑ NO

3. Do you have red or blond hair, blue or green eyes, and a light complexion?
    ❑ YES   ❑ NO

4. Are you heavily freckled with no atypical moles?
    ❑ YES   ❑ NO

5. Do you have a personal history of non-melanoma skin cancer?
    ❑ YES   ❑ NO

6. Do you have family members (parent, child, brother, sister) who have had skin cancer?
    ❑ YES   ❑ NO

7. Have you had intermittent exposure of normally covered skin to strong sunlight?
    ❑ YES   ❑ NO

8. Have you had one blistering sunburn under the age of 20?
    ❑ YES   ❑ NO

9. Have you used tanning beds 10 times or more in a year under the age of 30?
    ❑ YES   ❑ NO

10. Do you fail to use at least SPF 15 sunscreen when outdoors?
    ❑ YES   ❑ NO

11. Do you live in a high altitude area (8,500 feet or more above sea level)?
    ❑ YES   ❑ NO

If you answered "Yes" to any of the questions, your lifetime risk for melanoma is high.

Sources: Melanoma Education Foundation and The American Cancer Society.

Studies show that more than 1 million new cases of skin cancer will be diagnosed in the United States this year and that over 10,000 deaths will be traced to skin cancer in the same time period. Exposure to the sun is the major risk factor associated with the development of skin cancer, especially the deadliest skin cancer, melanoma. Approximately 28 million Americans visit tanning booths each year, and many assume that tanning booths are safer than regular sun exposure. Is this a correct assumption?

In fact, tanning booths are not safer than the sun. Booth equipment doesn't emit much UV-B light, which is what causes surface damage and sunburns. Instead, booths emit mostly UV-A light, which penetrates deeper into the skin and can damage internal organs or a person's DNA. UV-A exposure can increase the risk of melanoma.

A case in point. Anna Tremblay was a student at James Madison University in Virginia. She used tanning booths frequently, feeling it was a "social thing to do." Just before her senior year, she noticed a mole on her lower hip. After a trip to the dermatologist and a biopsy, she was diagnosed with melanoma.

Anna then had surgery to remove a large section of tissue from the area around the melanoma as well as other "suspicious" areas on the waist. According to Anna, her whole midsection "was just completely cut up. It was horrible." In the next four years she had two other melanomas diagnosed and treated. The good news is that Anna is a cancer survivor— however, because of her overuse of tanning booths, she now has to visit a dermatologist every six months for the rest of her life.

According to The Skin Cancer Foundation,

- UV light is a proven human carcinogen;
- exposure to tanning beds before age 35 increases melanoma risk by 75 percent;
- people who use tanning beds are 2.5 times more likely to develop squamous cell carcinoma; and
- occasional use of tanning beds almost triples the chances of developing melanoma.

Yes, tanning booths can be found anywhere—spas, shopping malls, hotels. Just because they are abundant doesn't mean they are safe. For years the American Cancer Society and other groups have been very vocal regarding the dangers of tanning booths. Finally, there has been a response. President Bush signed the Tanning Accountability and Notification Act (TAN Act), which gives the Food and Drug Administration the authority to regulate tanning equipment including language used on warning labels. Expect to see the perception of tanning booths as a safe way to procure a tan change to a high-risk behavior in the next few years.

There are signs and symptoms for the common sites for cancer. Through an understanding of the signs and symptoms and the early detection methods, you can reduce your risk of being a cancer-mortality number and increase the probability of a successful outcome with the cancer. Many cancers are a result of choices people make—diet, smoking, sun exposure, and use of certain medications. Knowing the long-term effect of your health choices and acting appropriately can significantly reduce your risk.

➤ Cancer Treatment

Cancerous tissue must be removed in some manner. Surgery is the chief option for excising both the cancer and surrounding tissue. Once the cancer is removed, then a radiation and/or chemotherapy regime is instituted in order to prevent it from growing back.

Chemotherapy simply means "chemical therapy," or the use of a variety of anticancer drugs. Some cancers do not require surgery and can be cured with just chemotherapy, whereas other cancers require both surgery and "chemo." There are many categories of anticancer drugs, some of which are quite toxic and have a very narrow margin of safety. The whole emphasis of chemotherapy is to kill new cancer cells before the cancer reoccurs.

Chemotherapy is hard on the body. Although drugs are becoming more precisely targeted, they often kill all fast-growing cells in a body, not just the cancerous ones. (People on chemotherapy sometimes lose their hair, because scalp cells are fast growing.) Chemotherapy also can suppress the immune system and leave a person open to infection. Further, it can cause nausea and weakness.

Radiation therapy is the last component of cancer treatment. Similar to chemo, the goal of radiation treatment is to destroy both cancer cells and cells that divide rapidly, which could be cancer cells. This treatment increases the likelihood that cancer cells remaining after surgery will be destroyed along with any cells that might become cancerous. In addition to killing cancer cells, radiation can help to reduce symptoms if a cancer cure is not possible.

Although there have been many remarkable advances in cancer treatment, there is no guarantee that surgery, chemotherapy, and radiation will be effective with everyone. What has been described is the conventional approach, and the implementation of this treatment protocol requires the clinical judgment of physicians and the decision of the patient. Cancer is such a serious condition that there is wisdom in getting a second opinion—

Chemotherapy is the use of numerous drugs to kill cancer cells.

Radiation treatment exposes cancer-ridden body areas to radiation doses to kill cancerous cells.

Health & the Media Quack Cancer Treatments

Amigdalina (amygdalin) has often been referred to as Vitamin B17. However, it is not really a vitamin but a chemical found in the pits of apricots and other fruits. *Laetrile* is the common term for the drug form of the chemical. Because Laetrile produces cyanide, which is a poison that kills cells, it has been marketed (particularly in Mexico) as a cancer cure. Amygdalin was first used as a cancer treatment in Russia in the 1840s. But modern studies show no scientific or clinical evidence that Laetrile cures cancer. Nonetheless, some people diagnosed with cancer are tempted to try Laetrile despite the numerous studies indicating it won't work.

Why are people susceptible to this quack drug? Some people do not research treatments before embracing them, so they remain ignorant of the science and evidence. This makes them easy prey for those who continue to market Laetrile therapy. Others may have tried traditional cancer therapies but remain uncured. People who are desperate to extend their life may try almost any treatment if they think it gives them even the tiniest chance for improvement. Still others are drawn to the idea that "natural" or "simple" cures like Laetrile, a drug derived from plants, must be better than invasive surgery or the arduous regimens of radiation or chemotherapy. So for a variety of reasons, quack drugs like Laetrile continue as cancer treatments.

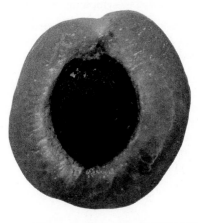

not just about the diagnosis but also before committing to an aggressive treatment protocol. Finally, and most importantly, early detection is critical to increase the options for less intense treatment and survival.

✓ NEED TO KNOW

More people are surviving cancer. Key to survival are the effect treatment modalities available—surgery, chemotherapy, and radiation. Although these modalities are not pleasant, they are effective in treating cancer. There is much more hope for surviving cancer than just there was just a few years ago.

Each type of cancer discussed has implications for early detection. Unfortunately, some kinds of cancer do not have symptoms until the cancer is advanced. Further, pain is a symptom of advanced cancer, so pain is not an early warning sign and should not be considered one. Figure 9.10 shows the array of cancer screenings available, when they should be done, and the appropriate age group.

To make cancer symptoms easy to remember, the American Cancer Society created the acronym CAUTION. If any of the symptoms below are noticed for at least two weeks, then a follow-up medical evaluation should be undertaken. CAUTION stands for

Changes in bowel or bladder habits, like bloody stool/urine, or painful elimination
A sore that doesn't heal—a sign of skin cancer
Unusual bleeding or discharge—possibly a symptom of cervical or bladder cancer
Thickening or lump in the breast or elsewhere
Indigestion or difficulty in swallowing—digestive-tract cancer symptoms
Obvious change in color of a wart or mole—a key sign of skin cancer
Nagging cough or hoarseness—symptoms of lung or throat cancer

Increasing the options to prevent cancer focus mainly on the choices people make that affect risk. These choices are related to tobacco use, diet, and exposure to environmental carcinogens.

Tobacco is related to most cases of lung, mouth, and throat cancer, so abstaining from tobacco would be a significant effort in reducing the risk of respiratory cancers. Diets high in saturated fat and red meat increase the risk of cancer of the colon, so moderation in intake of saturated fats and red meat will reduce one's risk of cancer of the colon. Environmental carcinogens range from ultraviolet light to industrial chemicals, and reducing exposure will reduce risk.

✓ **NEED TO KNOW**

There is not always a clear way to prevent cancer because we do not know with confidence what is related to the development of certain cancers. Just as important as prevention is early detection. CAUTION provides a simple framework for a basic set of symptoms that might indicate cancer. Learn and apply them. It may save your life.

FIGURE 9.10   RECOMMENDED CANCER SCREENINGS

Site & Recommendation

Breast

◆ Yearly mammograms are recommended starting at age 40. The age at which screening should be stopped should be individualized by considering the potential risks and beneﬁts of screening in the context of overall health status and longevity.

◆ Clinical breast exam should be part of a periodic health exam about every 3 years for women in their 20s and 30s and every year for women 40 and older.

◆ Women should know how their breasts normally feel and report any breast change promptly to their health care providers. Breast self-exam is an option for women starting in their 20s.

◆ Screening MRI is recommended for women with an approximately 20%-25% or greater lifetime risk of breast cancer, including women with a strong family history of breast or ovarian cancer and women who were treated for Hodgkin disease.

Colon & Rectum

Beginning at age 50, men and women should begin screening with 1 of the examination schedules below:

◆ A fecal occult blood test (FOBT) or fecal immunochemical test (FIT) every year

◆ A flexible sigmoidoscopy (FSIG) every 5 years

◆ Annual FOBT or FIT and flexible sigmoidoscopy every 5 years*

◆ A double-contrast barium enema every 5 years

◆ A colonoscopy every 10 years

> *Combined testing is preferred over either annual FOBT or FIT, or FSIG every 5 years, alone. People who are at moderate or high risk for colorectal cancer should talk with a doctor about a different testing schedule.

Prostate

◆ The PSA test and the digital rectal examination should be offered annually, beginning at age 50, to men who have a life expectancy of at least 10 years. Men at high risk (African American men and men with a strong family history of 1 or more first-degree relatives diagnosed with prostate cancer at an early age) should begin testing at age 45. For both men at average risk and high risk, information should be provided about what is known and what is uncertain about the benefits and limitations of early detection and treatment of prostate cancer so that they can make an informed decision about testing.

(continued)

FIGURE 9.10   RECOMMENDED CANCER SCREENINGS (continued)

Uterus

◆ **Cervix:** Screening should begin approximately 3 years after a woman begins having vaginal intercourse, but no later than 21 years of age. Screening should be done every year with regular Pap tests or every 2 years using liquid-based tests. At or after age 30, women who have had 3 normal test results in a row may get screened every 2 to 3 years. Alternatively, cervical cancer screening with HPV DNA testing and conventional or liquid-based cytology could be performed every 3 years. However, doctors may suggest a woman get screened more often if she has certain risk factors, such as HIV infection or a weak immune system. Women aged 70 and older who have had 3 or more consecutive normal Pap tests in the last 10 years may choose to stop cervical cancer screening. Screening after total hysterectomy (with removal of the cervix) is not necessary unless the surgery was done as a treatment for cervical cancer.

◆ **Endometrium:** The American Cancer Society recommends that at the time of menopause all women should be informed about the risks and symptoms of endometrial cancer and strongly encouraged to report any unexpected bleeding or spotting to their physicians. Annual screening for endometrial cancer with endometrial biopsy beginning at age 35 should be offered to women with or at risk for hereditary nonpolyposis colon cancer (HNPCC).

Cancer-related Checkup

◆ For individuals undergoing periodic health examinations, a cancer-related checkup should include health counseling and, depending on a person's age and gender, might include examinations for cancers of the thyroid, oral cavity, skin, lymph nodes, testes, and ovaries, as well as for some nonmalignant diseases.

◆ American Cancer Society guidelines for early cancer detection are assessed annually in order to identify whether there is new scientific evidence sufficient to warrant a reevaluation of current recommendations. If evidence is sufficiently compelling to consider a change or clarification in a current guideline or the development of a new guideline, a formal procedure is initiated. Guidelines are formally evaluated every 5 years regardless of whether new evidence suggests a change in the existing recommendations. There are 9 steps in this procedure, and these "guidelines for guideline development" were formally established to provide a specific methodology for science and expert judgment to form the underpinnings of specific statements and recommendations from the Society. These procedures constitute a deliberate process to ensure that all Society recommendations have the same methodological and evidence-based process at their core. This process also employs a system for rating strength and consistency of evidence that is similar to that employed by the Agency for Health Care Research and Quality (AHCRQ) and the US Preventive Services Task Force (USPSTF).

Source: American Cancer Society, Cancer Facts and Figures, 2008. Atlanta: American Cancer Society, Inc.

Alliance for Cervical Cancer Prevention
    http://alliance-cxca.org
American Cancer Society
    www.cancer.org
American Institute for Cancer Research
    www.aicr.org
American Medical Association
    www.ama-assn.org/
American Public Health Association
    www.apha.org
Centers for Disease Control
    www.cdc.gov
Harvard Center for Cancer Prevention
    www.diseaseriskindex.harvard.edu/
Medline Plus Cancer Information
    www.nlm.nih.gov/medlineplus/cancers.html
National Comprehensive Cancer Network
    www.nccn.org
Skin Cancer Organization
    www.skincancer.org

Knowing the Language

Basal cell carcinoma
Biopsy
Cancer
Carcinogen
Carcinoma
Chemotherapy
DNA
Dysplasia
Leukemia

Lymphoma
Melanoma
Metastasis
Mutation
Oncogene
Radiation therapy
Sarcoma
Squamous cell carcinoma
Staging

Understanding the Content

1. What is meant by *cancer* and *metastasis*?
2. Where are the most common sites where cancer occurs, and what are the major risk factors for each site?
3. What are the major methods used to treat cancer? Are they successful?
4. How can cancer be prevented?
5. What does the acronym CAUTION mean?

Selected References

Exploring Ideas

1. Why is it that when people hear the word *cancer*, they think immediately of death?
2. What sites of cancer do college-age students risk? What can be done to reduce risk?
3. What steps should be taken after a person is diagnosed with cancer?
4. Is there a role for complementary and alternative medicine in cancer treatment, and if so when?
5. Do you think the statement is true that if a person lives long enough he or she will most likely develop cancer? If so, why would this be true?

Selected References

American Academy of Dermatology. The Darker Side of Tanning. 2004. **www.aad.org/public/publications/pamphlets/sun_darker.html**

American Cancer Society (ACS). *Cancer Facts and Figures.* Atlanta, GA: American Cancer Society, 2005.

ACS. *Cancer: What Causes It. What Doesn't.* Atlanta, GA: American Cancer Society, 2006.

Callee EE, et. al. Overweight, obesity, and mortality from cancer in a prospectively studied cohort of U.S. adults. *New England Journal of Medicine* 348: 1625–1638, 2003.

Chao A, et. al. Meat consumption and risk of colorectal cancer. *Journal of the American Medical Association* 293 (2): 172–182, 2005.

Christenson LJ, Borrowman TA, Vachon CM, Tollefson MM, Otley CC, Weaver AL, Roenigk RK. Incidence of basal cell and squamous cell carcinomas in a population younger than 40 years. *Journal of the American Medical Association* 294 (6), 2005.

Curry SJ, Byers T, Hewitt M, eds. *Fulfilling the Potential of Cancer Prevention and Early Detection.* Washington, DC: National Academic Press, 2003.

Elmore JG, et. al. Screening for breast cancer. *Journal of the American Medical Association* 293 (10): 1245–1256, 2005.

Fung T, et. al. Major dietary patterns and the risk of colorectal cancer in women. *Archives of Internal Medicine* 163 (3): 309–314, 2005.

Matias KP. Studies of the viral origins of some cancers lead to new prevention, treatment strategies. *OncoLog* 39 (1), 2004.

Raloff J. Sun struck: Data suggest skin cancer epidemic looms. *Science News Online* 168 (7), Aug. 13, 2005.

Ruckington C, Straus JJ. *The Encyclopedia of Cancer.* New York: Facts on File, 2005.

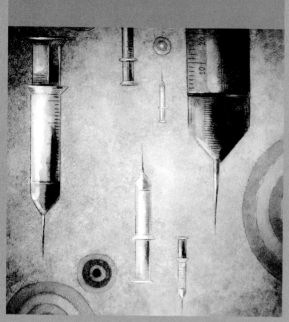

Good health is a serious business. Like life itself, it has to be worked at and it takes on added meaning with effort.

— NORMAN COUSINS

Chapter 10

DIABETES

In this chapter, we focus on what public health experts describe as the fastest growing chronic disease among Americans today—diabetes. The metabolic syndrome associated with diabetes, heart disease, and obesity is also discussed, because it demonstrates the interrelatedness of these multiple chronic conditions and the across-the-board impact that lifestyle can have.

DIABETES IS DISABLING, deadly, and on the rise. New evidence indicates that one in three Americans born in 2000 will develop diabetes. Due to the rapid rise in prevalence—a tripling over the past three decades—and the dire prediction for further increases, an expanded look at this disease called *diabetes* is warranted. An understanding of diabetes is important because it may well affect our personal health or the health of those close to us. Moreover, facing the challenges of diabetes today provides a striking example of how lifestyle, medicine, and technology converge in 21st-century American society.

The Greeks described the disease as a "melting down of the flesh and limbs into urine." Indeed, the symptoms of diabetes have been recognized for centuries. Early records describe a puzzling and deadly condition that caused intense thirst, excessive urine production, and a wasting away of the body. And, oddly, the urine of those afflicted was sweet. Thus, the full medical term, *diabetes mellitus,* comes from the Latin words meaning "siphon" (in reference to excessive urine output) and "sweet like honey," respectively.

Little was understood about the cause of diabetes until the late 19th century, when the pancreas, a little-known organ, was discovered to play a central role. Experiments involving the removal of the pancreas from dogs resulted in diabetes, confirming the relationship between the organ and the disease. The focus then shifted toward identifying a substance in the pancreas that could be the key to solving the diabetes puzzle. This led to the discovery of insulin in 1921. For this remarkable scientific achievement, Canadian researchers Frederick G. Banting and John Macleod were awarded the 1923 Nobel Prize in Medicine.

Subsequent events continued to advance our understanding and treatment of diabetes. Soon after the discovery of insulin, Eli Lilly and Company started commercial production of insulin from the pancreases of animals. Concurrently, home testing kits for sugar (glucose) in the urine were developed. Yet, it would be the 1950s before it was fully realized that diabetes could be caused in two ways. This finding spurred the discovery of (non-insulin) drugs to lower blood glucose levels. In the 1970s, treatment innovations included blood glucose meters and insulin pumps. They were followed in the early 1980s by the commercial production of bioengineered "human" insulin.

Despite these major advances in treating the disease, diabetes among Americans has skyrocketed. Researchers agree that these rising numbers are due to the widespread combination of over-eating and physical inactivity among a large proportion of the population. This "fattening of America" is clearly triggering the onset of diabetes along with increasing risk for heart disease and stroke. Related to these changes, a pattern of chronic disease risk factors has been recognized and in recent years has come to be known as the *metabolic syndrome.*

In large part, diabetes, like atherosclerosis, is an unintended consequence of our technologically advanced, affluent society where food is plentiful and daily physical demands are nearly non-existent. For those with diabetes, the disease is not reversible or curable. Thankfully though, it is highly treatable. And for those without diabetes, the key concept is prevention. Let's learn about diabetes and see what we can do to turn the tide, both for ourselves and society.

➤ Diabetes

Diabetes is the seventh leading cause of death in the United States, behind heart disease, cancer, stroke, lower-respiratory-tract disease (primarily tobacco-related emphysema), unintentional accidents (primarily motor vehicle accidents) and Alzheimer's disease. Nearly 8 percent of the population has diabetes (about 24 million people), with about the same number of males and females being affected. Of these, about 25 out of 100 are undiagnosed. That translates into nearly 6 million people who have the disease but are unaware of it. The risk for early death among people with diabetes is at least two times that of people without diabetes.

Among Americans age 20 or older, nearly 11 percent have diabetes. As shown in Figure 10.1, the prevalence of diabetes increases with age. For those 60 and older, the prevalence is nearly 24 percent. Risk of diabetes is also associated with race/ethnicity, as illustrated in Figure 10.2. Mexican Americans and Blacks are about one and a half to two times more likely to have diabetes than Asian Americans and Whites of similar age, and Native Americans are over two times more likely.

Just what is diabetes? **Diabetes** is a group of disorders in which there is a defect in the transfer of glucose (sugar) from the bloodstream into cells. This leads to abnormally high levels of blood glucose, which is known as **hyperglycemia** (*hyper-* means "high" or "elevated"; *glycemia* refers to glucose in the blood). Blood glucose levels are controlled by **insulin,** a hormone produced by the pancreas that helps move glucose from the blood into the cells of muscles and other tissues.

PANCREAS, METABOLISM, AND DIABETES

The pancreas, sandwiched between the stomach and the spine, is an oblong gland about the size and shape of a flattened banana. Part of it lies behind the stomach, and the other part is nestled in the curve of the small

Diabetes—or technically *diabetes mellitus*—is a group of disorders characterized by hyperglycemia resulting from defects in insulin production, insulin action, or both. **Hyperglycemia** is high blood glucose levels and is the hallmark of uncontrolled diabetes. **Insulin** is a hormone produced in the pancreas that helps glucose pass into the cells where it can be used for energy.

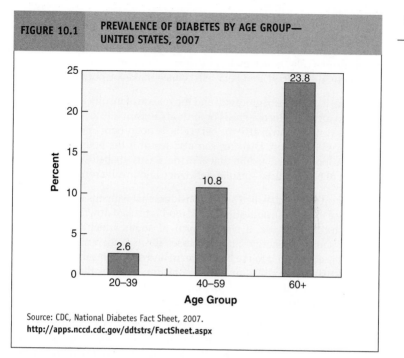

FIGURE 10.1 PREVALENCE OF DIABETES BY AGE GROUP—UNITED STATES, 2007

Source: CDC, National Diabetes Fact Sheet, 2007.
http://apps.nccd.cdc.gov/ddtstrs/FactSheet.aspx

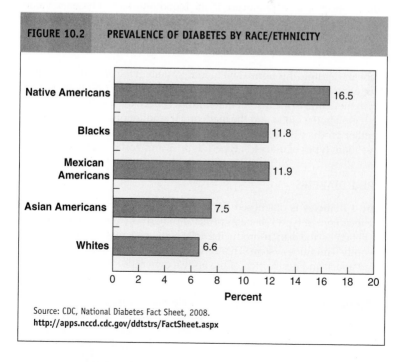

FIGURE 10.2 PREVALENCE OF DIABETES BY RACE/ETHNICITY

Source: CDC, National Diabetes Fact Sheet, 2008.
http://apps.nccd.cdc.gov/ddtstrs/FactSheet.aspx

intestine (duodenum). The pancreas makes hormones and enzymes that help the body digest and use food. Throughout the pancreas are clusters of cells called the *islets of Langerhans*. These islets are made up of two types of cells: alpha cells, which make glucagon, a hormone that raises the level of glucose in the blood, and beta cells, which make the hormone insulin.

Balancing the release of glucagon and the release of insulin into the bloodstream to regulate glucose needs of the body is normally an efficient physiological system. However, if the beta cells do not produce enough insulin, diabetes will develop. Diabetes can also result if the body does not respond properly to the insulin that is made. Lastly, diabetes can by a combination of both defects—insulin deficiency and insulin resistance.

To better understand diabetes, let's consider what happens when a person eats. Once in the gastrointestinal tract, food is broken down into constituents including glucose, a simple form of sugar which is the body's primary source of energy. Glucose passes through the wall of the intestine and is absorbed into the bloodstream and stimulates the beta cells in the pancreas to produce and release insulin. Insulin then allows the glucose to move from the blood into the cells. Once inside the cells, glucose is used for energy or stored until it's needed.

With this in mind, you might expect that the level of glucose in the blood would vary somewhat throughout the day. And indeed it does. It rises after a meal and returns to a baseline level within about two hours after eating. Once the level of glucose in the blood returns to a baseline value, insulin production decreases. Standard variation in blood glucose levels is within a narrow range of about 70 to 110 milligrams per deciliter (mg/dl) most of the time and up to 140 mg/dl following meals.

Diabetes disrupts this normal metabolic system. If the body does not produce enough insulin to move the glucose into the cells or if there is a defect in the action of the insulin that limits its effect, the resulting high level of glucose in the blood and the inadequate amount of glucose in the cells together produce the symptoms and complications of diabetes. There are three main types of diabetes: type 1, type 2, and gestational diabetes.

TYPE 1 DIABETES

Type 1 diabetes is diagnosed in children, teenagers, and young adults. The incidence of type 1 diabetes peaks at puberty. In this form of diabetes, the beta cells, the insulin-producing cells of the pancreas, are destroyed by the body's immune system. This abnormal autoimmune response—a targeted attack and destruction of the body's own cells—is linked to genetic

> **Type 1 diabetes** develops during childhood or young adulthood due to pancreatic beta cell destruction. This form includes cases due to an autoimmune process and those with an unknown etiology.

predisposition, but it may also be associated with environmental factors. Although pieces of the puzzle are coming together, the actual causes are not yet well understood. The eventual permanent destruction of all or nearly all of the beta cells typically leads to absolute insulin deficiency—that is, a complete inability to produce insulin. Most people who have type 1 diabetes develop it before age 25 and must take insulin for the rest of their lives. Due to the acute onset of symptoms (e.g., increased urination, increased thirst, unexplained weight loss), type 1 diabetes is nearly always diagnosed soon after symptoms appear. Although the preferred term is *type 1 diabetes,* this condition is also referred to as *insulin-dependent diabetes* or *juvenile diabetes.* From a public health perspective, it's important to note that only 5 to 10 percent of people with diabetes have this form of the disease.

TYPE 2 DIABETES

Type 2 diabetes usually develops in people older than 30 and becomes more common with age. It is by far the most prevalent type of diabetes—over 90 percent of all people with diabetes have type 2. In this type of diabetes, the pancreas continues to produce insulin, but the body develops what is known as *insulin resistance.* This is a condition in which the body's cells do not use insulin properly. Initially, the pancreas compensates by producing more insulin at higher than normal levels. Over time, however, the pancreas cannot supply enough insulin in response to meals. Excess body fat (adipose tissue) is the primary cause of insulin resistance and the chief risk factor for type 2 diabetes. It's estimated that 80–90 percent of people with type 2 diabetes are obese. This type of diabetes, like type 1, is also associated with a complex genetic predisposition and tends to run in families. In contrast to type 1 though, type 2 develops gradually. People can have high blood glucose levels for years—with ongoing damage to tissues—yet have no outward symptoms. The only way to tell is with regular screening for diabetes. Type 2 is also referred to as *non-insulin dependent diabetes* because insulin is usually not needed to treat the condition, at least initially. Historically, type 2 diabetes was commonly called *adult-onset diabetes* and known as a disease of middle age.

GESTATIONAL DIABETES

Gestational diabetes develops in about 4 out of 100 women during the late stages of pregnancy. It is more common among obese women, certain ethnic/racial groups (Black, Hispanic, Native American), and those with a family history. This form of diabetes is typically caused by the develop-

---

Type 2 diabetes, the most common form of diabetes, encompasses cases that range from an inability to make enough insulin (secretory defect) to an inability to use the insulin that is made (insulin resistance).

Gestational diabetes is diabetes that first appears during pregnancy; it affects about 4 percent of pregnant women.

ment of insulin resistance late in pregnancy. Gestational diabetes requires treatment to normalize the maternal blood glucose levels to avoid complications in the infant. Treatment usually consists of dietary changes and avoiding excess weight gain. Although gestational diabetes usually resolves after the baby is born, women who develop it are more likely to develop type 2 diabetes later in life. Following pregnancy, a small proportion of women with gestational diabetes (5–10 percent) are found to have type 2 diabetes and a larger proportion (40–60 percent) are at risk for developing type 2 diabetes within the next 5 to 10 years. For additional information on gestational diabetes, go to the American Diabetes Association's Web site (**www.diabetes.org/gestational-diabetes.jsp**).

PRE-DIABETES

Pre-diabetes is a condition that causes blood glucose levels to be higher than normal but not high enough for a diagnosis of diabetes. People with pre-diabetes are at increased risk for developing diabetes. This borderline condition is similar to the pre-hypertension category for blood pressure. The American Diabetes Association estimates that there are twice as many Americans with pre-diabetes as those with diabetes. Before people develop type 2 diabetes, they almost always have pre-diabetes. Recent evidence indicates that initial damage to the body, especially the heart and circulatory system, starts during pre-diabetes. However, not all individuals with pre-diabetes inevitably progress to diabetes. Interventions work. Improving diet, increasing physical activity, and losing weight can reverse pre-diabetes and delay or prevent diabetes. Being diagnosed with pre-diabetes represents an important crossroad at which a choice must be made. It is a last window of opportunity for true prevention, because once diabetes is developed, it doesn't go away.

✓ **NEED TO KNOW**

Diabetes is a group of metabolic diseases characterized by hyperglycemia resulting from defects in insulin secretion, insulin action, or both. Type 1 diabetes develops during childhood due to destruction of the beta cells of the pancreas. Lifelong insulin therapy is required. Type 1 accounts for 5–10 percent of all cases of diabetes. Type 2 diabetes generally appears during adulthood and is associated with weight gain and insulin resistance. It is by far the most common (over 90 percent of all cases). Pre-diabetes is a transitional condition in which the blood glucose level is higher than normal but not high enough for a diagnosis of diabetes. People with pre-diabetes are at high risk for developing type 2 diabetes. For these people, several lifestyle strategies are available to prevent or delay the onset of the disease.

Pre-diabetes is a borderline condition in which the blood glucose level is between normal and diabetic levels.

We all know individuals with diabetes. Yet, unless we live with a person who has diabetes or have it ourselves, it's difficult to fully appreciate the disease. People with diabetes may experience many serious, long-term complications. Some complications begin within months of the onset of diabetes, although most develop over a period of years. Nearly all complications are progressive. If not managed, diabetes can be extremely disabling in a number of ways.

DAMAGE TO BLOOD VESSELS

Uncontrolled diabetes damages both the small blood vessels (such as arterioles, capillaries, and venules) and the large ones (arteries and veins). Compounds accumulate within the tiny vessels that compromise the microvascular systems, causing them to thicken and leak. Blood flow is restricted, especially to the skin and nerves. High glucose levels also cause the levels of fats in the blood to rise, hastening atherosclerosis in the larger blood vessels. As a result, atherosclerosis occurs at younger ages and is at least twice as common in people with diabetes as in those without diabetes.

HEART ATTACK AND STROKE

Over time, elevated blood glucose levels and compromised circulation harm multiple organs, including the heart and brain. Angina, heart attack, stroke, and heart failure can result. Heart disease and stroke cause about two out of three deaths among people with diabetes.

EYE DISEASE AND BLINDNESS

Diabetic eye disease is the leading cause of blindness in adults. Complications from diabetes primarily result in damage to the retina (retinopathy) but also include cataracts and glaucoma. Diabetic retinopathy is caused by a breakdown of the small blood vessels in the retina. All three diabetic complications of the eye can result in loss of vision and eventually blindness.

KIDNEY DISEASE

Over 40 percent of all new cases of kidney disease are in people with diabetes. Diabetic kidney disease develops as the tiny blood vessels in the kidney are damaged and the system to filter the blood is slowly degraded. Eventually, this can lead to kidney failure requiring dialysis or kidney transplantation.

NERVE DAMAGE

In 60–70 percent of people with diabetes, high blood sugar and related metabolic factors lead to nerve damage (neuropathy). Although nerve problems can occur in every organ system, the most common is peripheral neuropathy, which causes pain, tingling, or numbness (loss of feeling) in the toes, feet, legs, hands, and arms. Blisters and sores may appear on numb areas of the foot because pressure or injury goes unnoticed. Peripheral neuropathy may also cause muscle weakness and loss of balance and coordination.

AMPUTATIONS

Poor circulation and nerve damage can lead to ulcers, infections, and poor wound healing. People with diabetes are especially likely to have skin break down and infections of the feet and legs. Such wounds typically heal slowly or not at all. More than half of all lower-limb amputations in the United States occur in people with diabetes.

The complications just highlighted are only the major ones. There are other outcomes, less vivid but still debilitating. Diabetes can also compromise immune function; flu- and pneumonia-related deaths are three times more likely among people with diabetes than those without diabetes. And there are gender-specific concerns such as pregnancy complications affecting women and their babies and the risk of impotence among men.

Although diabetes-related complications can be severe, they don't have to be. The more tightly a person with diabetes controls his or her blood glucose level in the blood (glycemic control), the less likely it is that these complications will develop or become worse. Early detection, comprehensive medical care, and vigilant self-management are proven strategies in preventing or minimizing complications. Regular medical exams should include careful screening for heart disease and stroke, eye disease, kidney disease, skin and foot infections, and nerve damage.

✓ **NEED TO KNOW**

Early diagnosis of diabetes is extremely important because medical complications from untreated diabetes are far-ranging and extensive. Over time high glucose levels in the bloodstream and insufficient levels in the cells can cause irreversible damage. Both microvascular and macrovascular systems are affected. Serious complications include heart disease, stroke, blindness, kidney damage, nerve damage, and lower limb amputations. The key to preventing or minimizing complications is to control blood glucose levels and associated risk factors such as hypertension, abnormal blood lipids, and overweight/obesity. Moreover, persons with diabetes should follow preventive care practices for their eyes, kidneys, and feet.

As previously mentioned, undiagnosed diabetes is common; as many as 25 percent of people with type 2 diabetes are unaware of their condition. Similar to high blood pressure or abnormal lipid levels, type 2 diabetes can be present for years before a person has symptoms. And when symptoms develop, they may be subtle. Increased urination and thirst are mild at first and gradually worsen over weeks or months. Eventually, the person experiences extreme fatigue, is likely to develop blurred vision, and may become chronically dehydrated. Sadly, even during the early stages of type 2 diabetes—before the symptoms arise—uncontrolled high blood glucose (hyperglycemia) causes microvascular disease (e.g., damage to the retinas and kidneys) and may cause or contribute to macrovascular disease (e.g., heart disease, stroke, peripheral vascular disease). Undiagnosed diabetes is a serious condition.

For apparently healthy adults, testing for diabetes is recommended for everyone age 45 and older, particularly if overweight (i.e., a BMI equal to or greater than 25). If results are normal, testing should be repeated every three years. However, for individuals with known risk factors for the development of diabetes, screening should begin earlier. Targeted testing is suggested for adults and children who are overweight and have one or more of the following risk factors:

- Habitual physically inactivity
- Parent or sibling with diabetes
- Previous diagnosis of pre-diabetes
- Member of high-risk ethnic/racial group—Asian American, Black, Hispanic, Native American, Pacific Islander
- High blood pressure
- Abnormal blood fats—HDL-cholesterol less than 35 mg/dl and/or triglycerides greater than 250 mg/dl
- Women who have been diagnosed with gestational diabetes or delivered a baby weighing more than nine pounds

Awareness and appropriate action are critical. In a recent study from Oregon, two out of three adults at high risk for developing diabetes reported being unconcerned about their risk for developing the disease and only one out of five had discussed their risk of diabetes with a health professional (Kemple, Zlot, Leman, 2005). These surprising findings indicate the need for increased recognition of future diabetes risk by high-risk individuals *and* health professionals.

To prevent or effectively treat diabetes, people must first be screened. The tests used to diagnose diabetes and pre-diabetes and the standard treatments for controlling the disease are reviewed in the next section.

Diabetes can be diagnosed by measuring blood glucose in one of three ways. The *fasting plasma glucose test* is the most common test. (Plasma is the fluid portion of blood after the cells are removed.) Fasting is defined as no caloric intake for at least eight hours. Typically a blood sample is drawn in the morning after an overnight fast. Normal fasting glucose levels range from about 70 to 99 mg/dl. Pre-diabetes or impaired fasting glucose is defined as 100 to 125 mg/dl. Diabetes is diagnosed based on a value of 126 mg/dl or above.

The second approach is to measure the *casual plasma glucose*. In this test, the blood sample can be taken at any time of day without regard to when the last meal was eaten. A diagnosis of diabetes is indicated if the glucose level is 200 mg/dl or above *and* the person has the classic symptoms of diabetes which are increased urination, increased thirst, and unexplained weight loss.

The third method is the *oral glucose tolerance test*. For this test, the patient reports to the lab after an eight-hour fast and drinks a glucose dose (75 grams dissolved in water). Two hours later a blood sample is collected. Diabetes is indicated if the two-hour value is 200 mg/dl or higher. Pre-diabetes or impaired glucose tolerance is indicated if the value is between 140 and 199 mg/dl. Regardless of the method used, if diabetes is diagnosed, it must be confirmed with a subsequent test on a separate day. Any one of the three methods can be used to confirm an initial positive diagnosis.

Of the three methods, the fasting plasma glucose test is the preferred method and most widely accepted. It's a routine measurement made on blood samples during annual physical exams. The test is easy to perform, relatively convenient for patients, and low cost. In contrast, the oral glucose tolerance test is not as widely used, as it's more burdensome to patients, more time consuming, and more costly. In certain cases though, it may be the preferred test.

CHALLENGE OF TREATMENT

The goal for successfully treating diabetes is to do what the body does naturally for most people—to maintain the proper balance between glucose and insulin. In diabetes the glucose-insulin synergy is impaired, either due to a lack of insulin being produced (insulin deficiency), an inability to effectively use the insulin (insulin resistance), or a combination of the two factors. Even with these limitations, the overall physiological processes remain operational. Food still makes the blood glucose level rise. Insulin and exercise make it fall. But the normal responsiveness and sensitivity to these variables are lacking.

Consequently, treatment of diabetes involves carefully controlling the type and amount, sequencing, and interaction among diet, exercise, and, for most people, drugs. Among adults with diagnosed diabetes, 14 percent take insulin only, 13 percent take both insulin and oral medication, 57 percent

| FIGURE 10.3 | TREATMENT WITH INSULIN OR ORAL MEDICATIONS AMONG ADULTS WITH DIAGNOSED DIABETES |

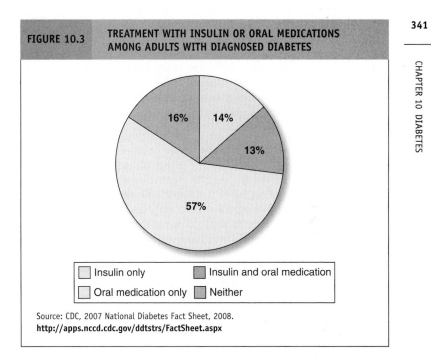

Legend:
- Insulin only
- Insulin and oral medication
- Oral medication only
- Neither

Source: CDC, 2007 National Diabetes Fact Sheet, 2008.
http://apps.nccd.cdc.gov/ddtstrs/FactSheet.aspx

take oral medication only, and 16 percent are treated without drugs (refer to Figure 10.3). With multiple factors to coordinate, it is easy to understand why diabetes self-management education is an integral part of medical care. The goal of diabetes treatment never stops. It is to keep blood glucose levels within the normal range as much as possible. If blood glucose levels are carefully controlled, complications are less likely to develop.

Keeping blood glucose levels from getting too high—hyperglycemia—is the primary challenge. But the problem with tightly controlling levels to prevent high blood glucose is that low blood glucose, or **hypoglycemia,** may occur. Most cases of low blood glucose—generally considered lower than 70 mg/dl—are caused by an "overshoot" or excessive effect of the insulin or oral medications taken to lower the blood glucose levels. Hypoglycemia is uncommon among people without diabetes.

Symptoms of hypoglycemia can begin slowly or suddenly and progress from mild discomfort to severe confusion to fainting or coma. Hypoglycemia should be treated immediately because prolonged hypoglycemia can cause brain damage. Symptoms are relieved within minutes of consuming sugar in any form such as a few ounces of fruit juice or a regular (not diet) soft drink or a few pieces of candy. Many people with diabetes carry these "quick-fix"

Hypoglycemia is low blood glucose levels and can occur as a side effect of diabetes treatment.

foods, glucose tablets, or foil packets of a glucose-containing liquid. Milk is actually better than juice or glucose because it has lactose, fat, and protein, and this combination not only raises blood sugar but also keeps it more stable over time. However, milk is not easily carried or always readily available. A doctor may prescribe a glucagon kit for those prone to hypoglycemia, as an injection will quickly raise one's blood glucose. Family, friends, and co-workers can be taught how to inject glucagon in an emergency.

Less frequent but even more dangerous is a condition called **ketoacidosis.** If glucose is not readily available to the body's tissues, fat is broken down as a source of energy, and ketones are produced as a by-product. If the body burns too much fat too quickly, ketones will accumulate in the bloodstream and make the body too acidic, upsetting normal chemical balance and leading to ketoacidosis. Untreated, this condition can lead to coma and death. Symptoms include excessive thirst and urination; nausea; vomiting; rapid, shallow breathing; stomach and chest pain; and fatigue. Hospital treatment involves intravenous administration of large amounts of fluids with electrolytes to replace those lost through excessive urination. Insulin is also generally given intravenously so that it works quickly and the dose can be adjusted frequently. Controlling blood glucose levels and replacing fluid and electrolytes usually allow the body to restore the normal acid-base balance.

MANAGING DIABETES

Diabetes is a complex disease and best treated with a team approach. Two key elements for optimally managing diabetes are patient education and a specialized medical team. People with diabetes benefit greatly from learning as much as possible about the disease—particularly, the practical, everyday steps that must be taken to control it. For example, self-testing of blood glucose is a daily routine. People with diabetes check their blood glucose level several times throughout the day using a drop of blood from a finger prick and a small, easy-to-use glucose monitor. Each test indicates the blood glucose level at that particular time and can guide the person's subsequent actions regarding eating, exercise, and medications.

A specialized medical team provides patient education along with medical care. If the person's primary care doctor does not have expertise and experience in treating diabetes, the person is typically referred to an endocrinologist, a physician specializing in the treatment of hormonal and metabolic diseases. Other members of a diabetes-care medical team often include a nurse practitioner or a physician's assistant, a dietitian, an exercise specialist, a pharmacist, and a mental health professional such as a social worker, a psychologist, or a counselor. Many are certified as diabetes

Ketoacidosis is a life-threatening condition requiring immediate treatment; it is typically associated with uncontrolled diabetes and characterized by accumulation of ketones in the blood and increased acidity of the blood.

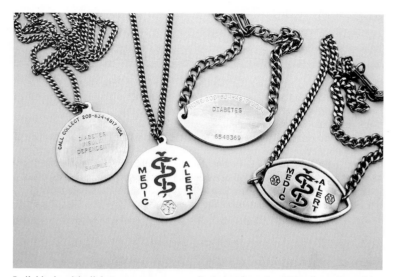

Individuals with diabetes may wear a medical alert bracelet. This allows for quick medical intervention in case the person is unable to give a medical history.

educators by the American Association of Diabetes Educators **(www .aadenet.org)**, a multidisciplinary professional organization that ensures the delivery of quality self-management training to diabetic patients.

An important marker of blood glucose management (glycemic control) is a blood test known as the *A1c*. This test indicates how well blood glucose has been controlled over the past several months. As glucose circulates in the blood, some of it spontaneously binds to hemoglobin A (the primary form of hemoglobin). Hemoglobin is the protein that carries oxygen in the red blood cells. Once the glucose is bound to the hemoglobin A, it remains there for the life of the red blood cell (about 120 days). The more glucose that is in the blood, the more that binds to hemoglobin A. This combination of glucose and hemoglobin A is called *A1c* or *hemoglobin A1c*. Measuring this compound reflects the overall blood glucose level over the previous two to three months. The A1c test helps the patient and doctor know if the treatment plan to control the diabetes is working or needs to be adjusted. A1c should be measured two to four times a year, and the goal is to have a reading that is less than 7 percent.

People with diabetes should let friends and co-workers know about their diabetes so that they are aware of the needs associated with diabetes management—such as dietary control, medications, and for some people, injections. Those with diabetes should also carry or wear a medical identification bracelet or tag to alert emergency workers and other health care professionals to the presence of diabetes. This information allows medical professionals to start life-saving procedures quickly and appropriately, whether treating a diabetes-related emergency or an injury or accident unrelated to the disease.

Health & the Media Ratcheting Up PSAs from Risk Awareness to Disease Management

Diabetes is now so widespread in the United States that PSAs such as this are designed for a broad audience—not just for people with diabetes but also their families and friends. Perhaps more than any other chronic disease, diabetes requires the individual's daily vigilance and appropriate actions to manage the disease. Using cartoonlike characters to catch the eye, this PSA is an example of how an information-dense message can be conveyed in a creative and engaging manner. The highlighted A, B, Cs combine the diabetes-specific measurement of A1c with measurements of blood pressure and cholesterol (which are discussed in Chapter 8, "Heart Disease and Stroke"), reinforcing the interrelatedness of the major cardiovascular and metabolic diseases.

Source: National Diabetes Education Program
http://ndep.nih.gov/diabetes/pubs/Ad_SuperHero.pdf

To deal with the complexities of diabetes, treatment and management should be individualized and address medical, psychosocial, and life-style issues. Acceptance of the disease and compliance with a management plan are not trivial issues. A team approach only works if the patient takes an *active role* in his or her care. In large degree, a person with diabetes is master of his or her fate. The actions a person chooses will determine how full a life he or she leads and to what degree disability is prevented.

Management of Type 1 Diabetes

Due to the lack of insulin production, type 1 diabetes is the most difficult form of diabetes to control. Type 1 is treated with insulin replacement along with a structured diet and physical activity regimen. Eating times, types and amounts of foods and beverages, and physical activity patterns should be consistent from day to day. Blood glucose is measured several times a day, and multiple insulin injections are necessary. Insulin can't be taken by mouth because the digestive juices destroy it. Most people find giving the injections simple and relatively painless because the needle is very small. Insulin is given at regular intervals, usually two to four times a day. Each injection may contain one type or a combination of different types of insulin—short-acting, intermediate-acting, or long-acting. As an alternative to injections, insulin pumps are increasingly being used. These pumps are small, computerized devices—about the size of a compact cell phone—worn outside the body (in a pocket, pouch, or on a belt). They provide continuous insulin delivery through a small, soft tube. Future prospects for treatment include the possibility of delivering insulin through an inhaler.

Breaking It Down "Human" Insulin— A First in Genetic Engineering

Since the discovery of insulin in 1921, a variety of insulins have been developed to meet the needs of people with diabetes. Harvesting pancreases from human corpses was not practical commercially, so insulin from the pancreases of cows and pigs was used instead. Both have "insulin activity" in humans because they are nearly identical to human insulin, differing in only one or a few amino acids (protein building blocks). However, even a slight difference is enough to elicit an allergic response in some people.

To overcome this problem, researchers looked for ways to make insulin that more closely resembled human insulin. Since the early 1980s, two methods have been used to make human insulin from nonhuman sources. One method involves the use of enzymes to convert insulin from pigs into human insulin by altering the one amino acid that is different. The second and more widely used method uses genetic engineering, or recombinant

(Continued)

DNA technology. Eli Lilly and Company marketed the first biogeneti-cally engineered synthetic human insulin in 1982.

Genetic engineering is the manipulation of the genetic material of cells in the laboratory to change hereditary traits or produce biological products. Techniques include isolating, copying, and multiplying DNA (genetic material); recombining DNA from different species; and transferring DNA from one species to another, bypassing the reproductive process. In this instance, bacteria are genetically altered to produce human insulin in large amounts. To provide a reliable source of human insulin, researchers obtain from human cells the DNA carrying the gene with the information for making human insulin. They then make a copy of this DNA and move it into a bacterium. As the bacterium grows in the lab, the microbe splits from one cell into two cells, and both cells get a copy of the insulin gene. As these two microbes grow, they divide into four, those four into eight, and so forth. And, remarkably, because the cells have a copy of the genetic "recipe card" for insulin, they produce insulin.

This synthesized human insulin is identical to the insulin naturally pro-duced in healthy humans. The recombinant DNA technology put to rest the fear that insulin production from animals would not be able to meet the need of the ever-increasing diabetic population. It had been forecast as early as 1976 that by the early 1990s demand would outstrip supply. Today, insulin from cows is no longer available and insulin from pigs is being phased out. The additional good news is that the cost of "human" insulin has remained similar to that of animal-derived insulin.

Genetic engineering is a controversial issue. And it should be. After all, genetic engineering provides the means to alter the normal biology of living organisms by increasing the yield of a crop species, introducing a novel trait, or producing a new protein. As such, it brings on a host of legal, regulatory, and ethical challenges. In the case of "human" insulin, there has been little debate. A major medical need was met, and no major side effects or long-lasting adverse events have been identified.

Currently, biotechnology products are regulated by the U.S. Department of Agriculture, the Environmental Protection Agency, and the Food and Drug Administration. Together, these agencies are empowered by law to use three criteria when assessing new products: safety, efficacy, and qual-ity. Is the product sufficiently safe for humans and the environment? Does the product work as intended? Can the quality of the product be assured? Other considerations include the potential or probable social and economic impacts of the product. Clearly, the more we know about biotechnology, the better prepared we are to make personal choices and provide input on policies about the use of new technologies and their products.

In the past, type 2 diabetes was sometimes considered the milder form of diabetes. This is no longer the case. Although most people with type 2 do not require insulin, the consequences of not controlling high blood glucose can lead to the same serious metabolic and tissue damage complications as type 1. Generally, type 2 can be controlled with diet and exercise, especially if detected early. When lifestyle measures don't provide adequate blood glucose control, then medication in tablet form is used. The different types of medicine work in one of several ways: helping the beta cells of the pancreas make more insulin, increasing the use of glucose and decreasing glucose production, slowing the absorption of glucose from the intestine, or stimulating insulin release from the pancreas. Over time, even a careful diabetes management plan (i.e., optimal diet, exercise, oral medication therapies) may not be sufficient to keep type 2 diabetes under control. If this occurs, then insulin injections may become necessary.

✓ NEED TO KNOW

The most widely-used criterion measure for diagnosing diabetes is a fasting blood glucose level equal to or greater than 126 mg/dl. Pre-diabetes is indicated when the fasting blood glucose level is in the borderline range of 100–125 mg/dl. Since as many as one out of four people with type 2 diabetes are undiagnosed, it's important to know the risk factors and be screened as appropriate. The goal of diabetes treatment is to keep blood glucose levels within the normal range. Hypoglycemia and ketoacidosis are related conditions that may occur with poor glycemic control. With the help of a diabetes health care team, a management plan addressing lifestyle, medical, and psychosocial issues is tailored to each individual. The key then becomes successful implementation and maintenance. In the final analysis, diabetes is about self-care.

➤ Prevention of Type 2 Diabetes

To date, there is no known method to prevent type 1 diabetes, although pancreatic islet transplantation shows promise and may become a viable option for selected patients within the next decade. In marked contrast to type 1, type 2 diabetes is largely a preventable disease. This is an important point to emphasize because the projected rise in type 2 diabetes is ominous. Unless population-wide lifestyle changes occur, public health experts forecast that approximately one out of three people born in the year 2000 will develop diabetes.

Responsibility to take action rests squarely on the shoulders of individuals and families. They need to avoid health-compromising habits and take the initiative to establish health-promoting practices. Once a person has diabetes, the decision to make smart choices seems so clear *in retrospect*. Humans, unlike most other animals, have the capacity to plan and set a course of action based on a plan. We should apply this capacity to our health and the prevention of disease just as we do in other aspects of our lives.

Be aware of the risk factors for diabetes and pre-diabetes, and be screened as appropriate. Remember that approximately one-fourth of all people with diabetes may be undiagnosed and that diabetes is occurring at earlier ages. Being overweight and having a family history of diabetes are the two most apparent risk factors. The relative risk for diabetes increases with increasing BMI. For the extended list of risk factors and guidelines for screening, refer to the earlier section "Diagnosis and Control."

What Is Your Risk? A New Phenomenon— Type 2 Diabetes in Young People

From the 1930s till the 1990s, if a child or young adult had diabetes, it was known that they had type 1 or what was then called *juvenile diabetes*. Type 2 or adult-onset diabetes was a disease of predominantly obese adults who were middle-aged and older; it was not seen in children or young adults. But then in the 1990s, a new trend emerged. Physicians began to occasionally diagnose type 2 diabetes in people in their 30s, 20s, and even occasionally in their teens. This was a startling observation. What was happening that could cause premature development of type 2 diabetes? Were these cases rare individual occurrences, or were they early indications of a troubling new trend?

The development of type 2 diabetes in children and young people is clearly linked to the obesity epidemic, which in turn is associated with poor dietary patterns and low levels of physical activity. As seen in Figure 10.4, the prevalence of children and adolescents who are overweight has tripled over the past three decades. Because about 90 percent of type 2 diabetes is attributed to weight gain, it is understandable that type 2 diabetes appears to be rising among U.S. youth. There is also evidence that exposure to diabetes in utero (gestational diabetes) may be a major contributor. Although the epidemiology of type 2 diabetes in youth is limited, clinical reports and regional studies indicate type 2 diabetes is being diagnosed more frequently in children and adolescents, particularly in Native Americans, Blacks, and Hispanics. The International Diabetes Federation states that type 2 diabetes in the young is a global phenomenon that is on the increase and affecting children in both developed and developing countries.

(Continued)

Another indicator of a national trend is the disproportionate rise in the prevalence of diabetes in young adults compared to middle-aged and older people. The estimated distribution of diabetes in 2007 was 2.6 percent among the 20–39 age group, which reflects an increase of 63 percent from the prevalence of 1.6 percent in this age group in 1990. By contrast, during the same 17-year period, the diabetes prevalence estimates for other age groups increased only slightly. Only a few chronic diseases among young adults have a higher prevalence. Asthma is a notable example, with about 11 percent of 20- to 39-year-olds affected. However, asthma is not on the rise and, generally speaking, the potential complications and consequences of diabetes are far more serious.

Despite extensive experience with and knowledge of type 2 diabetes among adults, we know little about the disease in children—its epidemiology, pathophysiology, and medical management. This presents a new challenge to researchers, health care professionals, and public health specialists as well as to individuals and their families. The medical scientists will continue to investigate this phenomenon and update us. In the meantime, the increase of premature diabetes among children, teenagers, and young adults can be combated with the same measures as those prescribed for middle-aged and older adults—regular physical activity, good dietary habits, and a healthy body weight.

Take the Diabetes Risk Test at **www.diabetes.org/risk-test.jsp**

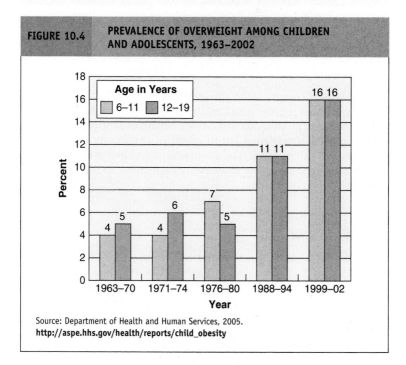

FIGURE 10.4 **PREVALENCE OF OVERWEIGHT AMONG CHILDREN AND ADOLESCENTS, 1963–2002**

Source: Department of Health and Human Services, 2005.
http://aspe.hhs.gov/health/reports/child_obesity

For those who already have been diagnosed with pre-diabetes, the potential to prevent the onset of diabetes with diet and exercise is promising. In a major three-year clinical trial known as the Diabetes Prevention Program, high-risk participants randomly assigned to a lifestyle intervention group reduced their risk of getting diabetes by 58 percent. The lifestyle intervention focused on healthful changes in diet and physical activity. For example, participants reduced intake of saturated fats and increased intake of whole grain foods. They also built up to and maintained physical activity at 30 minutes per day—through brisk walking or similar moderate-intensity exercise. In a second group, participants were treated with standard diabetes oral medication. They reduced their risk of getting diabetes by 31 percent—a nice reduction, but not as great as the reduction for those in the lifestyle intervention. Those in the lifestyle intervention group lost about 6 percent of their body weight compared to no weight loss among those in the medication group.

This large study was conducted at 27 centers nationwide and involved over 3,000 people with pre-diabetes. Participants ranged in age from 25 to 85 with an average age of 51, and nearly half were from minority groups that disproportionately develop type 2 diabetes. All were overweight, with an average BMI of 34. The structured lifestyle intervention worked as well in men as women, in all ethnic groups, and across the age range. The study ended a year early because the data clearly answered the main research question regarding the effectiveness of a lifestyle intervention to delay the development of type 2 diabetes. Ending a clinical trial study early due to excellent results is a highly unusual. While both the lifestyle and oral medication treatments were found to be effective, the lifestyle intervention (diet and exercise) was found to be better.

The best strategy for preventing pre-diabetes and type 2 diabetes is to eat properly, exercise regularly, and maintain a healthy weight. The overall health benefits of positive diet and exercise behaviors are truly astounding. Conversely, the detrimental health effects of chronically poor lifestyle habits are extensive as well. The multifactorial and global aspects of diet and physical activity on health are further illustrated in the next section on the metabolic syndrome.

✓ NEED TO KNOW

Type 2 diabetes is a largely preventable disease, yet its prevalence among Americans has been climbing steadily since the 1980s. Prevention depends primarily on awareness and proactive steps by individuals and families. If you know someone with advanced diabetes, your incentive to prevent diabetes may be particularly meaningful. The tools for prevention are readily available by incorporating a healthy diet and physical activity and maintaining a healthy weight. Even for those who are overweight and/or pre-diabetic, the potential to prevent or slow the progression to diabetes through lifestyle intervention is a real option. Research has convincingly shown that a reasonable program of proper diet and exercise substantially reduces the risk of getting diabetes.

➤ Metabolic Syndrome

The metabolic syndrome is a cluster of interrelated metabolic and cardio-vascular risk factors that appear to directly promote type 2 diabetes and atherosclerosis. Over the last few years, leading health organizations including the National Heart Lung and Blood Institute, American Heart Association, World Health Organization (WHO), and International Diabetes Association have issued official scientific statements to define and describe the metabolic syndrome and to provide up-to-date guidance on diagnosis and treatment.

WHAT IS THE METABOLIC SYNDROME?

Although it remains unclear whether the metabolic syndrome has a single cause, it appears that it can be precipitated by multiple underlying risk factors. The most important of these are abdominal obesity and insulin resistance. Other associated conditions include physical inactivity, hormonal imbalance, aging, and genetic or ethnic predisposition. Population studies show that the metabolic syndrome confers a twofold increase for heart disease and stroke, and in individuals without established type 2 diabetes, an approximate fivefold increase in risk for developing diabetes as compared with people without the syndrome.

Several different sets of criteria have been proposed over the past decade for diagnosis of the metabolic syndrome. The criteria most widely accepted are those adopted by the American Heart Association and the National Heart, Lung, and Blood Institute. As presented in Table 10.1, these include

TABLE 10.1	DEFINITION AND CRITERIA OF THE METABOLIC SYNDROME
Metabolic syndrome is defined as having three or more of the following five criteria:	
RISK FACTORS	**CRITERIA**
Abdominal obesity (waist girth)	> 40 inches for men, > 35 inches for women
Triglycerides	≥ 150 mg/dl
HDL cholesterol	< 40 mg/dl for men, < 50 mg/dl for women
Blood pressure	≥ 130/85 mm Hg
Fasting blood glucose	≥ 110 mg/dl

Reference: SM Grundy et al. *Circulation* 112: 2735–2752, 2005.

five common clinical measurements: waist circumference, triglycerides, HDL cholesterol, blood pressure, and fasting blood glucose. The presence of abnormalities in any three of these five measures constitutes a diagnosis of the syndrome.

Since the 1980s, substantial research has shown that accumulation of upper body fat (on the trunk)—also known as abdominal or visceral fat—is more highly associated with both type 2 diabetes and atherosclerosis than lower body fat (on the hips and thighs). For this reason, large waist circumference (i.e., greater than 35 inches for women and 40 inches for men) is used in lieu of a high BMI as a criterion for the metabolic syndrome.

The summary schematic in Figure 10.5 presents a simple depiction of a complex web of interactions and likely causal links among lifestyle factors, human physiology, and metabolic syndrome. The middle box reflects a biological "mixing pot"—still a scientific black box in many respects—where multiple physiological systems are attempting to adapt to health-compromising factors as well as to each other. Behaviors can be viewed as input; the biological "pot" is where compensatory interplay among systems and disease processes occurs; and the resulting related diseases that constitute the metabolic syndrome are presented as output. Over time, cascading and wide-ranging effects toward disease (or health) can result from basic lifestyle choices.

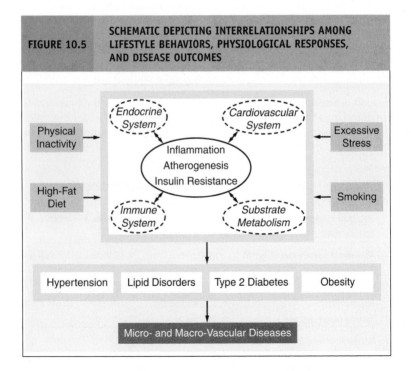

FIGURE 10.5 SCHEMATIC DEPICTING INTERRELATIONSHIPS AMONG LIFESTYLE BEHAVIORS, PHYSIOLOGICAL RESPONSES, AND DISEASE OUTCOMES

The primary goal in treating the metabolic syndrome is to reduce risk for atherosclerosis—namely, heart disease and stroke—and to decrease the risk for type 2 diabetes in people who do not yet have the disease. As in managing the diseases separately, the first-line approach is to reduce the major risk factors: reduce LDL cholesterol, blood pressure and blood glucose levels to the recommended goals, and if a smoker, to stop.

At age 27, Mike acknowledged that he was overweight but gave little thought to his overall health. After all, he was simply a big person, still relatively young, and busy with work and home activities. Then he volunteered to give blood during a blood drive at work and was turned away because of high blood pressure. Surprised by this, he saw his doctor who confirmed his hypertension and told him that his blood lipids were off the chart, too. His doctor was direct and to the point: "You need to lose 70 pounds. It's time to get serious about your health." Mike suddenly realized that his poor eating habits and his sedentary lifestyle had caught up with him, and he was at risk for heart disease and diabetes as well as many other diseases.

Whenever possible, initial treatments for metabolic syndrome should begin with lifestyle interventions—weight loss in overweight and obese people, a change in dietary patterns toward a prudent diet (low in saturated fats and refined sugars; high in whole grains, fruits, vegetables), and an increase in regular physical activity. Such changes will produce a reduction in all the metabolic syndrome risk factors simultaneously. The greatest benefit will be derived from consistent and lasting lifestyle intervention. As a second tier of treatment, an array of drug therapies are available for individual risk factors and are often used in combination with positive lifestyle modifications.

Mike decided to do something about his deteriorating medical condition and the inattention he had shown to his health. He made a promise to himself to turn his situation around. He started going to the gym regularly and made consistent adjustments in his diet, eating less processed foods and more fruits and vegetables. He relates, "I didn't cut out all the fun stuff; rather I just began to make better choices." These days, Mike feels healthier than he has in a long time. He is glad he finally recognized the need to take action and now would not have it any other way.

ONGOING PROFESSIONAL DEBATE

The definition of metabolic syndrome and the concept itself are still evolving. A consensus among the major professional societies has yet to be achieved. In a joint scientific review and position statement, the American Diabetes Association and the European Association for the Study of Diabetes report that too much essential information is missing to warrant the designation of the "metabolic syndrome" as a new syndrome and question the value of doing so. As an interesting aside, the American Diabetes Association recently proposed a similar concept of cardiometabolic health as a measure of a person's risk for diabetes and heart disease.

In contrast to the doubts of the American and European diabetes associations about the usefulness of the metabolic syndrome, the International Diabetes Federation, the American Heart Association, and the National Heart Blood Lung Institute are aligned in support of the concept. Their shared view is that early detection and intensive management of the metabolic syndrome are warranted. They contend that while no single treatment for the metabolic syndrome is yet available, lifestyle changes—such as improving diet and increasing physical activity—provide a solid basis for treatment. In addition, new drug treatments that would reduce several risk factors concurrently are under development and may have a significant impact on reducing both cardiovascular disease and diabetes in the years ahead.

These professional differences of opinion appear to be more about the interpretation and use of the concept than about its scientific basis. Regardless, further research will continue to shed light on our understanding and application of the metabolic syndrome to both personal and public health. In closing, the term *metabolic syndrome* describes a condition in which metabolic and atherogenic risk factors cluster in the same people more often than would be expected by chance. This provides a practical means for early detection of individuals at high risk for type 2 diabetes and cardiovascular disease and indicates an interaction among diseases once thought to be separate conditions.

In related initiatives, the American Cancer Society, American Diabetes Association, and American Heart Association have joined together to promote clinical and public health interventions that reduce prevalence of tobacco use, poor diet, and insufficient physical activity—the major risk factors for cardiovascular disease, diabetes, and cancer. Perhaps over the next decade, as research progresses and we learn more about the metabolic syndrome, professional organizations will reach consensus. Stay tuned. In the meantime, all are united in supporting prevention and early detection of chronic disease.

✓ NEED TO KNOW

The metabolic syndrome is a clustering of risk factors associated with diabetes and cardiovascular disease. The metabolic syndrome provides a striking example of the continuous interaction among circulatory, metabolic, endocrine, and immune systems in their adaptations to lifestyle behaviors. Our body's physiological systems do not operate separately. Rather, complex collective and compensatory influences are at work among them. Likewise, our health behaviors affect more than a single system or disease. Indeed, lifestyle habits have overall effects—for better or worse.

Diabetes
American Diabetes Association
www.diabetes.org
American Association of Diabetes Educators
www.aadenet.org
GlaxoSmithKline's Diabetes.com
www.diabetes.com
International Diabetes Federation
www.idf.org
Joslin Diabetes Center
www.joslin.harvard.edu/

Metabolic Syndrome
Mayo Clinic **www.mayoclinic.com/health/metabolic%20syndrome/
DS00522/DSECTION=1**
National Diabetes Education Program
http://ndep.nih.gov
National Heart, Lung, and Blood Institute, NIH
www.nhlbi.nih.gov/health/dci/Diseases/ms/ms_whatis.html

Knowing the Language

diabetes
gestational diabetes
hyperglycemia
hypoglycemia
insulin

ketoacidosis
metabolic syndrome
pre-diabetes
type 1 diabetes
type 2 diabetes

Understanding the Content

1. Where is insulin produced, and what is its role in the body?
2. Explain the differences among type 1 diabetes, type 2 diabetes, and pre-diabetes.
3. What are the risk factors for diabetes?
4. Define *metabolic syndrome* and the criteria for diagnosis.

Exploring Ideas

1. Type 2 diabetes is by far the most common form of the disease, yet it's largely preventable. Its prevalence in the population is at an all-time high and projected to rise even higher. Why is this happening, and what needs to be done to turn the tide?
2. Just as with high blood pressure and abnormal blood lipids, we should know the numbers that define the condition. What fasting

blood glucose levels define pre-diabetes and diabetes? What is the A1c measurement, and when is it used?

3. Explain how eating a healthy diet and exercising regularly lowers a person's risk for developing type 2 diabetes and the metabolic syndrome.

Selected References

American Diabetes Association. Diabetes Statistics
  www.diabetes.org/diabetes-statistics.jsp

American Diabetes Association. CheckUp America: Know Your Risk, Lower Your Risk for Diabetes and Heart Disease.
  www.diabetes.org/diabetes-prevention/check-up-america.jsp

American Diabetes Association. Clinical practice recommendations 2007. *Diabetes Care* 30: Supplement 1, 2007.
  http://care.diabetesjournals.org/content/vol30/suppl_1/index.shtml

American Diabetes Association. The Cardiometabolic Risk Initiative, 2006.
  www.diabetes.org/for-health-professionals-and-scientists/cardiometabolic-risk.jsp

Blaha M, Elasy TA. Clinical use of the metabolic syndrome: Why the confusion? *Clinical Diabetes* 24:125–131, 2006
  http://clinical.diabetesjournals.org/cgi/content/full/24/3/125

Centers for Disease Control and Prevention (CDC). *Health, United States,* 2007.
  www.cdc.gov/nchs/hus.htm

CDC. National Diabetes Fact Sheet, 2007.
  http://apps.nccd.cdc.gov/ddtstrs/factsheet.aspx

CDC. Diabetes Projects: Children and Diabetes.
  www.cdc.gov/diabetes/projects/diab_child.htm

Department of Health and Human Services. Childhood Obesity. 2005.
  http://aspe.hhs.gov/health/reports/child_obesity

Diabetes Prevention Program Research Group. Reduction in the incidence of type 2 diabetes with lifestyle intervention or metformin. *New England Journal of Medicine* 346: 393–403, 2002.
  http://content.nejm.org/cgi/content/full/346/6/393

Eckel RH, Kahn R, Robertson RM, et al. Preventing cardiovascular disease and diabetes: A call to action from the American Diabetes Association and the American Heart Association. *Diabetes Care* 29:1697–1699, 2006.
  http://care.diabetesjournals.org/cgi/content/short/29/7/1697

Eyre H, Kahn R, Robertson RM, et al. Preventing cancer, cardiovascular disease, and diabetes: a common agenda for the American Cancer Society, the American Diabetes Association, and the American Heart Association. *CA: A Cancer Journal for Clinicians* 54: 190–207, 2004.
  http://caonline.amcancersoc.org/content/vol54/issue4/

Grundy SM, Cleeman JI, Daniels SR, et al. AHA/NHLBI scientific

statement: Diagnosis and management of the metabolic syndrome. *Circulation* 112: 2735–2752, 2005.
http://circ.ahajournals.org/cgi/content/full/112/17/2735

International Diabetes Association. The IDF consensus worldwide definition of the metabolic syndrome, 2005.
www.idf.org/home/index.cfm?node=1429

International Diabetes Association. *Diabetes e-Atlas*
www.eatlas.idf.org/

Kahn R, Buse J, Ferrannini E, et al. The metabolic syndrome: time for a critical appraisal: joint statement from the American Diabetes Association and the European Association for the Study of Diabetes. *Diabetes Care* 28: 2289–2304, 2005.

Kemple AM, Zlot AI, Leman RF. Perceived likelihood of developing diabetes among high-risk Oregonians. *Preventing Chronic Disease* [serial online], November 2005.
www.cdc.gov/pcd/issues/2005/nov/05_0067.htm

Nobel Prize in Physiology or Medicine, 1923.
http://nobelprize.org/medicine/laureates/1923

Public Health Agency of Canada. The Many Faces of Diabetes—Mike's Story.
www.phac-aspc.gc.ca/ccdpc-cpcmc/diabetes-diabete/english/faces/mike.html

Sanders LJ. *The philatelic history of diabetes: In search of a cure.* Alexandria, VA: American Diabetes Association, 2001.

Steinberger J, Daniels SR. AHA Scientific statement: Obesity, insulin resistance, diabetes, and cardiovascular risk in children. *Circulation* 107: 1448–1453, 2003.

Weiss R, Dziura J, Burgert TS, et al. Obesity and the metabolic syndrome in children and adolescents. *New England Journal of Medicine* 350: 2362–2374, 2004.

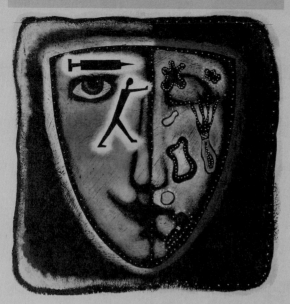

Epidemics have often been more influential than statesmen and soldiers in shaping the course of political history, and diseases may also color the moods of civilizations.

— RENÉ DUBOS

Chapter 11

INFECTIONS

The relationship between people and microbes has in part defined our world. Who hasn't heard of the Plague? The great influenza epidemic? HIV/AIDS? In Chapter 11 we examine all facets of the infectious disease process including signs, symptoms, treatment, risk factors, and risk reduction. At the end of the chapter, emerging issues, from new diseases to bioterrorism, will be explored.

Communicable Disease Process
PATHOGENS
MODE OF TRANSMISSION
PORTALS OF ENTRY AND EXIT
STAGES OF RESPONSE

Fighting Disease
IMMUNE SYSTEM
VACCINES
ANTIBIOTICS
ANTIVIRALS
PREVENTION

Common Bacterial Infections
STAPH INFECTIONS
STREP INFECTIONS

Common Viral Infections
INFLUENZA
MONONUCLEOSIS
HERPES 1
HEPATITIS

Common Fungal Infections

Sexually Transmitted Infections
CHLAMYDIA
GONORRHEA
PELVIC INFLAMMATORY DISEASE
SYPHILIS
HERPES 2
(HPV) HUMAN PAPILLOMA VIRUS
PREVENTION OF SEXUALLY TRANSMITTED INFECTIONS
HIV AND AIDS

Bioterrorism

> The fate of most microbes that invade us is quick death. Sometimes, though,
> a microbe finds in humans an ideal environment, with plenty of nourishment
> and mere Maginot resistance. And it has its own weapon; it can attack or
> elude white blood cells, produce toxins, and kill and feed on tissues anywhere
> from the toes to the depths of the brain. If it multiplies unhindered, it may kill
> the host. But should that happen before the germ finds transport to another
> home, the meeting becomes a dead end for host and parasite alike.

As the quote from Karlen's book describes, the world is filled with microbes that infect and sicken humans. Some cause illnesses that are easy to transmit but prove more annoying than serious. Others are life threatening but hard to catch. A few are unfortunately both deadly and easy to spread. An example of the last type of infection is the one that was responsible for the Influenza Pandemic of 1918, which is estimated to have killed tens of millions of people—more than died in World War I.

In the second half of the 20th century, the development of antibiotics greatly reduced the number of deaths from bacteria infections. But microbes have mutated and adapted defenses against many antibiotics in the past few decades. Each year approximately 18,000 Americans die from MRSA (methicillin-resistant *Staphylococcus aureus*), a common bacteria that has become resistant to antibiotics. Because of this resistance, the bacteria can multiply unhindered and may kill the host.

In this chapter we will discuss the communicable disease process and the human immune response that protects us. We will also describe some of the more common infections that affect people today.

➤ Communicable Disease Process

The common link shared by all communicable diseases is that they are caused by microorganisms called **pathogens,** *germs,* or *microbes*. Thousands of communicable diseases have been identified. The American Public Health Association publishes the *Control of Communicable Diseases in Man,* the definitive resource that describes all communicable diseases and all facets of the communicable disease process including transmission, prevention, and treatment.

Any communicable disease is defined by not only the pathogen responsible for the disease but also the process by which the pathogen can infect people. The communicable disease process involves pathogens, reservoir, modes of transmission, hosts, and stages of response (incubation,

Pathogens are microorganisms that cause communicable disease.

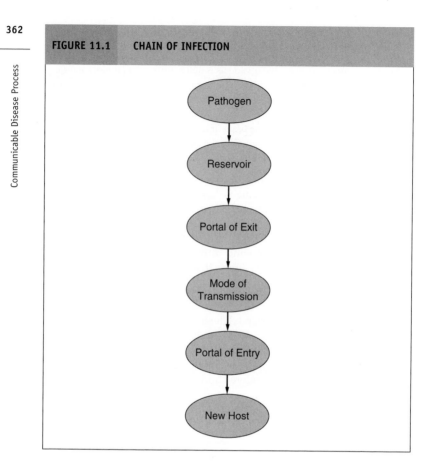

FIGURE 11.1   CHAIN OF INFECTION

prodromal, acute, and recovery). All communicable diseases follow the process shown in Figure 11.1.

PATHOGENS

Six major groups of pathogens cause communicable diseases. These include bacteria, viruses, fungi, rickettsia, metazoa, and protozoa. Most common diseases are caused by bacteria, viruses, and fungi. Pathogens are living organisms, and as such, must have a place where they can live and reproduce in their natural environment. This place is termed a *reservoir*. Not surprisingly, the reservoir for the most common diseases that affect people is the human body.

MODE OF TRANSMISSION

Infection occurs when a pathogen leaves the reservoir (that is, an infected person) and enters another person. This process is referred to as the *mode of transmission.* **Direct modes of transmission** are person to person via coughing, sneezing, or sexual contact. **Indirect modes of transmission** include vectors and vehicles. Vectors are insects, such as mosquitoes or ticks, that carry a pathogen. An insect that carries a pathogen bites a person in order to feed and as a result gives the person the pathogen that causes disease. Vehicles are substances like water and food. If a pathogen exists in the vehicle, it is consumed. Inanimate objects such as drinking glasses and eating utensils are also considered vehicles, since people can pick up pathogens from their contaminated surfaces.

PORTALS OF ENTRY AND EXIT

Pathogens require portals of entry and exit in order to infect a person and for that person to pass the infection to others. Portals include the nose, mouth, and reproductive system. The skin normally protects against infection, but when its surface is broken by a cut, scrape, or insect bite, then it too becomes a possible portal of entry. Finally, during sexual activity, pathogens can be transmitted from mucous membrane to mucous membrane.

STAGES OF RESPONSE

Once inside the body, pathogens have specific mechanisms of action on body cells. There are many variations within pathogen groups that result in differences in infection mechanisms. Some of these will be noted when discussing selected diseases. Regardless of the variations, there are four stages of response to any pathogen.

The first stage is called **incubation,** which is defined as the time between exposure to the pathogen and the onset of clinical symptoms. It is the time when the pathogen is reproducing in the system and doing whatever it uniquely does to take over the body.

After incubation, the infected person begins to experience early symptoms of the disease, called *prodrome* or the **prodromal stage.** During the prodromal stage, most people don't realize they are sick, and they tend to attribute the symptoms to something else—lack of sleep, allergies, or general tiredness. As the symptoms get more intense and the person begins to feel sick, the infection enters the peak, or **acute, stage.**

Direct mode of transmission is disease transmission through person-to-person contact. **Indirect mode of transmission** is disease transmission via food or insects.

Incubation is the time between exposure to a pathogen and the onset of the infection's symptoms.

The **prodromal stage** is the early symptoms of a disease. The **acute stage** is the period when a person is the sickest with an infection.

One of three things can happen after the acute stage: death (the pathogen wins), **recovery** (the person's immune response system wins), or relapse (the person begins to recover and then goes back into another acute stage). Relapse normally occurs if a person doesn't get the right amount of rest or stops taking prescribed medication too soon, allowing the pathogen to once again gain the upper hand.

✓ NEED TO KNOW

Most common infectious diseases are caused by bacteria, viruses, and fungi. Direct modes of transmission are person to person via coughing, sneezing, or sexual contact. Indirect modes of transmission include vectors (such as insects) and vehicle (such as food, utensils, or other objects). Stages of infection are incubation, when symptoms have not yet appeared; prodromal, when symptoms first begin to emerge; and acute, when the full-blown infection is obvious. The acute stage is followed by recovery if the host successfully conquers the infection, or by death if the pathogen completely overwhelms the host. In long-term infectious diseases, the acute stage may sometimes be followed by a series of partial recoveries and relapses to the acute stage.

➤ Fighting Disease

Our body interprets infection with a pathogen as an invasion and tries to fight. A war of sorts ensues, with the pathogen trying to multiply on one side, and the body trying to kill off the pathogens on the other. The most effective method of fighting infections is our own immune system. Other methods include drugs such as vaccines, antibiotics, and antivirals.

IMMUNE SYSTEM

The immune system continually guards against foreign substances called **antigens.** Pathogens are considered antigens. White blood cells called **leukocytes** are the most basic unit of the immune system. Phagocytes and lymphocytes are the two main types of leukocytes. **Phagocytes** will surround, engulf, and digest pathogens or other material that is recognized as being foreign to the body. Phagocytes can also be specialized.

Recovery is overcoming the infection and getting better.

An **antigen** is a foreign substance in the body that triggers the production of antibodies.

Leukocytes are white blood cells.

Phagocytes are white blood cells that surround and destroy foreign substances in the body.

For example, neutrophils are a type of phagocyte that primarily targets bacteria. A clinical application of this knowledge about different kinds of white blood cells is a blood test ordered by a physician to determine neutrophil count. If the count is higher than normal, it indicates a bacterial infection, which then has implications for the physician's recommendations about treatment.

Lymphocytes originate in the bone marrow, and they can stay in the bone marrow and develop into B lymphocytes, often referred to as **B cells.** T lymphocytes, or **T cells,** are those that leave the bone marrow and mature in the thymus gland. T cells and B cells work in partnership. If a pathogen invades the body, it is detected by the B cells, which produce antigen-specific **antibodies,** specialized proteins capable of destroying antigens. The T cells then destroy the pathogens.

The process of immunity is defined by lymphocytes and antibodies, but the broader types of immunity include activity immunity and passive immunity. In active immunity, the protection develops after direct exposure to the pathogen. Cells in our immune response recognize the pathogen if we are subsequently exposed, and that increases our body's capability to fight that particular type of infection. Passive immunity is a process by which people get antibodies from another source, such as when infants ingest them in breast milk. Passive immunity is short-lived.

VACCINES

Vaccines can be an effective way to prevent an infection. When people are vaccinated, they are given a weakened or dead form of the pathogen, and they develop an immunity to it through their body's formation of antibodies. Figure 11.2 shows the diseases for which vaccinations are available.

ANTIBIOTICS

As their name implies, **antibiotics** fight bacterial infections. They are antibodies that, once administered, either destroy the bacteria directly or

---

Lymphocytes are a type of white blood cell and are the most basic unit of immunity. **B Cells** are lymphocytes that produce antibodies. **T Cells** are small circulating lymphocytes that mediate immune response.

Antibodies are proteins that are produced to destroy antigens, including pathogens.

Vaccines are a treatment made from weakened or dead pathogens that allow the body to build up immunity against specific diseases.

Antibiotics are antibodies given as a drug that disrupt bacterial processes and stop an infection from growing.

FIGURE 11.2 ADULT IMMUNIZATION SCHEDULE

VACCINE ▼ / AGE GROUP ▶	19–49 Years	50–64 Years	≥ 65 Years
Tetanus, Diphtheria, Pertussis (Td/Tdap)[1],*	Substitute 1 dose of Tdap for Td		
Tetanus, Diphtheria, Pertussis (Td/Tdap)[1],*	1 dose Td booster every 10 yrs		
Human papillomavirus (HPV)[2],*	3 doses females (0, 2, 6 mos)		
Measles, Mumps, Rubella (MMR)[3],*	1 or 2 doses	1 dose	
Varicella[4],*	2 doses (0, 4–8 wks)		
Influenza[5],*	1 dose annually		
Pneumococcal (polysaccharide)[6,7]	1–2 doses		1 dose
Hepatitis A[8],*	2 doses (0, 6–12 mos or 0, 6–18 mos)		
Hepatitis B[9],*	3 doses (0, 1–2, 4–6 mos)		
Meningococcal[10],*	1 or more doses		
Zoster[11]			1 dose

For all persons in this category who meet the age requirements and who lack evidence of immunity (e.g., lack documentation of vaccination or have no evidence of prior infection)

Recommended if some other risk factor is present (e.g., on the basis of medical, occupational, lifestyle, or other indications)

*Covered by the Vaccine Injury Compensation Program.

VACCINE ▼ / INDICATION ▶	Pregnancy	Immuno-compromising conditions (excluding human immunodeficiency virus [HIV], medications, radiation)[3]	HIV infection[3,12,13] CD4 + T lymphocte count — <200 cells/µL	HIV infection[3,12,13] CD4 + T lymphocte count — ≥200 cells/µL	Diabetes, heart disease, chronic pulmonary disease, chronic alcoholism	Asplenia[12] (including elective splenectomy and terminal complement component deficiencies)	Chronic liver disease	Kidney failure, end-stage renal disease, receipt of hemodialysis	Health-care personnel
Tetanus, Diphtheria, Pertussis (Td/Tdap)[1,*]	1 dose Td booster every 10 yrs / Substitute 1 dose of Tdap for Td								
Human papillomavirus (HPV)[2,*]		3 doses for females through age 26 yrs (0, 2, 6 mos)							
Measles, Mumps, Rubella (MMR)[3,*]	Contraindicated	Contraindicated	Contraindicated		1 or 2 doses				
Varicella[4,*]	Contraindicated	Contraindicated	Contraindicated		2 doses (0, 4–8 wks)				
Influenza[5,*]	1 dose TIV annually				1 dose TIV annually	1–2 doses			1 dose TIV or LAIV annually
Pneumococcal (polysaccharide)[6,7]					1–2 doses				
Hepatitis A[8,*]						2 doses (0, 6–12 mos or 0, 6–18 mos)			
Hepatitis B[9,*]						3 doses (0, 1–2, 4–6 mos)			
Meningococcal[10,*]						1 or more doses			
Zoster[11]	Contraindicated	Contraindicated	Contraindicated				1 dose		

- For all persons in this category who meet the age requirements and who lack evidence of immunity (e.g., lack documentation of vaccination or have no evidence of prior infection)
- Recommended if some other risk factor is present (e.g., on the basis of medical, occupational, lifestyle, or other indications)

*Covered by the Vaccine Injury Compensation Program.

Report all clinically significant postvaccination reactions to the Vaccine Adverse Event Reporting System (VAERS). Reporting forms and instructions on filing a VAERS report are available at **www.vaers.hhs.gov**. Additional information about the vaccines in this schedule is available at **www.cdc.gov/vaccines**

Source: CDC.

block bacterial biological processes, causing the pathogens to self-destruct. Antibiotics are specific to certain types of bacteria, so a diagnosis must be made in order to prescribe the correct drug. It is also important that once an antibiotic is prescribed, the person takes the whole prescription in the course of treatment. If not, resistant strains of the bacteria can result. Resistance to antibiotics is becoming a serious problem because the altered bacteria cause infections that can become very virulent, difficult to treat, and deadly.

Some individuals are allergic to antibiotics, and their reaction to them can be life threatening. Physicians should ask any patient about known antibiotic allergies before prescribing an appropriate drug.

ANTIVIRALS

Antivirals are drugs that block the reproductive ability of viruses; they can be effective in treating certain viral conditions such as influenza. Use of antiviral drugs is tricky because in many instances there is a narrow therapeutic window for effectiveness at the very beginning of the infection. Most people don't visit their physician until they are very ill, when the use of antivirals is less effective, if not contraindicated.

PREVENTION

Vaccines, antibiotics, and antivirals are all valuable ways to prevent infections or lessen their intensity and duration. Good hygiene is also important in the prevention of infections. Perhaps the most important behavior one can perform to prevent disease is to wash hands frequently. Many of the more common pathogens are found on hands and thus are capable of being transmitted to other people. Additionally, maintaining a good lifestyle (such as exercising regularly, eating healthy foods, and getting enough sleep regularly) also helps keep the immune system in good shape, which in turn helps the body fight off infections.

NEED TO KNOW

The human immune system is by far the most effective tool for fighting off infections. White blood cells called B cells target antigens by creating antibodies, while other white blood cells (T cells) then destroy the pathogens. Vaccines are drugs that are administered to prevent infections. Antibiotics are drugs that kill bacteria, and antiviral drugs fight viruses. People who maintain good health habits and are well rested will usually have a better immune response against infections than people who are stressed or have unhealthy habits. All people can decrease the chance of infections by frequently washing their hands.

Antivirals are drugs that treat viral infections.

Health & the Media Hand Sanitizer Dangers

Can the alcohol in hand sanitizers cause poisoning? You may have heard a story about a little girl who was rushed to the emergency room after becoming lethargic and unable to focus her eyes. Tests failed to discover the problem until a preschool teacher reported that children witnessed the child licking hand sanitizer before falling ill. Blood alcohol tests then showed the girl had dangerously high levels of alcohol in her system. The story ends with strict cautions about how deadly hand sanitizer can be.

Although this tale was widely distributed via e-mail with enough factual errors (such as an impossibly high blood alcohol level) that led it to be classified as an urban myth, the basic premise behind the story is true. Hand sanitizers contain up to 65 percent alcohol, and if ingested in sufficient amounts, they can cause alcohol poisoning. Although this isn't an issue for adults, who understand that sanitizer is for washing and not drinking, accidental poisoning could occur with small children.

Although nonalcoholic versions of hand sanitizers are available, some doctors and health policy administrators caution strongly against using this type. In this case, the worry is that widespread use of these alternative sanitizers may help build drug-resistant "superbugs." (See this chapter's Breaking It Down box, "Superbugs," for more information on drug-resistant infections.) Alcohol-based sanitizers are believed to kill more types of bacteria than other types, and the mechanism by which they work does not create drug-resistant pathogens.

Given their ability to reduce the spread of gastrointestinal and respiratory illness and the fact their use doesn't increase drug-resistant microbes, getting rid of alcohol-based hand sanitizers entirely is probably too strong a reaction. They have their place in the fight against infections. However, keeping them out of reach of children and allowing children to use them only with adult supervision are wise practices.

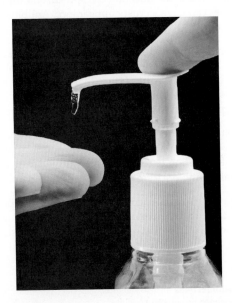

➤ Common Bacterial Infections

Bacteria are very simple pathogens. It should be noted that many bacteria do not cause disease and can even be beneficial to human health. Bacteria are single-celled plants that, after entering a body, divide until they reach sufficient numbers to cause symptoms. One cell becomes two, two cells then become four, four cells become eight, and so on until they reach billions and trillions. It is only after huge numbers of bacteria are present that a person becomes aware of the infection, because that is the point at which symptoms arise.

There are many common bacterial infections. Some will be covered in this section and some will be covered in the section "Sexually Transmitted Infections." Because most foodborne diseases (food poisoning) are bacterial, those diseases are discussed in Chapter 2.

STAPH INFECTIONS

Staph (staphylococcal) bacteria are common bacteria found on the skin and the membranes that line the nose and throat. In most instances the bacteria are harmless but if conditions are right, the bacteria can invade the body, secrete a toxin, and result in disease. Common **staph infections** include impetigo, boils, and cellulitis.

Impetigo is a contagious skin infection that can result when the staph bacteria invades the skins through a crack or broken area. During an impetigo infection, blisters can appear and the affected skin can become red. When the blisters burst, the infection can spread, and the area where the blister fluid dries can have a crusty appearance. Antibiotics can clear up the infection quickly.

Boils are inflamed, pus-filled lumps on the skin that are also caused by staph bacteria. Normally these lumps are infected hair follicles. To avoid spreading the infection, it is important that the boil not be burst. A hot compress can shrink the boil and facilitate drainage. In some instances antibiotics are prescribed to facilitate ending the infection.

Cellulitis is a staph infection of the skin and the tissues beneath. Usually the infection results from a wound. Cellulitis normally affects the neck, face, and legs. In addition to redness of the affected skin, fever and chills can result. Again, antibiotics are used to treat the infection.

Toxic shock syndrome is an uncommon staph infection, but because it is largely preventable and the people with the highest risk are young menstruating women, it warrants discussion. Typically toxic shock syndrome results when a woman inserts a tampon without first washing her hands.

Staphylococcal infections include cellulitis, impetigo, skin boils, and the much-feared, drug-resistant MRSA.

Pathogens capable of surviving antibiotics and other medications designed to kill them are called *superbugs*. Such pathogens, the most common of which is methicillin-resistant *Staphylococcus aureus* (MRSA), have the potential to become a significant medical and public health problem.

MRSA is colonized in approximately 1 percent of the population. The bacterium itself is not harmful unless it invades the skin or body organs and causes infection. There are about 90,000 reported infections each year. These bacteria are a real danger, because infection has a 20 percent mortality rate.

Until recently MRSA was a problem mostly found in hospitals and nursing homes, where approximately 85 percent of the reported cases originate. These settings are ideal for transmission because elderly and/or sick people tend to be more susceptible to infections. In the case of hospitals, invasive procedures such as surgery also provide an easy way for these bacteria to find their way into the body.

Although medical facilities are the riskiest locations for coming into contact with MRSA, infection can occur in any setting, especially where towels, soap, or equipment are shared by many. This is why we have seen outbreaks of MRSA in students at the same school, among U.S. soldiers returning from Afghanistan and Iraq, and even within the ranks of the St. Louis Rams football team.

MRSA is not the only superbug. Other strains of *Staphylococcus aureus* are becoming antibiotic resistant. *Enterococcus,* which is responsible for infections that range from the urinary tract to heart valves, and *Streptococcus pneumonia,* which can cause pneumonia and meningitis, are also developing tolerance to drugs that formerly killed them easily. There is also some evidence that the pathogens responsible for gonorrhea, salmonella, and *E. coli* disease are also becoming antibiotic resistant.

If more superbugs emerge, we could potentially see a new era where the leading causes of death will be communicable diseases, much as it was during the centuries before the modern advancements in medical care. In that event, medical efforts would shift to emphasizing the prevention of communicable diseases instead of chronic illnesses such as diabetes and heart disease. Further, if this scenario does play out, we could see decrease in both life span and life expectancy.

A hopeful point is the fact that superbugs were created through unintended consequences and sloppy practices that people can avoid, once they are aware of the dangers. This is a case where everyday actions by many will be a better defense than relying on science to create ever-stronger drugs to fight resistant, ever-stronger bacteria. Not sharing towels, washing hands frequently, taking the entire antibiotic prescription, and not insisting on antibiotics when the doctor says they are unnecessary are all ways that each of us can help prevent the emergence of new superbugs.

Staph bacteria on the hands is transmitted to the vagina via the tampon. If the staph grows in sufficient numbers, it can secrete a toxin that causes a sudden drop in blood pressure, high fever, skin rash, dizziness, disorientation, and possibly shock. The mortality rate is about 3 percent. Treatment is the same antibiotics used for other staph infections.

STREP INFECTIONS

Streptococcal (strep) **infections** are common, with the most common being the strep throat. One of the least common yet most highly publicized is flesh-eating bacteria. Strep throat usually starts one to five days after exposure, and its chief symptoms include fever, sore throat, and swollen neck glands. A simple throat culture can confirm the diagnosis, and antibiotics can be effective in treating the condition. In extreme or untreated cases, the initial strep infection can develop into a body rash known as scarlet fever, or turn into rheumatic fever, which causes heart problems.

Invasive Group A *Streptococcus* gets a lot of publicity because of its devastating and potentially disfiguring results. This kind of strep bacteria destroys fatty tissue and muscle, thereby gaining the nickname "flesh-eating bacteria." Usually the mode of transmission is an untreated skin wound. The wound becomes infected with strep, and tissue death occurs. Antibiotics can stop the infection, but any tissue that died will not grow back.

One in ten people carry the bacteria responsible for meningococcal meningitis or **bacterial meningitis.** The bacteria are transmitted by close contact between people, which is why outbreaks are known to happen in places such as college dorms. Some people have enough of an immune deficiency that the bacteria get into the bloodstream, affect the brain, and produce the symptoms associated with bacterial meningitis. These symptoms include severe headache, stiff neck, fever, frequent vomiting, and a rash. Fewer than 5 percent of victims will die. If the infection spreads, a condition called *septicemia* results, and the death rate can rise to around 20 percent or higher.

Bacterial meningitis and septicemia are very serious. When young people move into a college dorm or other setting where they come into close contact with a large number of people, they are at higher risk of exposure

✓ **NEED TO KNOW**

Bacterial diseases are common, although of all the types of bacteria only a relatively small number cause disease. Antibiotics treat bacteria infections. Bacterial meningitis is a life-threatening infection that sometimes breaks out in close living quarters like college dormitories. Fever, a stiff neck, vomiting, and a rash are symptoms of it. People can be vaccinated against bacterial meningitis.

Streptococcal infections include step throat and "flesh-eating" bacteria.

Bacterial meningitis is an infection that can affect the brain and is potentially fatal.

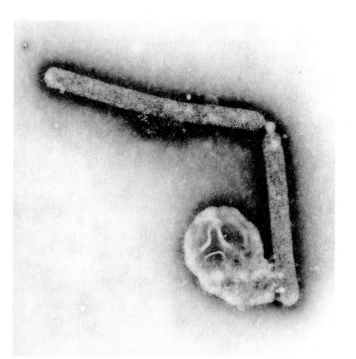

A virus as seen through a high-powered microscope.

to the bacteria. Vaccination is the best method of prevention. In addition, it is important to be aware of the symptoms so that medical attention can be sought before the symptoms get worse. Early medical attention with antibiotics can mean the difference between life and death.

➤ Common Viral Infections

Viruses are mysterious organisms. They are very simple—a strand of RNA or DNA wrapped in a protein coat. Viruses have the capability of invading the body and using the person's own cells as genetic material to replicate. This process baffles scientists, and because of its complexity, it has been difficult to medically intervene and rid the body of viruses in the way that antibiotics rid the body of bacteria. So the quality of the individual's immune response system, which can destroy the virus, is usually the key to dealing with viral infections. Examples of viral infections are the common cold, influenza, mononucleosis, herpes, and hepatitis. (Sexually transmitted viral infections will be covered later in the chapter.)

COMMON COLD

Over 100 different viruses can cause what we term the "common cold." Over 50 percent of colds are caused by rhinoviruses, which are viruses that are in the nose. It makes sense that the symptoms of a cold are a runny nose, nasal congestion, a sore throat, and sometimes a headache and fever.

Most adults have two to three colds each year. There is no cure for the common cold and since a healthy immune response system is very effective in eliminating the virus, the symptoms last about a week and they tend to be self-limiting. Since most cold viruses are transmitted by the hands, the most effective way to prevent the spread of the colds is to wash one's hands frequently and cover the mouth when sneezing or coughing.

INFLUENZA

Influenza, or the flu, spreads from person to person through coughing or sneezing. Shaking hands with an infected person is also a common mode of transmission; if people cough into their hand or wipe their nose, they can easily pass the virus on when they touch someone else. Influenza is similar to the common cold but the symptoms are usually more severe. The incubation period for influenza is usually one to three days, and the symptoms include headache, tiredness, body aches, fever, and chills. There is no cure for the flu. A person's natural immune response will be helped if the flu sufferer gets plenty of rest and drinks lots of fluids.

Flu vaccinations are an effective way to prevent the flu. The best time to get the vaccine is between October to mid-November because it takes about two weeks for the vaccination to develop protection against influenza. Influenza should be taken seriously because complications can result, including pneumonia and, in rare cases, paralysis.

MONONUCLEOSIS

Mononucleosis is a common viral infection that as many as 95 percent of adults in the United States will contract by the time they are forty years old. Epstein-Barr virus is the pathogen that causes mononucleosis. It is found in the saliva of the infected person and may be spread through direct contact, which is why it is nicknamed the "kissing disease."

Mononucleosis has a long incubation period. Approximately 30–50 days after exposure, the person can experience a fever, sore throat, swollen glands in the back of the neck, and tiredness. Symptoms can last anywhere from a week or two to several months. Although most people experience mono only once, it is possible for the virus to lie dormant and reactivate later, resulting in another episode of symptoms. As with influenza, treatment includes rest to help the immune system.

HERPES 1

The most common types of this virus are **herpes simplex virus 1 (HSV 1)** and herpes simplex virus 2 (HSV 2). HSV 1, or oral herpes, will be dis-

Herpes simplex virus 1 (HSV 1) infections are common incurable oral infections, and cold sores around the mouth and lips are the most typical symptom.

"Sexually Transmitted Infections."

The classic HSV 1 symptom is a cold-sore lesion on or near the mouth. The sores will appear for a week or two and then subside. The virus will the lie dormant and can reactivate at almost any time. The first outbreak of cold sores is usually the worst and most painful. HSV 1 is not dangerous unless one has a compromised immune system and the infection spreads and affects the nervous system. Medications are available to reduce the severity of the symptoms, but no medications exist that actually rid the body of the virus. To prevent the spread of herpes, limit saliva contact with an infected person, cover cold sores if possible, and wash hands often.

HEPATITIS

Hepatitis is a generic term meaning "inflammation of the liver." There are several types of the disease, categorized as A, B, or C, depending in part on the mode of transmission. Hepatitis A can be present in the feces and is normally contracted through eating food by prepared someone who is infected and did not wash his or her hands after using the bathroom. Hepatitis B and C are contracted through contact with infected blood via transfusions, dirty needles, or sexual intercourse.

Since hepatitis affects the liver, a key symptom is a yellowing of the skin and eyes called *jaundice.* Other symptoms include brown urine, diarrhea or light-colored stool, fever, loss of appetite, stomach pain, nausea, and fatigue. These symptoms usually begin about four weeks after exposure, can last for a long time, be quite intense, and are not usually self-limiting but do impair functioning. Hepatitis C victims can carry the virus the rest of their lives. Hepatitis is largely preventable. If restaurant workers wash their hands before touching food, risk of hepatitis A for customers is extremely low. Drugs are available to treat hepatitis, and vaccinations are available for hepatitis A and B.

Hepatitis B and C, which are the bloodborne forms of hepatitis, can be successfully prevented by using what are termed "universal precautions." All health care workers and many other workers are required to attend a workshop to learn these precautions.

Figure 11.3 lists the universal precautions. After reviewing the list, you can easily see that the main effort is to protect the portal of entrance—the skin and nose—from contact with blood products or body fluids. Adhering to universal precautions reduces risk by blocking the portal of entrance through use of masks, gloves, and protective clothing. If implemented correctly, these precautions will significant limit one's risk of bloodborne diseases.

Hepatitis is a generic term for an infection that causes inflammation of the liver.

FIGURE 11.3   UNIVERSAL PRECAUTIONS

1. *Use of gloves* to provide a barrier between the hands and potentially infectious body fluids or items contaminated with body fluids. Wash hands immediately after removing gloves.

2. *Wearing* face protection such as masks to prevent droplets of potentially infectious body fluids from being inhaled.

3. *Wearing* protective body clothing such as disposable laboratory coats when there is potential for body fluids to be splashed onto the body.

4. *Washing hands* thoroughly if there is contact with body fluids.

5. *Washing surfaces* that have been exposed to body fluids.

6. *Avoiding injuries* caused by potentially contaminated needles and any other sharp instruments.

7. *Placing* all used gloves and disposable items exposed to body fluids in a specially designated hazardous-materials container.

Bloodborne diseases such as Hepatitis B or HIV are best prevented by limiting exposure to potentially infectious body fluids, including blood, through following universal precautions. These precautions include three main practices: wearing a barrier between exposed skin and body fluids; washing hands; and placing exposed materials in a specially designated hazardous-materials receptacle.

✓ NEED TO KNOW

Options for treating viral diseases are limited. A healthy immune system and frequent hand washing are the best defense against viruses such as influenza. Avoiding contact with herpes sores is perhaps the best low-risk behavior to prevent a herpes 1 infection. Mononucleosis has been referred to as the "kissing disease," and the risk of getting it is increased by deep kissing with an infected person. However, many people get mononucleosis just through close person-to-person contact. Symptoms include sore throat, swollen glands, and extreme fatigue. Finally, to avoid contracting blood-borne diseases such as HIV and hepatitis, one should follow universal precautions. Universal precautions are based on three main practices: wearing a barrier between exposed skin and body fluids; washing hands; and placing exposed materials in a specially designed hazardous-materials receptacle.

➤ Common Fungal Infections

Fungi are pathogens capable of a wide range of infections, from minor annoyances like athlete's foot and ringworm to serious, life-threatening lung infections such as histoplasmosis.

Athlete's foot is caused by coming into contact with fungal spores commonly found on locker room floors (hence *athlete's foot*). Skin from an infected person is shed, and a barefoot person stepping on the infected skin runs a risk of also becoming infected. The key symptoms of athlete's foot are redness, itching, and cracking of skin, usually between the toes. Normally a topical antifungal medication can be applied and clear up the infection quickly. Prevention efforts include wearing flip-flops when walking on floors used by many barefooted people, especially in locker rooms, and keeping the feet dry.

Ringworm is a fungal infection normally confined to the scalp. The infection appears as a red circle on the scalp, and because it is raised, it looks like a worm. Direct physical contact with an infected person or animal is the chief method of developing the infection. Ringworm is highly contagious and can affect both children and adults. Once diagnosed, ringworm can be successfully treated with topical antifungal medications.

➤ Sexually Transmitted Infections

Sexually transmitted infections (STIs) are common diseases caused by bacteria or viruses. Pathogens can be transmitted through sexual activities such as vaginal intercourse, anal intercourse, or oral sex. The common STIs include chlamydia, gonorrhea, syphilis, herpes 2, and human papilloma virus (HPV).

CHLAMYDIA

Chlamydia is a type of bacteria found in infected body fluids from the penis or vagina. The bacteria is transmitted during sexual contact. Symptoms typically appear 7–30 days after exposure. They usually include a discharge from the penis, vagina, or rectum; cramps or pain in the lower abdomen in women; burning or itching around the opening of the penis; pain in the testicles; and painful urination. Many people with chlamydia do not have symptoms, but they can still spread the disease. Women who are asymptomatic might not be aware of the chlamydia infection until they experience pelvic inflammatory disease (PID). However, vaginal discharge with odor or bleeding between cycles can indicate infection, and a medical evaluation should be undertaken. Antibiotics can successfully treat chlamydia.

GONORRHEA

Gonorrhea, another sexually transmitted bacterial infection, is similar to chlamydia. The symptoms are virtually the same. However, symptoms usually appear sooner than chlamydia, 2–7 days after exposure. Untreated gonorrhea in women can lead to pelvic inflammatory disease. Vaginal discharge with odor or bleeding between cycles could indicate infection, and a medical evaluation should be undertaken. Gonorrhea can be successfully treated with antibiotics.

PELVIC INFLAMMATORY DISEASE

Pelvic inflammatory disease (PID) is a serious complication of untreated chlamydia and gonorrhea. When the disease is not treated, the bacteria can find their way to the cervix, uterus, fallopian tubes, and eventually the lower pelvic cavity. The symptoms of PID include lower abdominal pain and abnormal vaginal discharge, fever, pain in the right upper abdomen, painful intercourse, and irregular menstrual bleeding. PID causes more than 100,000 women per year to become infertile. Another complication of PID is ectopic pregnancy, where the fertilized egg implants in the fallopian tube or the ovary (see Chapter 5).

PID can be difficult to diagnose because the symptoms can be like those of many other diseases. Antibiotics can be used to treat PID, but any damage to pelvic structures will remain.

SYPHILIS

Syphilis is another sexually transmitted disease. Unlike chlamydia and gonorrhea, the signs and symptoms are dependent on which stage of syphilis the person is experiencing.

The first stage of syphilis is called the *Primary Stage*. An infectious, painless lesion or sore called a *chancre* appears at the point of sexual contact. The chancre will most likely appear 10–90 days after exposure and remain for an average of 21 days, after which it will heal and disappear naturally. Unfortunately, the healing doesn't mean the person is cured. It indicates he or she is moving into the *Secondary Stage* of the disease.

During the Secondary Stage, the bacteria spreads throughout the body, and a rash appears all over the body. This rash can look like a sunburn or take the form of wart-like bumps and white patches in the mouth. In addition to the rash, an infected person might also have a fever, swollen glands, sore throat, patchy hair loss, headaches, weight loss, and malaise. The rash and other symptoms can last 2–6 weeks and will disappear.

If untreated during the Primary and Secondary Stages, the bacteria will become even more disseminated and will damage body organs. This state is termed the *Latent Stage* and most often it has no symptoms. A

Pelvic inflammatory disease is a serious, painful condition often related to untreated chlamydia or gonorrhea.

person can be in the Latent Stage for years before there are symptoms of organ damage, such as, paralysis, blindness, and heart damage. This damage marks the last stage of syphilis, termed the *Tertiary Stage.*

The bacteria can be eliminated with antibiotics. At any stage in the infection, a person can receive the antibiotics and be cured. However, if organ damage occurs, it will not be reversed by antibiotic treatment.

HERPES 2 (GENITAL HERPES)

Herpes 2 is the sexually transmitted form of herpes. Approximately 2–12 days after exposure, a person develops small sores or lesions around either the external reproductive organs or the mouth, depending on the point of sexual contact and infection. These sores can be quite painful and will normally last for a week or two before disappearing. However, like herpes 1, when the sores disappear, it doesn't mean that the person is cured; rather, the virus has gone into dormancy and can reactivate at any time. There are medications that can limit the intensity or severity of the symptoms, but there is no cure—once infected, always infected. One out of every 12 Americans over the age of 12 is infected with herpes 2. Women with herpes 2 infections have a higher risk of cervical cancer and run the risk of not being able to vaginally deliver a baby, especially if there are active sores.

HUMAN PAPILLOMA VIRUS (HPV)

Human papilloma virus (HPV) is responsible for a condition commonly called *genital warts.* HPV is transmitted sexually, and the warts appear either externally or internally on the genitals between six weeks and eight months after exposure. In some instances people have the infection but never develop warts, leaving them unaware they have an STI. Approximately fifty percent of sexually active women will be infected with HPV at some point in their lives and as a result are at higher risk of cervical cancer. As with herpes 2, they may have difficulty with a vaginal delivery of a baby, depending on whether the warts are in the vagina. Genital warts are treated by applying medications to the warts which cause the warts to fall off, freezing the warts with liquid nitrogen, using electrical heat (cauterizing), or laser therapy.

A new vaccine is available to protect against HPV. Gardasil provides protection against four types of HPV, including two that are responsible for the majority of cases of cervical cancer. It is believed that most of the HPV infections that lead to cervical cancer are acquired shortly after women become sexually active. The Centers for Disease Control (CDC) recommends that all 11- and 12-year-old girls be vaccinated with Gardasil. The objective is to reduce cervical cancer, and if vaccination begins early, then the incidence of cervical cancer could be significantly reduced in the next 20–30 years.

Herpes 2 is an incurable viral infections; it is usually sexually transmitted, and lesions around the point of sexual contact are the most common symptom.

Two controversies arise from the CDC recommendation of Gardasil. First, the vaccine must be administered in three separate injections with a cost of around $350. Second, many ethical issues are raised in administering the vaccine to 11- and 12-year-olds. Some parents believe the vaccine is too new to recommend widespread use, because not all its side effects may yet be known. And some parents believe administering the vaccine may somehow encourage girls to have sex earlier than they would otherwise, because they feel it is safer. Despite these issues, since HPV can lead to more serious conditions, the vaccination will likely become common practice for girls and women.

PREVENTION OF SEXUALLY TRANSMITTED INFECTIONS

Sexually transmitted infections can be prevented in a number of ways. First, abstinence is the lowest-risk preventive behavior. Second, use of condoms greatly reduces rates of transmission. Condoms are not 100-percent protection against STIs, but they do provide a barrier that blocks the portals of entry and exit.

NEED TO KNOW

Sexually transmitted infections (STIs) are preventable. High-risk sexual choices can result in high risk for an STI. Condoms offer some protection. Pain upon urination, urethral or vaginal discharge, sores around the genital area, and pelvic pain all can be signs of an STI and require medical attention. Infertility can result from untreated STIs. A new vaccine offers some protection against the HPV virus, which is a leading cause of cervical cancer.

HIV AND AIDS

HIV and **AIDS** represent two ends of the same viral infection. Because this disease has such important life-and-death dynamics and is such a politically charged issue, we will discuss it independently of the common sexually transmitted infections.

The human immunodeficiency virus (HIV) is both the cause of acquired immunodeficiency syndrome (AIDS) and an infection itself. The term **HIV positive** is used for a person who has been shown to carry the virus

HIV is the human immunodeficiency virus. **AIDS** is the end-stage disease caused by HIV.

HIV positive is the term for a person who has the HIV infection but doesn't exhibit any symptoms yet.

but appears to have no symptoms; people whose infections have progressed to the point where they show symptoms are said to have AIDS. If the disease progresses, the person begins to experience fever, weight loss, swollen lymph glands, and white patches in the mouth.

HIV is transmitted through body fluids such as blood, semen, vaginal secretions, and breast milk of HIV-infected persons. Once in the body, HIV attacks the immune system's T cells (described in the "Immune System" section earlier in this chapter). HIV changes the way T cells function so that over time, the T cells stop sending messages to B cells to produce antibodies to fight infections. As the immune system become increasingly deficient because of a lack of antibodies, the infected person is susceptible to what are termed *opportunistic diseases* such as Kaposi's sarcoma, a skin lesion, and PCP (pneumocystis pneumonia).

The most common modes of transmission of HIV are dirty needles, anal intercourse, and high risk sexual practices where tissue is torn, allowing contaminated blood to enter another person's body. It can take between six weeks and six months after exposure for someone to test positive for HIV. People who feel fine despite being HIV positive can still pass the virus on to others.

Through medical interventions, people can live productive lives despite HIV infection. There are medications available that, if used at the appropriate time, can limit the reproductive capability of HIV and greatly prolong an infected person's life. If these drugs are not used, then most likely the infection will progress to AIDS.

What Is Your Risk? What Is Your Risk of Contracting an STI?

Young adults are at higher risk for getting STIs than any other age group. Although sexually active 15- to 24-year-olds represent 25 percent of the sexually active population, this group is responsible for 50 percent of all new cases of STIs. People who are sexually active and not in a monogamous sexual relationship with a non-infected partner are at risk of acquiring a sexually transmitted disease. Just how much they are at risk depends on their behaviors.

Abstinence is the most effective method to prevent an STI. Common sense tells us that. If one is not abstinent, then having sex in the context of a monogamous relationship with a non-infected partner is also low risk. After these two low-risk scenarios come a variety of behaviors that will lessen risk of infection. For example, "safer sex" practices such as using condoms, although not 100 percent effective, when used consistently and correctly, can greatly reduce one's risk of an STI. Modifying one's mood

(Continued)

through drug and alcohol use can impair judgment and increases risk of STI transmission. By remaining sober or straight, chances are better that low-risk behaviors will result.

Good communication skills are also important in reducing STI risk. Knowing one's limits and being able to communicate those limits to a sexual partner without fear of rejection or embarrassment is not only a sign of maturity but also a good risk-reduction strategy. If one can't communicate well with a partner about these issues, then perhaps it is a sign that one should hold off on having an intimate physical relationship until communication skills and maturity are better developed.

Young adults who choose to be sexually active can also decrease the risk of contracting and spreading STIs to others in several ways. Women in their mid-twenties or younger could get an HPV vaccination. And anyone who is sexually active in a non-monogamous relationship should be tested for chlamydia once a year.

Lastly, if you are diagnosed with an STI, notify your sex partners so that they can be tested as well. Doing so might feel uncomfortable or embarrassing, but it is the responsible and ethical thing to do. In the long run it could save many people possibly serious health complications.

The notion that HIV and AIDS is a "gay disease" is false. HIV can be contracted and transmitted to anyone, regardless of gender, race, sexual orientation, or level of wealth. However, HIV is a relatively difficult infection to acquire, and it is usually transmitted through high-risk behaviors such as sharing needles to take illegal drugs, anal intercourse (which can tear tissues), or frequent sexual activity with multiple partners. HIV/AIDS is preventable. The simple HIV Risk Assessment (Figure 11.4) is focused on behaviors that increase risk of HIV.

✓ **NEED TO KNOW**

HIV is a relatively difficult disease to get. It breaks down the human immune system over time. Most HIV infections are a result of sexual relations with an infected person or from sharing needles when using drugs. Fortunately being infected with HIV is not the "death sentence" it was years ago—but still, to take advantage of the life-saving medical interventions, a person should be diagnosed early.

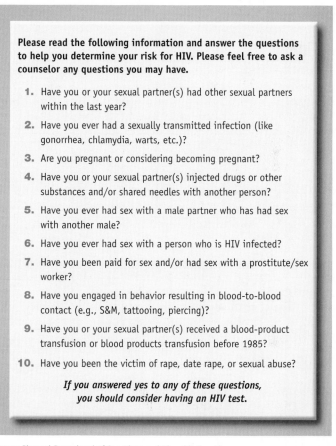

FIGURE 11.4   **HIV RISK ASSESSMENT QUESTIONNAIRE: SHOULD YOU GET AN HIV TEST?**

Please read the following information and answer the questions to help you determine your risk for HIV. Please feel free to ask a counselor any questions you may have.

1. Have you or your sexual partner(s) had other sexual partners within the last year?

2. Have you ever had a sexually transmitted infection (like gonorrhea, chlamydia, warts, etc.)?

3. Are you pregnant or considering becoming pregnant?

4. Have you or your sexual partner(s) injected drugs or other substances and/or shared needles with another person?

5. Have you ever had sex with a male partner who has had sex with another male?

6. Have you ever had sex with a person who is HIV infected?

7. Have you been paid for sex and/or had sex with a prostitute/sex worker?

8. Have you engaged in behavior resulting in blood-to-blood contact (e.g., S&M, tattooing, piercing)?

9. Have you or your sexual partner(s) received a blood-product transfusion or blood products transfusion before 1985?

10. Have you been the victim of rape, date rape, or sexual abuse?

If you answered yes to any of these questions, you should consider having an HIV test.

Source: Planned Parenthood of San Diego and Riverside Counties.

➤ Bioterrorism

Bioterrorism was once a term used primarily in science-fiction movies. In recent years, with highly publicized "weapons of mass destruction" and the anthrax deaths after September 11, 2001, bioterrorism has become a concept that is now well-integrated into our consciousness. It refers to the use of lethal pathogens in terrorism. The diseases of most concern in a bioterrorist context are anthrax, botulism, pneumonic plague, and smallpox. Figure 11.5 provides a clinical overview of the bioterrorist agents responsible for those diseases.

FIGURE 11.5 BIOTERRORIST AGENTS: WATCH FOR THESE SYMPTOMS

Disease	Signs & Symptoms	Incubation Time (Range)	Person-to-Person Transmission	Isolation	Diagnosis	Postexposure Prophylaxis for Adults	Treatment for Adults
Anthrax *Bacillus anthracis* A. Inhalation	Flu-like symptoms (fever, fatigue, muscle aches, dyspnea, nonproductive cough, headache), chest pain; possible 1-2 day improvement then rapid respiratory failure and shock. Meningitis may develop.	1 to 6 days (up to 6 wks)	None	Standard Precautions	Chest x-ray evidence of widening mediastinum; obtain sputum and blood culture. Sensitivity and specificity of nasal swabs unknown—do not rely on for diagnosis.	Prophylaxis for 60 days: Ciprofloxacin* 500 mg PO q 12h Or Doxycycline 100 mg PO q 12h Alternative (if strain susceptible and above contraindicated): Amoxicillin 500 mg PO q 8h "In vitro studies suggest that Levofloxacin 500 mg PO q 24h Or Gatifloxacin 400 mg PO q 24h Or Moxifloxacin 400 mg PO q 24h could be substituted	Inhalation anthrax Combined IV/PO therapy for 60d Ciprofloxacin 500 mg q 12h Or Doxycycline 100 mg q 12h, AND 1 or 2 additional drugs (vancomycin, rifampin, imipenem clindamycin, chloramphenicol, clarithromycin, and if susceptible penicillin or ampicillin
B. Cutaneous	Intense itching followed by painless papular lesions, then vesicular lesions, developing into eschar surrounded by edema.	1 to 12 days	Direct contact with skin lesions may result in cutaneous infection.	Contact Precautions	Peripheral blood smear may demonstrate gram positive bacilli on unspun smear with sepsis.	Recommendations same for pregnant women and immunocompromised persons	Cutaneous anthrax Ciprofloxacin 500 mg PO q 12h Or Doxycycline 100 mg PO q 12h Recommendations same for pregnant women and immunocompromised persons
C. Gastrointestinal (GI)	Abdominal pain, nausea and vomiting, severe diarrhea, GI bleeding, and fever.	1 to 7 days	None	Standard Precautions	Culture blood and stool.		
Botulism botulinum toxin	Afebrile, excess mucus in throat, dysphagia, dry mouth and throat, dizziness, then difficulty moving eyes, mild pupillary dilation and nystagmus, intermittent ptosis, indistinct speech, unsteady gait, extreme symmetric descending weakness, flaccid paralysis; generally normal mental status.	Inhalation: 12–80 hours Foodborne: 12–72 hours (2–8 days)	None	Standard Precautions	Laboratory tests available from CDC or Public Health Dept; obtain serum, stool, gastric aspirate and suspect foods prior to administering antitoxin. Differential diagnosis includes polio, Guillain Barre, myasthenia, tick paralysis, CVA, meningococcal meningitis.	Pentavalent toxoid (types A, B, C, D, E) 0.5 ml SQ may be available as investigational product from USAMRIID.	Botulism antitoxins from public health authorities. Supportive care and ventilatory support. Avoid clindamycin and aminoglycosides.
Pneumonic Plague *Yersinia pestis*	High fever, cough, hemoptysis, chest pain, nausea and vomiting, headache. Advanced disease: purpuric skin lesions, copious watery or purulent sputum production; respiratory failure in 1 to 6 days.	2–3 days (2–6 days)	Yes, droplet aerosols	Droplet Precautions until 48 hrs of effective antibiotic therapy	A presumptive diagnosis may be made by Gram, Wayson or Wright stain of lymph node aspirates, sputum, or cerebrospinal fluid with gram negative bacilli with bipolar (safety pin) staining.	Doxycycline 100 mg PO q 12 Or Ciprofloxacin 500 mg PO q 12h	Streptomycin 1 gm IM q 12h; Or Gentamicin 2 mg/kg, then 1.0 to 1.7 mg/kg IV q 8h Alternatives: Doxycycline 200 mg PO load, then 100 PO mg q 12h Or Ciprofloxacin 400 mg IV q 12h
Smallpox variola virus	Prodromal period: malaise, fever, rigors, vomiting, headache, and backache. After 2-4 days, skin lesions appear and progress uniformly from macules to papules to vesicles and pustules, mostly on face, neck, palms, soles, and subsequently progress to trunk.	12-14 days (7-17 days)	Yes, airborne droplet nuclei or direct contact with skin lesions or secretions until all scabs separate and fall off (3 to 4 weeks)	Airborne (includes N95 mask) and Contact Precautions	Swab culture of vesicular fluid or scab, send to BL-4 laboratory. All lesions similar in appearance and develop synchronously as opposed to chickenpox. Electron microscopy can differentiate variola virus from varicella.	Early vaccine critical (in less than 4 days). Call CDC for vaccinia. Vaccinia immune globulin in special cases—call USAMRIID 301-619-2833.	Supportive care. Previous vaccination against smallpox does not confer lifelong immunity. Potential role for Cidofovir.

Adapted from a chart developed by North Carolina Statewide Program for Infection Control Epidemiology (SPICE). Copyright 2003 by University of North Carolina at Chapel Hill.

Anthrax is a bacterial disease most associated with cows. When humans are infected by inhaling anthrax spores, they experience flu-like symptoms, and after a brief time period when they think they are recovering, they lapse into respiratory failure and shock. Unless there is medical intervention with high powered antibiotics, death is likely.

Botulism is a bacterial foodborne disease. Because we have such strict food preparation standards, botulism has not been a serious problem. As a terrorist weapon, the organism would infect a person and after incubation, dizziness, weakness, and paralysis would result. Unless botulism antitoxins are administered, death can result.

Pneumonic plague is also caused by bacteria. A few days after exposure, the victim can spike a high fever and have a cough, chest pain, nausea, and vomiting. In the advanced form, skin sores will appear. Unless antibiotics are administered, respiratory failure and death can result.

Smallpox was once thought to be eradicated—meaning that enough of the total world population had been immunized to stamp out all infections. But in a bioterrorist context, the smallpox virus can be disseminated through the air. If people breathe in the smallpox virus, they can develop it. Symptoms include fever, vomiting, headache, and skin sores. Unlike the bacterial diseases, there is no cure for smallpox. The quality of the individual's immune response is the key to surviving smallpox. There is a smallpox vaccine that is derived from the virus, but because the disease was thought to have been eradicated, only a small supply of the vaccine is available.

Experts disagree on the extent of the threat of bioterrorism. Many of the diseases discussed here are caused by organisms that are hard to deliver to infect large numbers of people. But that doesn't mean that the organisms can't be manipulated to become easier to deliver and even more lethal. Bioterrorism should be considered a real threat.

Dealing with bioterrorism requires a comprehensive plan with involvement from every segment of American society. In an October 2007 Homeland Security Presidential Directive (HSPD-21), a national strategy for preparedness was presented. This strategy includes four major components: biosurveillance, countermeasure stockpiling and distribution, mass casualty care, and community resilience.

Biosurveillance measures include focused national and international activities to monitor disease occurrence and distribution for those diseases that are likely to be a part of bioterrorism in both animal and human populations. Countermeasure stockpiling and distribution involves ensuring that appropriate vaccines and drugs are available in the case of a real or potential bioterrorism event. Mass casualty care is the mobilization of public health and medical systems to treat those affected by a bioterrorism disease outbreak. Finally, community resilience is activities that communities and social networks can undertake to lessen the risk and damage done in such outbreaks.

HSPD-21 is key to both prevention and intervention activities to both protect citizens from effects of bioterrorist activities and to mobilize public health and medical sectors to deal with a bioterrorist event. The odds are something will eventually happen, and the impact of that event will be directly related to the degree of preparedness of the affected nation, with the United States being a key target. The need for a comprehensive plan that addresses the four major components is paramount and requires cooperation from institutions and individuals.

✓ **NEED TO KNOW**

Manipulating lethal organisms for the purpose of bioterrorism is a real threat. Although there is very little that individuals can do to physically protect themselves, paying attention to Homeland Security warnings and threat levels are key to identifying people or groups who may be involved in harming others through biology. A bioterrorism event is likely to happen at some point. How severe the outcome of such an event will be directly related to how well the critical components of Presidential Directive HSPD-21 are implemented. Bioterrorism is a real threat, and we all have a role in prevention, especially in helping our respective communities be resilient.

American Medical Association
www.ama-assn.org/ama
American Public Health Association
www.apha.org
Centers for Disease Control
www.cdc.gov
Healthology
www.healthology.com/
Infectious Disease Society of America
www.idsociety.org/
Medline Plub (NIH)
www.nlm.nih.gov/medlineplus/infectiousdiseases.html
Medscape (WebMD)
www.medscape.com/infectiousdiseaseshome
National Foundation for Infectious Diseases
www.nfid.org/
National Institute of Infectious Disease
www.nih.go.jp/niid
World Health Organization
www.who.int/topics/en/

Knowing the Language

acute stage
AIDS
antibiotics
antibodies
antigen
antivirals
bacterial meningitis
B cells
direct mode of transmission
hepatitis
herpes 1
herpes 2
HIV

HIV positive
indirect mode of transmission
incubation stage
leukocytes
lymphocytes
pathogens
pelvic inflammatory disease
prodromal stage
recovery
staphylococcal infections
streptococcal infections
T cells
vaccines

Understanding the Content

1. Describe the communicable disease process using the following terminology: *pathogen, reservoir, mode of transmission, portal of entry, portal of exit, incubation, prodromal stage, acute stage, and recovery.*
2. What are the main mechanisms for fighting disease?

3. What is MRSA and why are most people at risk for it?
4. Why can PID be a problem associated with chlamydia and gonorrhea?
5. What is HPV and why should women be concerned about it?
6. What is the difference between HIV, HIV positive and full-blown AIDS?
7. What are the main bioterrorism agents of concern?

Exploring Ideas

1. Why should we be so concerned about "superbugs," and whose role is it to prevent the spread of these pathogens?
2. Should Gardasil be required for all girls beginning at ages 11 or 12? If so, why? If not, why not?
3. Should there be mandatory HIV testing to determine the extent of HIV infection? Why or why not?
4. What has been done since September 11, 2001, to prevent a bioterrorism event? Is America ready?

Selected References

American Public Health Association. *Control of Communicable Disease in Man* (17th ed.). Washington, DC: American Public Health Association, 2000.

Brown J. *Don't Touch That Doorknob.* New York: Warner Books, 2001.

Fauci AS. Emerging infectious diseases: A clear and present danger to humanity. *Journal of the American Medical Association* 292 (15): 1887–1888, 2004.

Garrett L. (2005). Probable cause. *Foreign Affairs* 84 (4) : 3–23, July/ August 2005. Centers for Disease Control. *Healthy People 2010*, 2000.

Garrett L. The lessons of HIV/AIDS. *Foreign Affairs* 84 (4): 51–65, July/ August 2005.

Harrison LH, Dwyer DM, Maples CT, Billmann L. Risk of meningococcal infection in college students. *JAMA* 281 (20): 1906–1910, May 26, 1999.

Karlen A. *Man and Microbes.* New York: Putnam, 1995.

Miller J, Engelberg S, Broad W. *Germs.* New York: Simon and Schuster, 2001.

Preston, R. *The Hot Zone.* New York: Random House, 1994.

The White House. Homeland Security Presidential Directive/HSPD-21. Released October 18, 2007
www.whitehouse.gov/news/releases/2007/10/print/20071018-10.html

World Health Organization. *The World Health Report 2004: Changing History.* Geneva: World Health Organization, 2004.

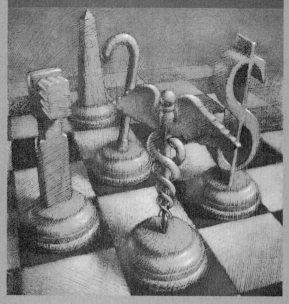

When it comes to your health, I recommend frequent doses of that rare commodity—common sense.

— VINCENT ASKEY, M.D.,

PRESIDENT,

AMERICAN MEDICAL ASSOCIATION

Chapter 12

HEALTH CARE FUNDAMENTALS

In this chapter, we describe the current health care system and its components. Because of the growing interest in health care options beyond those of mainstream medicine, a review of complementary and alternative medicine in addition to conventional Western medicine is included. We finish with an overview on the emerging concept of integrative medicine.

➤ **Organization of the U.S. Health Care System**

COMPONENTS AND LEVELS OF CARE

MAJOR CHALLENGES: CONTROLLING COSTS AND REDUCING ERRORS

➤ **Western Medicine**

PHYSICIANS: M.D.'s AND D.O.'s

DENTISTS

PODIATRISTS

OPTOMETRISTS

CLINICAL PSYCHOLOGISTS

ALLIED HEALTH CARE PROFESSIONALS

➤ **Complementary and Alternative Medicine (CAM)**

COMPARISON WITH WESTERN MEDICINE

NATIONAL CENTER FOR COMPLEMENTARY AND ALTERNATIVE MEDICINE

ALTERNATIVE MEDICAL SYSTEMS

MIND-BODY INTERVENTIONS

BIOLOGICALLY BASED THERAPIES

MANIPULATIVE AND BODY-BASED METHODS

ENERGY THERAPIES

BEING A CRITICAL CONSUMER OF CAM

➤ **Integrative Medicine**

EACH OF US has some familiarity with the U.S. health care system because we've all been patients. Most of you also have a family member or friend who works in health care. Yet, basic information on how the health care system works is only background noise for many of you, as your parents or family watch over your medical needs. You have had no compelling reason to understand the health care system. But the time is coming when you will. In contrast, some of you are already facing responsibility for your own health care. Perhaps you are a returning adult student, or you lost your coverage as a dependent on a parent's health insurance plan when you turned 18 or 21.

As the current or soon-to-be decision maker for your own health care, you need a working knowledge of the U.S. system to use it effectively. Our health care system is complex. For the uninformed, it can be confusing and downright overwhelming. In this chapter we present the fundamentals of the health care system to help prepare you to be your own advocate. We provide an overview of 21st-century medicine, explain the key players in conventional Western medicine, review the realm of complementary and alternative medicine (CAM), and end with a profile of a future system known as *integrative medicine*.

As a side note, we also provide a glimpse into potential occupations that may be appealing. Many of you may in fact eventually work in health care—either directly as a health care professional or indirectly in a health-related business. Among all jobs in the U.S. economy, those in the health care sector are expected to be among the fastest growing over the next decade.

➤ Organization of the U.S. Health Care System

COMPONENTS AND LEVELS OF CARE

The U.S. health care system is a multilevel, market-based network of individuals and organizations that provide and underwrite medical services. Our current system evolved from a simple two-party arrangement between a family doctor and a patient. In the old system, the patient would either go to the doctor's office for care, or the doctor would go to the patient in what was known as a "house call." Patients paid doctors directly, and those payments were sometimes in the form of goods or services (for instance, food from a farmer) instead of money. Over the decades, this simple practice of medicine steadily expanded to a system encompassing more complex care options. Today in addition to the general practitioner or family doctor, there are a myriad of physician specialists and allied health professionals, a multitude of high-tech instruments and specialized facilities for medical tests and procedures, and a wide array of third-party health care insurers that help patients pay for all those services.

In today's system, health care is described as being at one of three levels: primary, secondary, or tertiary. **Primary health care** involves diagnosis and treatment of common illnesses such as acne, influenza, high blood pressure, or depression. A family practice physician usually provides primary care; thus, he or she is known as the *primary care provider.* Your primary care provider orders standard tests such as urinalysis, blood tests, and X-rays to aid in diagnosis and treatment.

Health problems that are less common, more complex, or persistent may require **secondary care.** This is the realm of the specialist. There are several approaches to finding a specialist, but the typical route is a referral from your primary care provider. For example, a patient may visit his or her primary care physician to treat migraine headaches. If the migraines persist despite the primary care physician's best efforts, then the physician will likely refer the patient to a neurologist, a doctor who specializes in treating nervous system disorders.

The tests and therapies provided by secondary care may solve the health problem. But if they do not, then **tertiary care** can come into play. Tertiary care is the most complex set of medical services, involving many types of health care specialists and taking place at a medical center or specialized clinic. If, for instance, a neurologist is unsuccessful in helping the migraine sufferer, then he or she might consult with yet another specialist, such as an endocrinologist, and more complex tests might be ordered, such as an MRI (magnetic resonance imaging) to assess brain function.

MAJOR CHALLENGES: CONTROLLING COSTS AND REDUCING ERRORS

In terms of highly trained health professionals and cutting-edge medical technology, the United States is one of the top countries in the world. Yet, despite recognized excellence in medical resources, significant weaknesses exist in our health care system. First, the American approach to health care is the most expensive in the world. Medical economists fear that continuation of spiraling costs will have dire consequences and that policy changes are needed sooner rather than later. Second, the rate of preventable medical errors that result in illness, disability, or death is unacceptably high. What's being done to reduce medical mistakes? As consumers and citizens, these two major challenges warrant our attention.

Primary health care is the diagnosis and treatment of simple, routine illnessess.

Secondary care is the use of specialists for more complex or unusual conditions.

Tertiary care is the utilization of complex medical services and networks in order to diagnose and treat the most challenging medical conditions.

The major cost categories for health care are hospitals, physician and related clinical services, prescription drugs, and nursing home care. Predictably, hospital care and physician/clinical services account for over half of annual health care costs. Highly trained medical professionals justifiably earn high salaries, and state-of-the-art specialty equipment is extremely expensive to develop, manufacture, and maintain. The main concern is the *rate of rise* in the cost of health care. Health care spending has exceeded overall growth in the U.S economy in every recent decade. Put another way, for individuals and families, increases in the cost of health insurance and out-of-pocket medical expenses have consistently outpaced inflation and growth in workers' earnings.

Factors such as medical litigation, the aging population, and treatment for the uninsured contribute significantly to increasing health care costs. Today, physicians routinely carry malpractice insurance; high-risk specialists like obstetricians and surgeons pay malpractice premiums of over $100,000 per year. The costs that physicians must bear to practice medicine are ultimately passed on in patient fees. A second factor pushing health care costs higher is the "graying" of America—the fastest growing segment of our population is people over age sixty. The elderly require more health care services simply due to their age; consequently, as this proportion of the population increases, so do the total expenditures for medical care.

A third factor contributing to rising health care costs is the large number of uninsured persons: in 2006, approximately 47 million Americans, about one out of six, had no health care insurance. The uninsured generally do not seek medical care unless it is absolutely necessary, so most are treated at emergency rooms and the costs are underwritten with tax dollars. Currently, the availability of low-cost or free care to treat routine medical problems or conduct preventive screening is minimal. Limited services are provided through state, county, and city public health departments and benevolence organizations. Finding a solution to the uninsured problem is a major national challenge.

U.S. health care costs continue to escalate and show no sign of slowing down. (To follow national trends, refer to the ongoing Medical Expenditure Panel Survey [MEPS] within the Agency for Healthcare Research and Quality at **www.meps.ahrq.gov/mepsweb/**.) Nearly all Americans are concerned. Policy makers continue to debate options, but little real change is seen in the near future. Plainly, we should view health insurance as a necessity, not an option. Without it, medical care is not affordable. Information on how to select a health insurance plan is presented in the next chapter (see Chapter 13's section "Understanding Health Insurance").

Organization of the U.S. Health Care System

Medical Errors

We've read about the tragic cases. A woman dies from an overdose during chemotherapy. A man has the wrong leg amputated. An eight-year-old dies during "minor" surgery due to a drug mix-up. A comprehensive national study conducted in 1999 by the prestigious Institute of Medicine of the National Academy of Sciences found that medical errors were a leading cause of death and injury. Researchers estimated that between 44,000 and 98,000 Americans die in hospitals each year as a result of medical errors. Even with the lower estimate, deaths due to preventable medical errors exceeded deaths due to motor vehicle accidents (43,000), breast cancer (42,000), or AIDS (16,000).

Indeed, the problem is probably much larger. Hospital patients represent only a small proportion of the total number of people at risk. More medical care and increasingly complex care is provided in outpatient surgical centers, medical clinics, physicians' offices, and nursing homes. Retail pharmacies and home care are also settings for medical errors. Clearly, health care is not as safe as it should be. In stark terms, this landmark study demonstrated the need for initiating a comprehensive approach to improving patient safety.

As a result of national attention, significant steps have been taken to create safety systems within health care organizations from top to bottom. For example, many hospitals have gone to electronic patient records in which all medications are recorded and noted when administered; this minimizes errors due to illegible handwriting, paper records, and

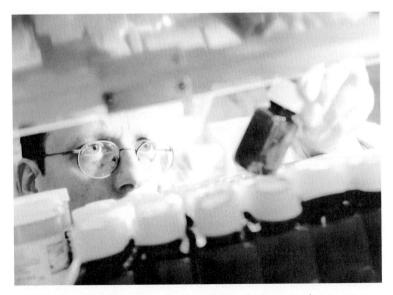

Receiving the wrong drug or the correct medication at the wrong dose are examples of preventable medical errors.

different personnel across shifts. Yet, despite reforms to improve health care services, progress has been slow. Fundamental change takes time and commitment by all stakeholders. Knowing that preventable medical errors are *not* a rare occurrence should reinforce our commitment to being active, engaged partners in our own treatment and medical management. Tips on preventing medical errors, especially those related to medicines and hospital stays, are presented in the next chapter (see Chapter 13's sections "OTC and Prescription Medicines" and "Medical Tests and Procedures").

With regard to the U.S. health care system, there are two clear messages for the individual consumer: (1) have adequate health insurance, and (2) be vigilant for medical errors. At the societal level, Americans should support policies to provide health care that is cost effective, safe, and equitable.

✓ **NEED TO KNOW**

The U.S. health care system is a complex, market-based network of individuals and organizations. Medical care is provided at three levels: primary, secondary, and tertiary. Controlling health care costs and reducing medical errors are major challenges. In the American system both health insurance and vigilance are fundamental to receiving quality health care.

➤ Western Medicine

Health care in the United States is predominantly in the form of Western medicine—that is, science-based medicine that was largely developed in Europe and North America (the Western world). *Western medicine,* also known as *conventional medicine* or *biomedicine,* can be defined as medicine practiced by mainstream medical doctors and allied health professionals. To maintain a high standard of care, these health care professionals adhere to strict educational and licensing criteria. As consumers of health care, we need to have some familiarity with how doctors and allied health care workers are trained and credentialed.

When the call goes out over the plane's intercom, "Is there a doctor on board?" you can be sure the attendant is calling for a physician, not a college professor. Yet, general knowledge about health care doctors other than physicians and dentists—such as podiatrists, optometrists and clinical psychologists—is fairly limited. In each case, these doctors can function as independent health care practitioners and must be licensed to practice. A brief review of the training, specializations, and overlap among these mainstream health care doctors is provided next.

There are two types of **physicians:** the M.D.—doctor of medicine—and the D.O.—doctor of osteopathic medicine. Both M.D.'s and D.O.'s are trained to use all the tools of modern health care including a vast array of medical tests, drugs, and surgery to diagnose and treat illnesses and injuries. In 2004, there were an estimated 850,000 active physicians (about 800,000 M.D.'s and 50,000 D.O.'s) in America. About one third are women.

M.D.'s and D.O.'s are much more similar than different. The main distinction is that osteopathic medicine places special emphasis on the body's musculoskeletal system, preventive medicine, and holistic care. As a result, D.O.'s are more likely than M.D.'s to be primary care doctors and practice family medicine, internal medicine, pediatrics, or obstetrics/gynecology. D.O.'s are often referred to as *osteopaths,* which is a shortened term for *osteopathic physician.*

Physician Education
Medical education typically extends 7–11 years beyond the undergraduate degree. This is divided between four years of medical school and three to seven years of postgraduate medical education (referred to as *residency*). Most of the first two years of medical school is spent in laboratories and classrooms taking core science courses such as anatomy, biochemistry, physiology, microbiology, pathology, and pharmacology as well as courses in human behavior, medical ethics, and medical law. During years three and four, students learn to take medical histories, examine patients, and diagnose illnesses under the supervision of physicians in hospitals and clinics. Students learn acute, chronic, rehabilitative, and preventive care in broad areas of medicine such as internal medicine, surgery, psychiatry, obstetrics/gynecology, pediatrics, and geriatrics.

Physician Specialties and Board Certifications
Following medical school, almost all physicians enter a residency in a major hospital or medical center. A residency is graduate medical education in a specialty that takes the form of paid on-the-job training. Residencies and additional training commonly last from three to seven years. This advanced training prepares doctors for board certification in a specialty. This process is overseen by the American Board of Medical Specialists, which comprises 24 specialty boards, ranging from anesthesiology to radiology.

Board certification is not just a topic of interest among physicians—it's also relevant to consumers who want quality health care. Simply put, it's

A **physician** is either a doctor of medicine (M.D.) or a doctor of osteopathy (D.O.). Nearly all physicians trained and licensed in the United States have three or more years of residency training following graduation from medical school.

TABLE 12.1   **EXAMPLES OF PHYSICIAN SPECIALTIES**

PRIMARY CARE	MEDICAL SPECIALTIES	SURGICAL SPECIALTIES
Family Medicine	Dermatology	Colon & Rectal Surgery
Internal Medicine*	Emergency Medicine	Neurological Surgery
Pediatrics*	Ophthalmology	Orthopedic Surgery
Obstetrics & Gynecology	Otolaryngology (ear/nose/throat)	Plastic Surgery
	Psychiatry	Thoracic Surgery
	Urology	Vascular Surgery

*Within both internal medicine and pediatrics, physicians can pursue additional training in subspecialties such as cardiovascular disease, pulmonary disease, oncology, infectious disease, and endocrinology.

Source: American Board of Medical Specialties
www.abms.org/Who_We_Help/Physicians/specialties.aspx

best to select a doctor who is board certified whenever possible. Board certification attests to the highest level of training in a specialty area. A few familiar medical specialties are highlighted in Table 12.1. These can be broadly grouped as primary care specialties, medical specialities, and surgical specialties. In most cases, we are referred to medical and surgical specialists by our primary care doctor. The eye specialist (ophthalmologist) and skin specialist (dermatologist) are two who many of us have already visited. And, we may have been seen by an emergency-medicine physician when we went to the ER (emergency room/department) after an accident or for a severe sudden-onset illness. You can determine if a physician is board certified via the medical specialty Web sites (see "Web Site Resources" at the end of the chapter).

Primary Care Physicians

The **primary care physicians** are our family or personal doctors. Most specialize in family medicine, internal medicine, pediatrics, or obstetrics-gynecology. They are skilled at diagnosing and treating common medical problems. Equally important, they know when to refer us to a medical or surgical specialist. In this role, they serve as gatekeepers and guides to a vast array of medical specialists and resources. In fact, some insurance plans require that people always see their primary care physician first (except for emergencies) before seeking other care.

A **primary care physician** is the front-line doctor (an M.D. or D.O.) who spends most of his or her time diagnosing and treating common and routine illnesses and diseases. Most specialize in family medicine, internal medicine, pediatrics, or obstetrics-gynecology.

Even if you can go directly to a specialist, there are good reasons to have a primary care physician. People without medical training have limited skills in diagnosis and knowing when to see which specialist. We should recognize our limitations and rely on our primary care doctors for their expertise (see Chapter 13's section "Caring for Yourself"). Plus, if a serious problem requires seeing several doctors, being able to rely on a primary care doctor to coordinate care and integrate findings is invaluable.

The aim is to have a primary care physician with whom you've established a relationship over a period of years—a doctor who knows you well, provides ongoing medical care, refers you to specialists as needed, interprets results, and generally advises you on medical matters. In addition to being board certified, it's important to select a primary care doctor who is a good communicator and with whom you feel comfortable. A solid patient-doctor relationship is based on confidence and trust.

Doctors specializing in internal medicine (internists) focus on the primary care of adults, particularly the diagnosis and (nonsurgical) treatment of diseases of the internal organs. They are trained to solve diagnostic problems in which multiple illnesses and diseases may be occurring at the same time. They also are trained to advise people on disease prevention, women's health, substance abuse, and mental health, as well as common problems of the eyes, ears, skin, nervous system, and reproductive organs. Although their focus is on the internal organs, they do treat the whole person. (Do not confuse internists with interns, who are doctors in their first year of residency training.)

Just as internists specialize in adult medicine, pediatricians are the primary care specialists in the medical care of infants, children, and adolescents. Obstetricians and gynecologists are trained in the medical and surgical care of the female reproductive system and associated disorders. They are also trained and often serve as primary care physicians for women.

✓ NEED TO KNOW

Most 21st-century physicians (M.D's or D.O's) are highly trained specialists with three or more years of training beyond medical school. Adults should have a primary care physician who is a family medicine specialist or an internist. Women may elect to rely on their obstetrician/gynecologist as their primary doctor. Infants, children, and adolescents should be seen by a pediatrician or family medicine specialist. To receive the best medical care, consumers should seek out physicians who are board certified. Finally, it's important to select a primary care doctor who is a good communicator and with whom you feel comfortable.

An anonymous woman tries to disentangle a shopping cart from an interlocked row of them outside a suburban store. She is frustrated and angry. She becomes even more exasperated when another shopper enters the frame, calmly unhooks a cart, and glides smoothly on her way. Watching this TV advertisement unfold, it might look like the woman is experiencing little more than a normal bout of tension or stress. But the folks at the drug company Lilly know better. This woman may need a powerful antidepressant because she is suffering from a severe form of mental illness known as PMDD. "Think it's PMS? It could be PMDD," intones the voiceover.

Not everyone agrees with the drug company's assessment. This example was taken from the book *Selling Sickness: How the World's Biggest Pharmaceutical Companies Are Turning Us All into Patients* (2005). Authors Roy Moynihan and Alan Cassels argue that the pharmaceutical industry is no longer focused on selling cures for disease, but rather on marketing drugs to the masses. They provide persuasive evidence that the big drug companies now influence all facets of medication use—research, approval, marketing, and the doctors and their patients.

Selling Sickness is just one of the current books to delve into this remarkable entanglement of capitalism, medicine, and culture. When the arthritis pain drugs Celebrex and Vioxx were recalled from the market because of reports that they increased the risk of heart disease, troubling questions arose. Were these drugs prematurely pushed through the approval process in the rush to get them to market? The intrusion of drug companies into the practice of medicine has been described as scandalous and fraudulent. Even those who are sympathetic to the drug companies recognize that the situation is—at the very least—troubling and problematic. Consumers should be alert and concerned.

A few statements of fact: Many prescription drugs are truly life-saving and life-sustaining in their ability to help cure or manage specific diseases and illnesses. For some medical conditions, compelling evidence from years of careful research has shown that specific drug therapies are effective and safe. Examples include statin drugs to manage high cholesterol and synthetic insulin for type 1 diabetes. Drugs are also often expensive, and all have side effects.

So what's the problem? Through strategic and systematic corporate sponsorship, drug companies have undue influence in the promotion and sales of prescription drugs. To begin with, a large proportion of research at medical schools is funded by drug companies. Less noticeable because it's omnipresent is the benefactor role of drug companies in the lives of physicians from medical school till retirement. Such support pervades

(Continued)

both medical education (medical school, residency training, and continuing education) and clinical practice. Drug companies sponsor all sorts of educational and social events from luncheons for medical students to lavish seminars for physician specialists. Drug company representatives who regularly visit physicians to present new products have an array of thank-you gifts and favors to bestow.

But of all the inroads to influence forged by the drug companies, perhaps the most far-reaching is direct marketing to the public. Through slick "awareness-raising" campaigns, the drug industry has capitalized on the American illusion that we can have it all—eternal youth, beauty, sexual desire, enhanced intellect, and continual happiness—by taking a pill. This has led to the creation or exaggeration of medical conditions such as PMDD (premenstrual dysphoric disorder, a severe form of premenstrual syndrome), motivational deficiency disorder, adult-attention-deficit-disorder, social anxiety disorder, female sexual dysfunction, and erectile dysfunction. Doctors are no longer just subliminally conditioned to prescribe drugs. They are now confronted by patients who saw an advertisement and subsequently ask for, and sometimes demand, the new drug.

The goal of for-profit companies is to increase sales, often aggressively within the limits of the law. In their ambition, drug companies have steadily pushed the envelope to broaden the base of potential clients beyond those who are sick to the healthy too. This has required new corporate strategies aimed at creating markets for their products. Roy Moynihan asks, only somewhat tongue-in-cheek, "Is the goal of pharma [the drug industry] a disease for every pill?"

In today's world, many factors influence how doctors prescribe drugs to their patients. We must remember that doctors are human just like the rest of us. They are not immune from influences inherent in the system of medical training and practice. The influence of drug companies is another compelling reason to select your doctor with care. Find one who accepts you as not just a patient, but as a partner in your own health care. And before asking your doctor for that new medicine you saw advertised, do your homework on the drug and its targeted medical condition. You may be just fine without it.

DENTISTS

Nearly every reader has visited a dentist within the last year or two. In America, we are fortunate to have regular access to dentists to help ensure good oral health. **Dentists** prevent, diagnose, and treat problems with teeth and with mouth tissue. They commonly remove tooth decay,

A **dentist** is a doctor of dental surgery (D.D.S.) or dental medicine (D.M.D.), whose practice includes problems with teeth and gums and other aspects of oral health.

fill cavities, interpret X-rays, straighten teeth, and repair or replace damaged or diseased teeth. They also perform corrective surgery on gums and supporting bones to treat gum diseases. They provide instruction on oral hygiene including diet, brushing, flossing, and the use of fluorides, as well as administer anesthetics and write prescriptions. In 2006, there were about 161,000 active dentists.

As with medical school students, most students who are admitted to dental school hold an undergraduate degree. Dental school is typically four academic years. During the last two years, students treat patients in dental clinics, under the supervision of licensed dentists. Most dental schools award the degree of Doctor of Dental Surgery (D.D.S.). The rest award an equivalent degree, Doctor of Dental Medicine (D.M.D.). A major difference between the education of a physician and a dentist is the extent of postgraduate education. For medical school graduates, a three-year residency is standard. In contrast, most dental school graduates go straight into practice after graduation. Most become general practitioners, handling a variety of dental needs. Only about one in eight new graduates enroll in postgraduate programs to prepare for a dental specialty. Orthodontists who straighten teeth with braces or retainers constitute the largest group of specialists. Oral and maxillofacial surgeons, who operate on the mouth and jaws, and periodontists, who treat gums and bone supporting the teeth, are two other types of specialists.

PODIATRISTS

A **podiatrist** is to the foot what a dentist to the mouth. The podiatrist—or doctor of podiatric medicine (D.P.M.)—specializes in the prevention, diagnosis, and treatment of foot and ankle disorders. A podiatrist makes independent judgments, prescribes medications, and performs surgery. The foot may be the first area to show signs of serious conditions such as diabetes or heart disease. In this role, podiatrists often become a vital link in the patient's health care team.

Although podiatry has been a recognized medical practice for nearly a century, the profession remains poorly understood. Most foot and ankle problems are treated by primary care physicians or orthopedic surgeons (M.D.'s/D.O.'s). Although podiatrists are foot and ankle specialists, there is substantial overlap in medical care of foot injuries by physicians and podiatrists. Because there are only about 15,000 podiatrists nationwide, many Americans simply do not have access to podiatric care.

The medical training to become a podiatrist is similar to that for an M.D. or D.O. The curriculum leading to a D.P.M. is four years long. The first two years are classroom instruction and laboratory work; they are followed by

A **podiatrist** is a doctor who holds a Doctor of Podiatric Medicine (D.P.M.) degree and whose practice focuses on medical problems of the foot and lower leg.

two years of supervised clinical rotations. Graduation from podiatric medical school is followed by a two-year residency in a hospital-based program.

OPTOMETRISTS

Doctors of Optometry (O.D.'s) are health care professionals for the eye. The primary function of **optometrists** is correcting what are known as *refractive errors*. A refractive error is due to the eye not bending light correctly, resulting in a blurred image. Refractive errors are the most common eye disorders, and they include nearsightedness, farsightedness, and astigmatism. Optometrists prescribe corrective lenses both in the form of glasses and contact lenses. In addition they counsel people regarding their visual needs and associated surgical and nonsurgical options related to their occupations, avocations, and lifestyle.

Optometric Education
A four-year curriculum leads to the O.D. degree. Nearly all O.D.'s enter the workforce immediately following graduation. A small percentage complete an optional one-year residency in a specific area of practice.

Optometry versus Ophthalmology
Both optometrists and ophthalmologists are referred to as "eye doctors." Indeed, there is overlap in the services they perform. But there are differences as well. An ophthalmologist is a physician, with 8 or more years of education beyond college (medical school, and at least four years of specialty training), who performs a full range of eye-related medical care, including surgery. In comparison, an optometrist generally has four years of education beyond college (four-year professional degree in optometry) and mainly examines eyes, prescribes corrective lenses, and advises on nonsurgical management of certain eye problems. As a final note, let's consider the optician. An optician is a technician licensed to fit and dispense eyeglasses and contact lenses according to a written prescription from an ophthalmologist or optometrist. The training and certification of opticians vary widely from state to state.

CLINICAL PSYCHOLOGISTS

Clinical psychologists are mental health practitioners. They work closely with physicians, often referring patients to each other. Clinical psychologists constitute the largest specialty group within the broad field of

---

An **optometrist** holds an O.D. degree and is primarily trained to evaluate refractive errors and prescribe corrective glasses or contacts.

A **clinical psychologist** holds a Ph.D. or Psy.D. in clinical psychology and provides psycho-socio-behavioral therapies to help people adjust to or overcome emotional problems or mental illnesses.

psychology. Most of them help mentally and emotionally disturbed people adjust to life, and others assist medical and surgical patients in dealing with illnesses or injuries. For example, in physical rehabilitation centers, clinical psychologists can be found treating patients with spinal cord injuries, chronic pain or illness, stroke, and neurological conditions.

Clinical psychologists work with individuals of all ages from infants to older adults, as well as families, groups, and organizations. They use a wide range of assessments and interventions to promote mental health and to alleviate discomfort and maladjustment. Interventions are directed at preventing and treating emotional conflicts, personality disturbances, and psychopathology. Common interventions include psychotherapy, psychoanalysis, behavior therapy, marital and family therapy, group therapy, biofeedback, cognitive retraining, social learning approaches, and environmental consultation and design. Many clinical psychologists are also involved in research, teaching and supervision, program development and evaluation, and public policy.

Doctoral Education in Clinical Psychology

A doctoral program in clinical psychology—leading to either a Ph.D. or Psy.D. degree—takes five to seven years and requires substantial course work in personality and psychopathology and a one-year internship. The American Psychological Association accredits clinical psychology doctoral programs. All states require a license to practice clinical psychology.

Clinical Psychologist versus Psychiatrist

As between optometrists and ophthalmologists, overlap exists between clinical psychologists and psychiatrists. The main difference is that psychiatrists are physicians who can order medical tests to assist in diagnoses and prescribe medications for treatment. Although the clinical psychologist's training is firmly rooted in psychology and the psychiatrist's in medicine, both are experts in mental health and, in fact, often work together in complementary fashion on health care teams in hospitals and clinics.

✓ **NEED TO KNOW**

Along with the familiar physician (M.D., D.O.), a number of other doctors provide health care services. In addition to the dentist (D.D.S., D.M.D.), there are the doctoral-level professions of podiatrist (D.P.M.), optometrist (O.D.), and clinical psychologist (Ph.D., Psy.D.). Understanding the similarities and differences between these three professions versus the physician specialists of orthopedist, ophthalmologist, and psychiatrist, respectively, is important in making decisions about health care needs related to the foot, eye, and the mind.

In conventional Western medicine, complex illnesses are treated and managed by medical teams led by physicians. The health care team contains a mix of allied health care professionals depending on the patient's particular medical condition. There are over 50 recognized allied health professions. They range from audiologists (hearing) and prosthetists (artificial limbs) to technologists trained in specialized medical services from medical imaging to surgery. As mentioned in the chapter introduction, many of you will eventually work in health care—as doctors, allied health care professionals, or employees in a health-related business. Knowing that job growth in the health care sector is projected to remain strong, you may wish to investigate related educational programs and career paths. Four allied health professionals that you—as a patient—are likely to interact with are the registered nurse, physician assistant, physical therapist, and registered dietitian.

Registered Nurses

Registered nurses (R.N.'s) constitute the largest health care profession, with 2.4 million jobs in the United States. Most R.N.'s work as staff nurses, providing health care services to patients under the direction of physicians and other health care practitioners. Round the clock, nurses are the true front-line care givers. In the hospital or clinic, when a doctor orders a treatment or test, it's the nurse who typically administers or supervises the procedure. Basic duties include checking vital signs, dressing wounds, administering treatment and medications, educating and reassuring patients, and providing support to patients' family members. Additionally, R.N.'s record medical histories and symptoms, help to perform diagnostic tests and analyze results, and assist with patient follow-up and discharge. In some cases, R.N.'s direct health screenings, immunization clinics, blood drives, and public seminars on various medical conditions.

There are three main paths to becoming an R.N.: a bachelor's of science degree in nursing (B.S.N.), an associate degree in nursing, and a diploma. In 2006, over 700 colleges offered the bachelor's degree (typically a four-year program), about 850 community and junior colleges offered the associate degree (two to three years), and only about 70 hospital-based programs offered the diploma (about three years). Generally, licensed graduates of any of the three types of educational programs qualify for entry-level positions as staff nurses. Accelerated B.S.N. programs also are available for people who have a bachelor's or higher degree in another field. In 2006, about 200 of these programs were available.

A **registered nurse** is a graduate of a nursing school (diploma, associate degree, or undergraduate degree who has passed the licensing exam for the R.N. credential.

Some R.N.'s choose to become advanced practice nurses by obtaining a master's degree in one of four areas—as a nurse practitioner, clinical nurse specialist, nurse anesthetist, or nurse midwife. Nurse practitioners provide basic preventive health care to patients and increasingly are serving as primary and specialty care providers in medically underserved areas. Clinical nurse specialists provide direct patient care and expert consultations in a particular nursing specialty (related to a disease, a body organ or system, or a patient population). Nurse anesthetists administer anesthesia, monitor the patient's vital signs during surgery, and provide post-anesthesia care. Nurse midwives provide primary care to women, including gynecological exams, family planning advice, prenatal care, assistance in labor and delivery, and neonatal care.

Physician Assistants

Physician assistants (P.A.'s) are health professionals licensed to practice medicine with a physician's supervision. Within the physician–P.A. relationship, P.A.'s can have significant autonomy in medical decision making and provide a broad range of diagnostic and therapeutic services. P.A.'s can take medical histories, perform physical exams, order and interpret laboratory tests, diagnose and treat illnesses, counsel patients, assist in surgery, and set fractures. In nearly all states they can prescribe medicines under the supervision of an M.D. or D.O.

Most P.A. programs consist of a two-year master's program. All programs emphasize primary care. Nearly all successful applicants already have a bachelor's degree. P.A.'s often have prior experience as registered nurses, while others come from varied backgrounds, including military corpsmen/medics and allied health occupations such as respiratory therapists, physical therapists, and paramedics. Many P.A.'s obtain additional training in a primary care specialty—family medicine, internal medicine, pediatrics, or obstetrics and gynecology. Others may opt for specialty fields, such as cardiovascular surgery, orthopedics, or emergency medicine.

Physical Therapists

Under the guidance of a physician, **physical therapists** (P.T.'s) provide treatments that help restore function, improve mobility, relieve pain, and prevent or limit permanent physical disabilities of people suffering from injuries or disease. Their patients range from accident victims with fractures and injuries to the spine and head to people with disabling

A **physician's assistant** is a health care professional trained to provide routine primary care to patients under the supervision of a physician.

A **physical therapist** is a health care professional who holds a degree in physical therapy and generally works in rehabilitation medicine helping patients restore musculoskeletal function.

conditions such as low-back pain, arthritis, stroke, and cerebral palsy. P.T.'s most commonly provide care in hospitals, clinics, and private offices. There are over 100,000 P.T.'s working in the United States. Throughout most of the rest of the world, physical therapists are known as physiotherapists.

There are about 200 U.S. programs awarding the doctor of physical therapy (D.P.T.). The degree transitioned from a master's (M.P.T.) to a doctorate over a 10-year period starting in the late 1990s. Nearly all programs require applicants to have an undergraduate degree with a core set of science courses. D.P.T. programs are three to four years with clinical internships interspersed throughout. P.T.'s can enter the workforce as generalists and treat patients with a wide range of conditions, or they can specialize in areas such as pediatrics, geriatrics, orthopedics, sports medicine, neurology, and cardiopulmonary rehabilitation.

Registered Dietitian

Registered dietitians (R.D.'s) are food and nutrition experts who typically work in one of four areas: clinical, community, management, or consultant dietetics. Clinical dietitians provide nutritional services for patients in institutions such as hospitals and nursing care facilities. They confer with doctors and other health care professionals to coordinate medical and nutritional needs for patients. Over half of all full-time R.D.'s work as clinical dietitians. Community dietitians work in public health clinics, home health agencies, and HMOs, where they counsel individuals and groups on nutritional practices to prevent disease and promote health. Management dietitians oversee large-scale meal planning and preparation in places such as school and company cafeterias. Consultant dietitians work on a contract basis for individual clients or organizations such as wellness programs, sports teams, supermarkets, and nutrition-related businesses.

To be eligible for the R.D. exam, the standard route is to complete an accredited bachelor's degree in nutrition/dietetics. There are over 200 bachelor's and master's degree programs in the United States. The curriculum includes course and laboratory work in all four dietetics practice areas as well as an approved internship. R.D.'s are trained to translate the science of nutrition into practical solutions across the lifespan and for a variety of diseases and conditions. There are over 50,000 practicing full-time R.D.'s. Many pursue additional graduate training to prepare for advanced clinical positions, or to work in public health, or research. Given the current diet-related health problems faced by Americans, the value of a dietitian in advising patients and working with other health care professionals to coordinate medical care has never been greater.

A **registered dietitian** is a food and nutrition expert who holds a degree in dietetics and has passed the national R.D. exam.

For additional information on these and other types of allied health care professions, see the Web sites listed at the end of the chapter. Related to both consumer information and career prospects, it should be noted that competition is keen, and educational standards are continually increasing for allied health care professional preparation programs. As with health care doctors, the job opportunities in allied health careers are excellent, and future demand is projected to remain high.

✓ **NEED TO KNOW**

A patient's needs may require the expertise of a health care team that includes one or more physicians and a mix of allied health care professionals. The team approach is particularly important in diagnosing, treating, and managing complex illnesses. As a consumer, it's important to understand how these supporting professionals contribute to patient care. The training and roles of allied health care professionals—such as nurse, physician's assistant, physical therapist, and dietitian—are varied and multifaceted and continue to evolve over time.

➤ Complementary and Alternative Medicine (CAM)

In addition to conventional or Western medicine, to which most of us are accustomed, there is a wide variety of other approaches to health care collectively referred to as **complementary and alternative medicine (CAM).** Chiropractic and acupuncture are two well-known examples. CAM practices are based on principles quite different from those of mainstream Western medicine. For this reason, CAM is also known as *nonconventional medicine. Complementary medicine* specifically refers to practices used at the same time but not necessarily in conjunction with conventional medical practices, whereas *alternative medicine* refers to practices used instead of conventional treatments.

COMPARISON WITH WESTERN MEDICINE

The fundamental differences between Western medicine and CAM are summarized in Table 12.2. The foundation of Western medicine is science,

Complementary and alternative medicine (CAM) is a group of diverse medical and health care systems, practices, and products that are not currently considered to be part of Western or conventional medicine.

TABLE 12.2	COMPARISON OF BASIC PRINCIPLES: WESTERN MEDICINE vs. ALTERNATIVE MEDICINE	

PRINCIPLES OF WESTERN MEDICINE	PRINCIPLES OF ALTERNATIVE MEDICINE
Rooted in the scientific method and guided by empirical evidence from research	Often rooted in traditional medicine based on ancestral practices
Illness has a physical cause due to pathogens, environment, lifestyle, genetic factors, aging	Illness is due to an imbalance in the person or between the individual and others
Diagnosis of illness is based on established signs and symptoms that occur across patients	Illness is different in each person; evidence is case-based
Focus is to heal via outside intervention as with drugs and/or surgery	Focus is on helping the body's capacity for self-repair
Use of specialists and advanced technology to diagnose and treat illness	Based on metaphysical premises that may not be testable

the scientific method is the discovery and accumulation of knowledge through systematic and rigorous research. In contrast, CAM practices are often rooted in culture-specific traditions and medical customs passed down across generations. CAM practices, also referred to as *traditional medicine*, are still widely used in parts of Asia, Africa, and Latin America.

The Western medicine approach involves the diagnosis and treatment of illness within a biomedical framework using highly trained specialists and advanced technology. Western medicine focuses on curing illness and disease through drugs and surgery, based on objective scientific evidence. In contrast, CAM is generally case-based rather than research-based and often has spiritual or metaphysical underpinnings that are not readily testable by the scientific method. For most forms of CAM, illness is thought to be caused by an imbalance within the individual or between the individual and others, and treatment is directed toward assisting the body's innate capacity for self-repair and restoration of balance.

Thus, the very nature of CAM—where interpretation of similar symptoms, diagnosis of illness, and prescribed treatments may vary widely from one patient to the next—make CAM practices difficult if not impossible to study using the scientific method. Standard research methods typically involve studying hundreds of subjects with the same illness to test the effectiveness of a given treatment.

Western medicine is evidence-based medicine and the bedrock for health care in the 21st century. However, CAM is routinely used by significant segments of our population, and some CAM practices may provide healing benefits for certain patients. A recent survey found that more than 40 percent of American adults reported using some form of CAM on a regular basis. Patients' perceptions about limitations in Western medical care are reflected in their increasing expenditures for alternative treatments. About half of these costs are paid out of pocket because insurance companies do not authorize payment for most CAM therapies.

As strong as Western medicine is, it cannot answer all our questions about health and disease. Even the foremost medical researchers agree on this point. And, conversely, as unproven as CAM appears to those who understand the world through science, the fact remains that some alternative therapies help people get better. The difficulty is in reconciling our inability to prove cause and effect between certain CAM practices and what appears to be a potent benefit.

With that in mind, we should remain open to the possibility that CAM offers beneficial treatments, yet always examine specific practices based on their own merits and evidence. As consumers of health care, our challenge is to do our homework on the effectiveness and safety of a CAM practice and to investigate the practitioner's qualifications and experience *before* making a decision about treatment.

NATIONAL CENTER FOR COMPLEMENTARY AND ALTERNATIVE MEDICINE

In 1998 the National Institutes of Health (NIH) created the National Center for Complementary and Alternative Medicine (NCCAM) in response to the growing interest in alternative medicine and the need for an objective resource for information and guidance on these diverse practices. The primary objectives of the NCCAM are twofold: to investigate alternative healing practices in the context of rigorous science and to disseminate authoritative information to the public and professionals.

The NCCAM has developed a category system to organize the large number of assorted practices and treatments within alternative medicine. We will follow this system and provide examples of common therapies within each category. The NCCAM organizes alternative medicine into five major categories: alternative medical systems, mind-body interventions, biologically based therapies, manipulative and body-based methods, and energy therapies. From the onset, it should be recognized that these are broad domains and that overlap exists.

For the most popular forms of alternative medicine, we will also describe educational and licensing requirements. In contrast to Western medicine,

FIGURE 12.1   ORGANIZATION OF ALTERNATIVE PRACTICES

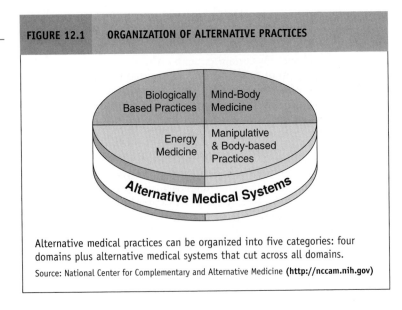

Alternative medical practices can be organized into five categories: four domains plus alternative medical systems that cut across all domains.

Source: National Center for Complementary and Alternative Medicine **(http://nccam.nih.gov)**

professional preparation programs for practitioners of alternative medicine are generally much less rigorous and systematic. Practice standards and credentialing are often lacking or not uniform.

ALTERNATIVE MEDICAL SYSTEMS

Alternative medical systems are integrated systems of medical care that are separate from the Western medical system. Traditional Chinese medicine and homeopathic medicine are two examples. Alternative medical systems vary widely from each other because each is based on its own unified body of thought and practice that reflects unique historical origins and underlying philosophies. As illustrated in Figure 12.1, the domain of alternative medical systems can cut across the other four categories. To illustrate, traditional Chinese medicine utilizes specific treatments based on qi (pronounced chee and roughly translated as "life" or "vital energy"), herbs, and Chinese massage that are also considered modalities within energy therapies, biologically based therapies, and manipulative therapies, respectively.

Traditional Chinese Medicine and Acupuncture

Traditional Chinese medicine is a system of medicine that has been practiced in China for over 3,000 years. A fundamental principle is that to remain healthy, harmony must be maintained within the body and between the body and nature. This view is represented in the distinctive yin-yang theory that encompasses the concepts of opposites, interdependence, and change. This theory and its many associated concepts (beyond the scope of this brief overview) reflects a coherent, well-developed

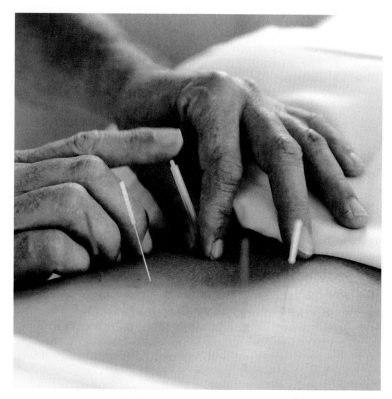

An acupuncturist carefully places needles in the body.

medical system and a wide variety of therapeutic methods. Traditional Chinese medicine continues to be widely practiced in China today alongside Western medicine.

In the Western world, **acupuncture** is the best known of the traditional Chinese medicine treatments. Acupuncture is the practice of inserting small needles into carefully selected points along the body's energy pathways. Needles are positioned just under the skin or deeper into the muscle and then either manually rotated or electrically stimulated. Acupuncture treatment is based on the belief that by adjusting the body's *qi*, or vital energy, healing can occur.

Acupuncture has been most thoroughly studied as a potential treatment for two conditions: low back pain and nausea/vomiting. Systematic

Acupuncture is an alternative medicine procedure used in or adapted from traditional Chinese medicine in which specific body areas are pierced with fine needles to treat a variety of illnesses.

reviews of multiple studies indicate acupuncture is more effective for relief of low back pain than no treatment or sham (pretended) treatment. Moreover, when acupuncture is added to conventional therapies, it relieves pain and improves function better than conventional therapies alone. Yet, all effects are small. Multiple studies have also assessed whether acupuncture can be used reduce nausea and vomiting (typically postoperative or following chemotherapy). Overall results indicate that acupuncture can be effective, particularly on the first day.

Practitioners of acupuncture are known as *acupuncturists*. The National Certification Commission for Acupuncture and Oriental Medicine has been providing bona fide certification in acupuncture since 1985. These certificates are accepted for licensure in about 40 states. Refer to the Commission's Web site to find a certified acupuncturist and for information on state licensure **(www.nccaom.org).**

Homeopathy

Homeopathy is another example of an alternative medical system. Homeopathy is based on the "law of similars." This refers to the observation that medicines can produce in healthy people the same symptoms they cure in the sick. This concept—also known as "like cures like"—was derived from simple trial and error or empirical observations. Homeopathic treatment was developed. This involves giving extremely dilute medicines to trigger the patient's innate ability to heal. Homeopathic medicines are natural remedies derived from animal, plant, and mineral sources and are sold as over-the-counter products.

Homeopathy was developed over 200 years ago in Europe by Samuel Hahnemann, a German physician. His followers immigrated to the United States in the mid-1800s and established the American homeopathic movement, which flourished for several decades. However, the tide turned in the first half of the 20th century. As medical science (Western medicine) grew and more and more modern drugs were discovered, homeopathy lost its appeal.

Even though all formal degree programs were disbanded by 1950, homeopathy has persevered over the decades and still has its advocates. Seminars and courses continue to be offered by homeopathic interest groups. A resurgence of interest in homeopathy has occurred in recent years as part of the broader interest in self-care and alternative medicine. Because there is no federal licensure exam, the current practice of homeopathy is generally limited to medically licensed physicians (M.D.'s, D.O.'s) who use selected homeopathic remedies along with conventional medical treatments.

The scientific basis and medical effectiveness of homeopathy remain dubious. Although there may be instances in which "like cures like," the concept does not qualify as a universal principle. A limited number of studies have evaluated homeopathic treatments. Few carefully controlled randomized studies have been conducted due to the lack of positive findings from smaller studies. Systematic reviews of homeopathic treatments find no conclusive evidence of effectiveness for any specific medical condition. Although the risk of serious side effects from using highly diluted homeopathic remedies appears low, there is no compelling theory or solid evidence to support their use.

MIND-BODY INTERVENTIONS

The overarching premise of mind-body treatments is that a potent connection exists between our mind and our physical health. This view is readily acceptable to many people. As discussed in Chapter 6, "Manage Stress," and Chapter 7, "Mental Health and Disorders," the reciprocal mind-body link is well established and is a reflection of our holistic nature. Our thoughts and emotions can affect our physical health, just as physical illness can affect our thinking and feelings. Several mind-body interventions such as psychotherapy, biofeedback, and hypnosis have been carefully studied and systematically developed and are now recognized by many experts as mainstream Western medicine practices.

Most mind-body interventions, however, are still placed under the umbrella of CAM practices. Movement therapies are a grouping that includes tai chi and yoga as well as less familiar movement pattern/postural awareness regimens like the Alexander technique and the Feldenkrais method. They are used to reduce stress and treat a variety of disorders from asthma to osteoporosis. Creative therapies are another grouping; these interventions typically use art, dance, or music as a means to treat people with communication or psychological disorders. Spiritual healing is a third grouping in which practitioners and in some cases laypeople use purposeful focused intention to help cure another person; faith healing and intercessory prayer are examples, respectively.

Meditation is one of the oldest and most widely practiced mind-body therapies. Meditation and its different forms evolved from Eastern religions. During meditation one focuses on breathing or on a mantra (a single word or syllable) and is taught to disregard other thoughts and emotions. Meditation is a self-administered tool for mental and physical relaxation that gives a sense of control and autonomy. It should be practiced daily to fully accrue its benefits. Meditation is taught by various groups such as Transcendental Meditation as well as by psychologists and other health care professionals.

Although anecdotal reports are persuasive and meditation appears to be safe and pose little risk, systematic reviews show that the scientific evidence is weak or insufficient to demonstrate therapeutic effectiveness for any specific health condition. Many people practice meditation simply as a lifestyle choice—not to treat a specific medical condition but rather because meditation imparts a sense of relaxation and self-awareness. Aspects of meditation are closely related to other mind-body therapies including deep breathing, progressive muscle relaxation, and yoga.

BIOLOGICALLY BASED THERAPIES

A biologically based therapy uses specific compounds, foods, or special diets—typically derived from natural sources—to treat an illness or disease. Examples include using aloe to treat a burn or consuming ginger to alleviate nausea. These therapies are referred to as biologically based because the use of the compound or food is believed to have a positive physiological effect in treating a given medical condition. Of all the CAM categories, biologically based therapies may be the broadest, with several hundred treatments including but not limited to the use of plant-based products (herbals or botanicals), animal-based products, vitamins, and minerals. The vast majority of therapies involve the ingestion of a specific compound.

A recent survey by the NCCAM reported that about one in five American adults use natural products. Echinacea, ginseng, ginkgo, garlic, and glucosamine were the most popular. The top 10 natural medicines, their typical uses, and level of evidence are summarized in Table 12.3. Note that for half of the natural remedies, evidence of effectiveness is mixed or uncertain; that is, some studies have found positive effects while others show no benefit. For ginger, glucosamine, and soy, the level of evidence to treat specific conditions is promising, but more research is needed. Finally, there is good evidence that fish oils lower cardiovascular risk and

TABLE 12.3   POPULAR NATURAL MEDICINES USED BY AMERICANS

NATURAL PRODUCT	COMMON CONDITION TREATED	EVIDENCE
Echinacea	prevent/treat colds, flu, infections	mixed
Garlic supplements	prevent/treat infections	mixed
Ginger supplements	prevent/treat nausea & vomiting	promising
Ginkgo	memory loss, variety of illnesses	mixed
Ginseng	reduce susceptibility to illness	mixed
Glucosamine	joint pain, osteoarthritis	promising
Fish oils (omega-3 fatty acids)	circulatory disorders	good
Peppermint	digestive disorders	mixed
Soy supplements	menopause hot flashes, high cholesterol	promising
St. John's wort	depression	good

Based on information from Ernst E et al., *Desktop Guide to Complementary and Alternative Medicine* (2006); Medline Plus (www.nlm.nih.gov/medlineplus/druginformation.html); and the National Center for Complementary and Alternative Medicine (http://nccam.nih.gov)

St. John's wort is effective in treating mild to moderate depression. However, not a single natural medicine among the 10 most popular has compelling evidence to support its use.

Several key points are important to keep in mind when thinking about using a biologically based therapy. These CAM products are chemically active and can interact with other compounds, foods, and drugs. For this reason, you would be wise to first discuss the pros and cons of any natural product with your doctor, especially if you are on medications, including birth control pills, or have a chronic health condition. Also, be aware that nearly all of these natural products are classified as dietary supplements, not as drugs (see the section "Dietary Supplements" in Chapter 2). Consequently, the purity, effectiveness, and safety of the compound must always be questioned. As a reminder, conventional medicines—both over-the-counter and prescription—go through a rigorous drug approval process by the FDA before they go to market, but this is *not* the case for dietary supplements, so it is buyer beware.

In the United States, herbalists and practitioners of other biologically based therapies have no standardized training or certification, and most are not medically qualified. Hundreds of natural products have been studied. For nearly all, evidence of effectiveness is negative or insufficient; for a few, evidence is mixed or promising. General contraindications are pregnancy and lactation. Additional precautions should be taken by people on medications or with chronic health conditions. Individual biologically based therapies should be thoroughly investigated for proof of effectiveness and safety.

MANIPULATIVE AND BODY-BASED METHODS

In the United States, the three most common types of manipulative and body-based methods (manual therapies) are osteopathic manipulation, chiropractic adjustment, and therapeutic massage. In manual therapy, practitioners use their hands to manipulate the patient's soft tissues (primarily muscle and adipose tissue) and musculoskeletal joints, including the spine. The techniques and uses of these three manual therapies vary somewhat with the type of practitioner—osteopath, chiropractor, or massage therapist.

As described earlier in this chapter, the osteopath or D.O. goes through training similar to the M.D.—both are physicians (Western medicine). A notable difference though is that osteopathic medicine emphasizes manipulative techniques as a key part of medical training and an important clinical skill, particularly in the diagnosis and treatment of musculoskeletal problems. In general, osteopathic manipulative treatment is broadly accepted as part of conventional Western medicine. In contrast, chiropractic adjustment and therapeutic massage are still considered alternative practices.

Chiropractic

The health care philosophy of chiropractic is centered on the body's inherent recuperative abilities and embraces a holistic view of the patient's well being. A chiropractor, also known as a doctor of chiropractic (D.C.) primarily works with people whose health problems are related to the body's muscular, nervous, and skeletal systems, especially the spine. Chiropractors believe that interference with these systems impairs normal functions, lowers resistance to disease, and can cause pain. Chiropractic was established in 1895 by D. D. Palmer and is now practiced worldwide.

Chiropractors take medical histories, conduct clinical exams, and often use X-rays. The most common treatment procedure is known as *chiropractic adjustment*, also called *spinal manipulation*. Chiropractic adjustment—manipulating the patient's joints, particularly the spine—is used to reduce pain and restore joint function. This procedure seldom causes discomfort, and people often report improvements in their symptoms immediately following treatment. Chiropractors do not perform surgery or prescribe drugs but often recommend changes in lifestyle—in eating, exercise, and sleeping habits. As needed, chiropractors refer patients to mainstream physicians (M.D.'s or D.O.'s).

In the United States, a standardized curriculum must be followed to become a chiropractor. The D.C. degree is awarded after completion of a four-year course of study at one of the 17 accredited chiropractic programs in the country. At least two years of undergraduate education is required for entry, although many applicants enter with an undergraduate degree. During the first two years, students complete classroom and laboratory work in basic sciences, while the last two years provide clinical training with emphasis in manipulation and spinal adjustment. All states have licensing boards for chiropractic, and many health insurance companies provide coverage for chiropractic care.

There are over 50,000 chiropractors across the United States. The majority are solo practitioners. Seeing a chiropractor—particularly for a back, neck, or pain-related problem—is not an unusual event. It's estimated that one in ten American adults visited a chiropractor within the last year. Chiropractic is also gaining acceptance among Western medicine practitioners, and some physicians refer patients to chiropractors for treatment of back pain.

A **chiropractor** typically works with people whose health problems are associated with the muscular, nervous, and skeletal systems, especially the spine. Chiropractic adjustment is a common treatment to relieve neck and back pain. The effectiveness of such treatment holds promise, but conclusive evidence is lacking.

Many studies have been done on chiropractic and back pain. Findings are mixed—some researchers report positive effects, and others found no benefit. As is common in research on alternative practices, many of these studies are not well designed, which limits the interpretation of findings. Moreover, back pain is difficult to study because the cause is often never known, and in most cases the condition resolves within several weeks regardless of the treatment. Overall the evidence to support the use of chiropractic adjustment as an effective treatment for back pain is not convincing; spinal manipulation is no more or no less effective than conventional treatments. Use of chiropractic for other conditions is even less compelling.

Several precautions should be noted. Due to high-speed manipulations of some adjustment techniques, people with osteoporosis should not undergo chiropractic treatments. Also, damage to the arteries that run along the vertebrae is a potential serious risk during spinal adjustment, but this appears to be a rare risk for healthy people.

Therapeutic Massage

Therapeutic massage, or massage therapy, is one of the most popular forms of CAM. The central principle of therapeutic massage is that the body's soft tissues will function optimally when the circulatory and lymphatic systems are unimpeded. There are different types of therapeutic massage (for example, Swedish, shiatsu, neuromuscular). Most involve similar manual techniques such as stroking, kneading, and stretching, and these are often combined during a treatment session. Therapeutic massage is generally used to treat joint and muscle pain and to reduce high stress levels.

A client usually sees a therapist with a diagnosis—and often a referral—from a physician or with a self-diagnosis or symptom. Therapists take a brief medical history to rule out contraindications such as skin infections, acute inflammations, or recent injuries and may ask questions to better understand the diagnosis or health complaint. During the session, the therapist requests feedback as to how much pressure is preferred. Palpation, or touch, is fundamental to therapeutic massage and allows the therapist to identify areas of muscle tension or fluid accumulation with appropriate amounts of pressure for each individual, while also conveying a sense of caring.

In the United States, considerable variability still exists from school to school regarding the length and amount of training and from state to state regarding licensing. However, the National Certification Board for Therapeutic Massage, established in 1992, has become the leading organization in setting professional standards and administering written competency exams—over 90,000 people have been certified. When provided by a qualified therapist, therapeutic massage appears to be beneficial for musculoskeletal pain and for anxiety and depression. The evidence is promising but not unequivocal. Direct risks are minimal.

ENERGY THERAPIES

Energy therapies include a variety of alternative treatments based on the use, modification, or manipulation of energy fields. This category is the most controversial of the five NCCAM categories due largely to the untestable premises upon which many of the therapies are based. Most energy therapies assume that matter and energy are similar and that matter is simply a denser form of energy; matter is readily perceived whereas energy is not, yet it is present. Some energy therapies are associated with traditional Asian medicine; others draw upon modern physics-based principles of energy.

Energy therapies can be divided into two groups. Veritable (or bioelectromagnetic) energy therapies use electromagnetic or mechanical forces in unconventional ways to treat patients. They are referred to as *veritable* (meaning "real") because they involve specific, measurable wavelengths and frequencies. Examples include magnetic therapy, light therapy, and sound energy therapy. In comparison, putative energy (or biofield) therapies are based on theorized energy or life forces emanating from the body. These energies are known as *putative* (meaning "reputed" or "supposed") because they are unmeasurable; biofields are simply assumed to exist. Examples are *qi gong* from China, Reiki from Japan, and Therapeutic Touch (laying-on of hands).

Qualifications of practitioners or healers vary widely. Some practices have credentialing or training programs; others do not. Some practitioners of energy therapy believe that all people have the capacity to be healers; others regard the ability to use healing energies as a gift given only to people who are unusually spiritual.

Based on systematic reviews of research, none of the energy therapies have been found to be effective in treating medical conditions. Extra precautions should be taken to carefully assess potential risk and benefit for any of the energy therapies.

BEING A CRITICAL CONSUMER OF CAM

If you are considering using a nonconventional medical treatment, it's especially important to know how to get reliable and credible information. Compared to Western medicine, alternative medicine is generally unregulated. Thus, misinformation, misleading claims, and outright hoaxes abound. The key is to sort the honest and credible practitioners from the modern-day quacks. Use the following tips to assess information on alternative medicine practices and products found on the Internet:

1. Who runs the Web page? Is it a credible professional (.org), educational (.edu), or governmental group (.gov)? Or a business set up to market a product (.com)? Generally, the .edu, .gov, and .org sites are more trustworthy than the .com sites.

Health & the Media *Patent Medicines*

So-called patent medicines (protected by a patent or trademark and available without a doctor's prescription) were common following the Civil War. The illustration here is an example of a patent medicine trade card—an early form of advertising that extended the reach of peddlers and medicine shows. At county fairs and frontier settlements, doctors and druggists—often with suspect credentials—engaged in aggressive selling. Many were talented entertainers capable of wowing audiences with enthralling oratory and theatrics. Ayer's Sarsaparilla could "improve the complexion, purify the blood, and make the weak strong." Quackery continues today. Many ads, across all media—print, radio, TV, and the Internet—still use unsubstantiated claims of healing and generalized health benefits. Satisfaction "guaranteed," of course.

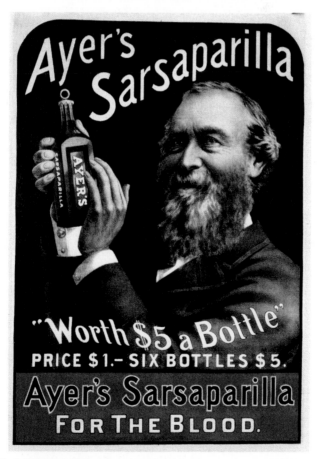

Source: Classic Poster Reproduction

http://www.ricsartshop.com/page/BPS/PROD/law/law0006

2. Be wary of sites that diagnose illnesses or suggest an individual course of treatment. These services should only be provided by a medical professional who knows the patient's medical history and has performed a proper examination.
3. Be suspicious of quasi-scientific statements that go against common sense or known health principles. Discount any treatments or products that make claims about miracle cures.
4. Don't rely on a single Web site for the final word. Always cross-check your information on multiple independent Web sites known to be reputable. For example, use the following Web sites as a starting point or to verify information from other sources:

NCCAM: **http://nccam.nih.gov**
Quackwatch: **www.quackwatch.org**
Office of Dietary Supplements: **http://ods.od.nih.gov/**
Food and Drug Administration: **www.fda.gov**

Remember, in order to investigate bona fide treatment options to a troubling health problem, seek solid information. Some advertisements are easy to discard as misleading, but others are more sophisticated and subtle. Convincing claims or personal success stories are not a substitute for scientific evidence. It is fair and appropriate to approach CAM practices with a healthy dose of skepticism. While some CAM approaches may be beneficial, you must take the time to separate the credible from the suspect. As always, your best guide to optimizing your health is accurate and trustworthy information.

What Is Your Risk? How Vulnerable Are You to Quackery?

Americans spend unknown amounts of money on health quackery. What is your risk of being mislead? The following 10 true-or-false questions are a simple way to estimate your risk of "being taken" by modern-day health hucksters.

Answer all 10 questions and then score as indicated below.

1. Quackery usually appears as outlandish approaches so it is easy to identify.	True	False
2. Most diseases are caused by faulty nutrition or can be remedied by taking supplements.	True	False
3. Anecdotes and testimonials are helpful in selecting health products and services.	True	False
4. I'm impressed when a person uses medical terms or language.	True	False
5. Drug companies and the medical profession conspire to suppress medical information.	True	False

6. There are many sound "secret cures" available for diseases and conditions.   True   False

7. Herbal remedies can cure most medical problems.   True   False

8. Some products can be effective against a wide range of unrelated diseases.   True   False

9. I "think for myself" and am not easily influenced by the wisdom of the scientific community.   True   False

10. If my doctor isn't going to help me, I will find my own solution.   True   False

Scoring: If you answered True to any question, you are at risk of being duped by someone practicing unconventional medicine in a fraudulent or inappropriate manner.

Adapted from Barrett S. Ten Ways to Avoid Being Quacked. **www.quackwatch.org**

✓ NEED TO KNOW

Complementary and alternative medicine (CAM) encompasses a multitude of diverse treatments and approaches to healing that are outside conventional medicine. The National Center for Complementary and Alternative Medicine organizes CAM into five categories: alternative medical systems, mind-body interventions, biologically based therapies, manipulative and body-based methods, and energy therapies. Even though many Americans regularly use CAM, fundamental questions about the risks and benefits of many CAM therapies are yet to be answered. Continued research on CAM practices is needed. The bottom line is to be a careful consumer.

➤ Integrative Medicine

Integrative medicine is the blending or combining of aspects of conventional Western medicine with those of complementary and alternative medicine (CAM). It's based on an awareness and appreciation of the strengths and weaknesses of both Western medicine and CAM. For example, in conventional medicine, the system of medical referral—being passed from specialist to specialist and having to undergo multiple tests—can be extremely frustrating for patients, especially if they're not getting better. People can begin to feel that they are simply "cases" or "specific conditions" rather than living, breathing individuals with their own unique histories and complex lives. Understandably, many people turn to CAM practitioners, who are known for holistic and patient-centered approaches. CAM practitioners tend to listen and get to know their patients better than mainstream physicians who work within a more regimented, time-constrained system.

Integrative medicine is a growing movement within health care that carefully selects and combines the most appropriate treatments from both realms of medicine, recognizing that neither Western medicine nor CAM has all the answers. Medical schools used to dismiss or ignore CAM, but now that has changed. The Consortium of Academic Health Centers for Integrative Medicine includes over 30 leading academic medical centers in the country such as Harvard, Duke, UCLA, and the Mayo Clinic. The Consortium's mission is to advance health care by educating medical students and physicians about integrative medicine and conducting research on CAM practices to better determine which treatments are effective or hold promise.

Prominent physicians Ralph Snyderman and Andrew Weil succinctly describe the appeal of integrative medicine for patients:

> Most Americans who consult alternative providers would probably jump at the chance to consult a physician who is well trained in scientifically based medicine and who is also open-minded and knowledgeable about the body's innate mechanisms of healing, the role of lifestyle factors in influencing health, and the appropriate uses of dietary supplements, herbs, and other forms of treatment, from osteopathic manipulation to Chinese and Ayurvedic medicine. In other words, they want competent help in navigating the confusing maze of therapeutic options that are available today, especially in those cases in which conventional approaches are relatively ineffective or harmful.

As an example, low back pain is a widespread health problem, affecting up to one out of three adults in a given month. Conventional medicine is important in identifying serious, underlying problems such as a herniated disc, rheumatoid arthritis, infection, fracture, or cancer. If no underlying cause can be determined—which occurs in a large percentage of cases—conventional medicine has little to offer the patient. Yet, there is promising evidence that acupuncture can relieve pain and improve function. In a clinic that practices integrative medicine, the doctor would discuss acupuncture as a possible treatment and arrange for treatments if requested.

Integrative medicine reaffirms the importance of the doctor-patient relationship, focuses on the whole person—not just a specific condition or disease—and makes use of all appropriate curative *and* preventive approaches. It is likely that integrative medicine will become the mainstream medicine of the future.

✓ NEED TO KNOW

Integrative medicine is based on a holistic view of patient care and the promotion of optimal health. Integrative medicine neither accepts Western medicine nor rejects CAM uncritically; instead it brings together practices from both, based on good science and the needs of the patient. Integrative medicine is a powerful movement in modern medicine and is being promoted as a new model at leading academic medical centers across the country. Integrative medicine may become the mainstream medicine of the future.

Medicine—M.D.'s and D.O.'s

American Medical Association
www.ama-assn.org
American Osteopathic Association
www.osteopathic.org
Association of American Medical Colleges
www.aamc.org
American Association of Colleges of Osteopathic Medicine
www.aacom.org
American Board of Medical Specialties
www.abms.org
Specialty Boards, American Osteopathic Association
www.do-online.org/index.cfm?PageID=crt_memboards

Dentistry

American Dental Association
www.ada.org
American Dental Education Association
www.adea.org

Podiatry

American Podiatric Medical Association
www.apma.org
American Association of Colleges of Podiatric Medicine
www.aacpm.org

Optometry

American Optometric Association
www.aoa.org
Association of Schools and Colleges of Optometry
www.opted.org/default.cfm

Clinical Psychology

American Psychological Association, Division of Clinical Psychology
www.apa.org/divisions/div12/homepage.html
National Register of Health Service Providers in Psychology
www.nationalregister.org/designate_stsearch.html

Nursing

American Nurses Association
www.nursingworld.org
American Nurses Credentialing Center
www.nursecredentialing.org/
Guide to Nursing Education and Careers
www.allnursingschools.com/faqs
National League for Nursing Accrediting Commission
www.nlnac.org/Forms/directory_search.htm

Physician Assistant
American Academy of Physician Assistants
www.aapa.org
Physician Assistant Education Association
www.paeaonline.org/

Physical Therapy
American Physical Therapy Association
www.apta.org
Physical Therapy Programs (accredited PT schools by state)
**www.apta.org/AM/Template.cfm?section=PT_Programs&template=/
aptaapps/accreditedschools/acc_schools_map.cfm&process=3&type=PT**

Dietetics
American Dietetic Association
www.eatright.org
Commission on Dietetic Registration
www.cdrnet.org

Complementary and Alternative Medicine

National Center for Complementary and Alternative Medicine (NCCAM)
http://nccam.nih.gov
National Certification Commission for Acupuncture and Oriental Medicine
www.nccaom.org
American Chiropractic Association
www.amerchiro.org
Council on Chiropractic Education
www.cce-usa.org
American Massage Therapy Association
www.amtamassage.org
National Certification Board for Therapeutic Massage and Body Work
www.ncbtmb.com
Medline Plus: Drugs, Supplements, and Herbal Information
www.nlm.nih.gov/medlineplus/druginformation.html
NCCAM: Herbs at a Glance
http://nccam.nih.gov/health/herbsataglance.htm

General
Agency for Healthcare Research and Quality
www.ahrq.gov
Cochrane Reviews (evidence-based reviews of medical interventions)
www.cochrane.org/reviews
Consortium of Academic Health Centers for Integrative Medicine
www.imconsortium.org
Explore Health Careers
http://explorehealthcareers.org
Food and Drug Administration
www.fda.gov

Health Professions, American Medical Association
   www.ama-assn.org/ama/pub/category/10481.html
Office of Dietary Supplements
   http://ods.od.nih.gov
Quackwatch
   www.quackwatch.org

Knowing the Language

acupuncture
chiropractor
clinical psychologist
complementary & alternative
   medicine (CAM)
dentist
integrative medicine
optometrist
physical therapist

physician
physician assistant
podiatrist
primary care physician
primary health care
registered dietitian
registered nurse
secondary health care
tertiary health care

Understanding the Content

1. Define and provide examples of primary, secondary, and tertiary health care.
2. Identify and discuss two of the major challenges facing our current health care system.
3. Define and contrast Western medicine with complementary and alternative medicine (CAM).

Exploring Ideas

1. Western medicine is often referred to as evidence-based medicine. Explain what is meant by this statement. For example, consider the centrality of the scientific method, how physicians and allied health professionals are trained in comparison with CAM practitioners, and the role of clinical trials in advancing medical knowledge.
2. Assume one of your parents has a recurring medical problem and the doctors have been unable to effectively treat it. Your parent now wants to try a CAM approach that was recommended by a neighbor. What advice would you give? List and explain the steps you would take to check out this CAM practice or product.
3. Explain the concept of integrative medicine. How does it differ from Western medicine? What changes need to occur if integrative medicine is to become widely accepted?

Selected References

Agency for Healthcare Research and Quality. Evidence-based Practice Reports for complementary and alternative care and dietary supplements.
www.ahrq.gov/clinic/epcindex.htm#complementary

Agency for Healthcare Research and Quality. Medical Expenditure Panel Survey.
www.meps.ahrq.gov/mepsweb/

Center on Budget and Policy Priorities. More Americans, including more children, now lack health insurance, August 31, 2007.
www.cbpp.org/8-28-07health.htm

Cochrane Reviews.
www.cochrane.org/reviews

Duke Integrative Medicine. What is integrative medicine?
www.dukeintegrativemedicine.org/about/about_im.aspx

Ernst E, Pittler M, Wider B. *Desktop Guide to Complementary and Alternative Medicine: An Evidence-based Approach* (2nd ed.). Philadelphia: Mosby, 2006.

Helfand WH. *Quack, Quack, Quack: The Sellers of Nostrums in Prints, Posters, Ephemera, & Books.* Falls Village, CT: Winterhouse Editions, 2002.

Henry J. Kaiser Family Foundation. Health Care Costs: A Primer, August 2007.
www.kff.org/insurance/7670.cfm

Institute of Medicine. *Complementary and Alternative Medicine in the United States.* Washington, DC: National Academies Press, 2005.
http://newton.nap.edu/catalog/11182.html

Kohn L, Corrigan J, Donaldson M (eds). *To Err Is Human: Building a Safer Health System.* Washington, DC: Institute of Medicine, National Academies Press, 2000.
http://newton.nap.edu/catalog/9728.html

Leape LL, Berwick DM. Five years after *To Err Is Human*. What have we learned? *JAMA* 293: 2384–2390, 2005.

Medline Plus: Herbs & Supplements, 2008.
www.nlm.nih.gov/medlineplus/druginformation.html

Micozzi M. *Fundamentals of Complementary and Integrative Medicine* (3rd ed.). St. Louis: Saunders, 2006.

Moynihan R, Cassels A. *Selling Sickness: How the World's Biggest Pharmaceutical Companies Are Turning Us All into Patients.* New York: Nation Books, 2005.

National Center for Complementary and Alternative Medicine.
http://nccam.nih.gov

Office of Dietary Supplements.
http://ods.od.nih.gov/

Snyderman R, Weil A. Integrative medicine: Bringing medicine back to its roots. *Archives of Internal Medicine* 162: 395–397, 2002.
www.bravewell.org/content/pdf/14_Snyderman_Weil_Article.pdf

University of Arizona Program in Integrative Medicine. What is integrative medicine?
http://integrativemedicine.arizona.edu/about/definition.html

U.S. Department of Labor, Bureau of Labor Statistics. Occupational Outlook Handbook.
www.bls.gov/search/ooh.asp?ct=OOH

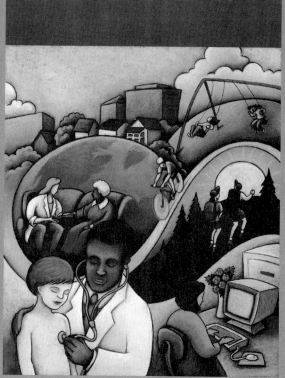

A hospital should also have a recovery room adjoining the cashier's office.

— Francis O. Walsh

Chapter 13

HEALTH CARE DECISION MAKING

In Chapter 12, we described the structure of the U.S. health care system and types of medical care available. This leads us to the question, How can we effectively use such information to navigate the system? In this chapter, we address this question by reviewing recommendations on medical self-care, the patient-doctor relationship, and health insurance. We end this last chapter by revisiting two recurrent themes central to optimal health: health literacy and preventive health care.

➤ **Caring for Yourself**

SIGNS AND SYMPTOMS

DIAGNOSING COMMON MEDICAL PROBLEMS

HANDLING MEDICAL EMERGENCIES

OTC AND PRESCRIPTION MEDICINES

COSMETIC SURGERY AND BODY ART

➤ **Developing a Patient-Doctor Partnership**

FINDING THE RIGHT DOCTOR

COMMUNICATING WITH YOUR DOCTOR

MEDICAL TESTS AND PROCEDURES

KEEPING MEDICAL RECORDS

➤ **Understanding Health Insurance**

HEALTH INSURANCE TERMINOLOGY

PRIVATE HEALTH INSURANCE: FEE FOR SERVICE AND MANAGED CARE

PUBLIC HEALTH INSURANCE: MEDICARE AND MEDICAID

CHOOSING AN APPROPRIATE PLAN

➤ **Striving for Optimal Health**

STAYING INFORMED

PRACTICING PREVENTION

ACCIDENTS are a part of life. During a pickup soccer game, Zoey, a 25-year-old part-time college student, severely twisted her ankle. Her friend took her to a nearby urgent care clinic directly afterwards, but as the weeks went by, the ankle remained swollen and painful. She finally concluded that she needed medical follow-up. But Zoey's college was 800 miles from her family home, so she was essentially on her own, and she was unsure of what to do next. How would she find a doctor? Should she see a primary care doctor or a specialist? And what about the cost? She knew it would be expensive. She already owed several hundred dollars for the visit to the urgent care clinic.

Dealing with the aftermath of an accident can sometimes be more difficult than the accident itself. Zoey's situation is not uncommon. The particulars of injuries and illnesses are different but the challenges are similar. They all have to do with making decisions about our own health care. How much can we do on our own? How do we determine when and if we need to use the health care system? How do we go about finding the right doctor?

Then there are the financial-reality questions about cost and health insurance. What are the health insurance options, and what particular type of plan is the right one for us? This chapter will help to answer these questions. Key information and resources for making informed choices about self-care, medical care, and health insurance are provided to help you navigate the health care and insurance systems.

➤ Caring for Yourself

Medical self-care is the steps and actions you take to optimize your health and to self-treat common illnesses and injuries. When motivated consumers have access to clear, simple health information, many health problems can be prevented or treated effectively and inexpensively without a visit to the doctor's office. Consequently, in this section, we'll focus on medical self-care as it relates to self-recognition of emergent signs and symptoms, and making decisions about self-treatment or seeing a health care professional. There are two key aspects of self-care: first, we must be sensitive to signs and symptoms, and second, we need to know how to acquire the relevant information.

SIGNS AND SYMPTOMS

The terms *sign* and *symptom* are similar but not synonymous. A **sign** can be measured objectively, usually by a health care provider during a physical

> **Medical self-care** is decisions and actions that an individual can take to cope with a health problem—in particular, informed steps that one can take without seeing a health care practitioner.
>
> A **sign** is a result of injury or illness and can be measured objectively by a health care provider.

exam. For example, heart rate, respiratory rate, body temperature, and blood pressure are standard vitals signs. Elevated blood pressure is a sign of possible heart disease. On the other hand, a **symptom** is a person's subjective perception, such as nausea or knee pain. Signs and symptoms are used together in recognizing and diagnosing medical conditions.

Being sensitive to signs and symptoms is sometimes referred to as "listening to your body." Being attuned to changes in your body is central to medical self-care because you are the best judge of what is normal and routine for you and what is not. It's important to pay attention to your intuition or premonitions that something is not right—as mentioned in Chapter 11 ("Infections"), *prodrome* is a medical term for patients' feelings or early symptoms indicating the onset of an illness. For example, most of us have a sense that we are coming down with a cold a day or two before the signs and symptoms are clearly recognizable. The true story of Carolyn Benivegna in the "Breaking It Down" box demonstrates the importance of knowing and listening to your body and following your intuition.

> A **symptom** is a result of injury or illness that is subjectively perceived by the patient.

Breaking It Down When Diagnosis Is a Long and Winding Road

Carolyn, an extremely healthy and health-conscious middle-aged woman became alarmed when her abdomen suddenly enlarged and she began experiencing bouts of constipation and bloated abdomen. She soon discovered that getting a good diagnosis is not always a straightforward process. It can take a combination of luck and perseverance.

She first went to her primary care doctor. Because her symptoms seemed to be intestinal, Carolyn was referred to a specialist of the digestive system—a gastroenterologist. He ran tests to determine whether there was a bacterial infection. After ruling that out, he diagnosed her with irritable bowel syndrome. Irritable bowel syndrome (IBS) consists of several symptoms at the same time; for example; abdominal pain, constipation, diarrhea, and abdominal swelling often occur together. Yet, this didn't seem right to Carolyn: "I guess I would have accepted this diagnosis had it not been for my enlarged abdomen. I swear to you, it looked like I was four to five months pregnant! I therefore insisted on more tests." The doctor ordered X-rays, which also found nothing. Carolyn was again assured she had irritable bowel syndrome and was encouraged to go on her scheduled month-long trip to Europe. But she remained worried:

"I couldn't wear any of my slacks or shorts because I couldn't get them buttoned. I *knew* something was radically wrong. I *insisted* on more tests."

Carolyn's doctor reluctantly scheduled a CAT scan (computerized axial tomography). This test showed an abnormal buildup of fluid in her abdomen. This finding suggested that Carolyn was indeed correct—she did *not* have IBS. Finally, a special blood test gave her a diagnosis: she had primary peritoneal cancer, a cancer involving the membrane that surrounds the organs in the abdomen and pelvis. In this case, the correct diagnosis was elusive because peritoneal cancer is closely related to ovarian cancer, yet Carolyn no longer had her ovaries (previously removed during a complete hysterectomy). Therefore, her doctors initially overlooked this type of cancer as a possible cause of her bloating and intestinal problems.

Carolyn's message is clear and direct: "I have learned that each of us must take *total* responsibility for our own health care." She knew her body well enough to realize that something serious might be wrong, and she pushed for more tests when she felt the doctor was missing something. The correct diagnosis was a direct result of her perseverance. Her actions led to getting life-saving treatment sooner rather than later. Carolyn's story is not typical, but it's not rare, either. The main point is not that the doctor misdiagnosed her illness, but rather that Carolyn and her doctor worked *together* to solve the mystery of her illness.

You know yourself—or should know yourself—better than anyone else. Pay attention to physical and mental changes and communicate with your doctor.

Adapted from Johns Hopkins Pathology, Personal Stories: Carolyn Benivegna **www.ovariancancer .jhmi.edu/stories2.cfm?personID=15**

DIAGNOSING COMMON MEDICAL PROBLEMS

To adequately address the topic of common medical problems requires the power of the Internet. Several excellent online resources are available to help us identify appropriate next steps when interpreting signs and symptoms. Two resources that are highly reputable, time-tested, and designed for the layperson are the American Academy of Family Physicians Web site **(www.familydoctor.org)** and the *Merck Manual* online medical library **(www.merck.com/mmhe/index.html)**. Both Web sites are comprehensive, regularly updated, and known for their ease of use.

The familydoctor.org Web site has a page that is organized alphabetically by symptoms—over 40 of the most common—from abdominal pain to urination problems **(http://familydoctor.org/online/famdocen/home/ tools/symptom.html)**. Clicking on any symptom generates a decision chart that provides guidance on a course of action. Decision charts are easy to follow and logically step through the decision-making process.

FIGURE 13.1   A DECISION CHART FOR HEADACHES

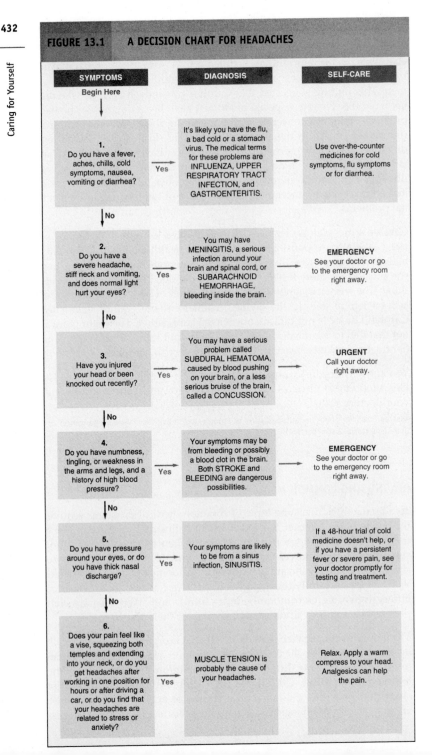

SYMPTOMS	DIAGNOSIS	SELF-CARE

Begin Here

1. Do you have a fever, aches, chills, cold symptoms, nausea, vomiting or diarrhea? — Yes → It's likely you have the flu, a bad cold or a stomach virus. The medical terms for these problems are INFLUENZA, UPPER RESPIRATORY TRACT INFECTION, and GASTROENTERITIS. → Use over-the-counter medicines for cold symptoms, flu symptoms or for diarrhea.

No ↓

2. Do you have a severe headache, stiff neck and vomiting, and does normal light hurt your eyes? — Yes → You may have MENINGITIS, a serious infection around your brain and spinal cord, or SUBARACHNOID HEMORRHAGE, bleeding inside the brain. → **EMERGENCY** See your doctor or go to the emergency room right away.

No ↓

3. Have you injured your head or been knocked out recently? — Yes → You may have a serious problem called SUBDURAL HEMATOMA, caused by blood pushing on your brain, or a less serious bruise of the brain, called a CONCUSSION. → **URGENT** Call your doctor right away.

No ↓

4. Do you have numbness, tingling, or weakness in the arms and legs, and a history of high blood pressure? — Yes → Your symptoms may be from bleeding or possibly a blood clot in the brain. Both STROKE and BLEEDING are dangerous possibilities. → **EMERGENCY** See your doctor or go to the emergency room right away.

No ↓

5. Do you have pressure around your eyes, or do you have thick nasal discharge? — Yes → Your symptoms are likely to be from a sinus infection, SINUSITIS. → If a 48-hour trial of cold medicine doesn't help, or if you have a persistent fever or severe pain, see your doctor promptly for testing and treatment.

No ↓

6. Does your pain feel like a vise, squeezing both temples and extending into your neck, or do you get headaches after working in one position for hours or after driving a car, or do you find that your headaches are related to stress or anxiety? — Yes → MUSCLE TENSION is probably the cause of your headaches. → Relax. Apply a warm compress to your head. Analgesics can help the pain.

↓ No		
7. Do you have intense, throbbing, one-sided headaches often with nausea or vomiting, and is the pain preceded by seeing flashing lights or spots? —Yes→	These are symptoms of MIGRAINE headaches. Often there's a family history of migraines. →	Make an appointment to see your doctor. A number of prescription medicines can be used to stop these headaches before or after they start.
↓ No		
8. Do your headaches occur after you read or watch a video screen closely? —Yes→	These headaches may be related to EYE PROBLEMS. →	See an optometrist or ophthalmologist for an eye exam to see if you need glasses.
↓ No		
9. Do you get headaches, weakness or shakiness if you miss a meal? —Yes→	Your headaches may be from HYPOGLYCEMIA (low blood sugar). →	Eat six small meals a day and avoid foods containing a lot of sugar.
↓ No		
10. Are you trying to cut down on caffeine, alcohol or some other drug? —Yes→	WITHDRAWAL headaches will usually last a few days. →	Use simple analgesics for the discomfort. The symptoms should fade. Don't restart your habit.
↓ No		

Pain in one area or multiple areas of the head sometimes is accompanied by other symptoms. There are many causes for headaches.

For more information, consult your doctor. If you think the problem is serious, call your doctor right away. This tool is for general educational purposes only. It is not a substitute for medical advice. Always consult your family doctor with questions about your individual condition and circumstances.

Source: American Academy of Family Physicians **www.familydoctor.org**

For example, a decision chart for headaches is presented in Figure 13.1. Following the first column under the heading of symptoms, one can scan down and follow the Yes or No branches to a probable diagnosis (second column) and then to a self-care action (third column), such as "Use an over-the-counter medicine," "Call your doctor," or "Go to the emergency room." Embedded in the Web site's decision chart are links to descriptions of the possible conditions that may be causing your symptoms.

The Merck Web site provides the online version of the *Merck Manual of Medical Information,* 2nd Home Edition. The *Merck Manual* goes back to 1899, when a reference guide was published for physicians and pharmacists. The home edition is a plain-language version of the classic medical reference text for people with an interest in health care but no medical training. It is organized alphabetically into over 20 sections, including accidents and injuries, digestive disorders, ear-nose-throat disorders, infections, men's health issues, mental health disorders, and women's health issues. Nearly all sections have illustrated subsections on the biology of the particular topic along with specific descriptions of related illnesses and conditions including symptoms, diagnosis, and treatment.

Lastly, we would be remiss if we did not recommend *Take Care of Yourself: The Complete Illustrated Guide to Medical Self-Care* by Donald Vickery, M.D. and James Fries, M.D. This is arguably the finest concise book on medical self-care for the consumer. These physician-authors pioneered the use of decision charts in medical self-care. As was illustrated by Figure 13.1, a decision chart (or flow chart) is a graphical representation of a process that shows a start point, end points, and the logical steps and possible branches in between. Decision charts originated in the fields of business (quality control) and computer science (programming). As applied to medical self-care, decision charts help us make informed decisions about treatment based on interpretation of signs and symptoms.

Drs. Vickery and Fries are nationally recognized for their leadership in educating and empowering everyday folks about their own health care. *Take Care of Yourself* is one of the few books whose impact has been systematically evaluated in randomized studies. Use of this book in community and worksite studies improved health status and reduced doctor visits and medical expenditures. For readers who are parents, see the similarly acclaimed *Taking Care of Your Child* by pediatrician Robert Pantell along with Dr. Fries and Dr. Vickery.

HANDLING MEDICAL EMERGENCIES

A final point on coping with medical problems is to consider what you would do in case of an emergency such as a heart attack, a serious fall, or a poisoning. Does the 9-1-1 system operate in your location? Where is the closest emergency room? Is your doctor's phone number readily accessible or programmed into your phone? Do you know CPR (cardiopulmonary resuscitation)? Emergencies require prompt action, so knowing what steps to take is crucial.

If you do not know CPR, or if it has been a few years since your last course, we strongly recommend that you take a course. A basic course includes information and practice on how to assist an unconscious or choking person—an infant, child, or adult—and how to use an automatic external defibrillator (AED). Even better, take a first aid course that, in addition to CPR, teaches basic skills to treat wounds and bleeding, injuries to bones and joints, extremes of hot and cold, and poisoning, bites, and stings.

In any serious accident, assume the victim is in shock to some degree.

Shock is a condition of general weakness caused by physical trauma such as loss of blood (internal or external bleeding) or extreme pain or fear. People in shock may feel faint, giddy, anxious, or restless. They may feel sick, may vomit, and may lose consciousness. To assist a person in shock, take the following steps:

- Lay the person down and raise the feet above the level of the head.
- Treat obvious wounds and loosen tight clothing.
- Minimize any movement if serious neck or spine injuries are suspected.
- Cover the person with a blanket or coat and keep him or her as comfortable as possible.
- Check pulse and breathing every few minutes.
- Stay with a person in shock, because constant reassurance is extremely important.

Remember, emergencies will occur. How well we deal with them depends largely on knowing what actions to take. For further information, refer to the Mayo Clinic First Aid Guide or go to the Merck Manual Web site and click on the "Accidents and Injuries" section. (The URLs are in "Web Site Resources" at the end of this chapter.)

OTC AND PRESCRIPTION MEDICINES

The medicines we buy at the local pharmacy or drugstore are either **over-the-counter (OTC) drugs** or **prescription (Rx) drugs.** Both types are approved and regulated by the Food and Drug Administration (FDA). OTC or non-prescription medicines are those stocked on the store shelves and readily available for consumers to select and buy for self-care purposes. In contrast, the sale of prescription drugs—generally more potent, specialized, and expensive—is more tightly regulated. Typically a medical doctor writes a prescription for a specific drug to treat a particular patient. Prescriptions are filled by a pharmacist, who issues the drug with specific instructions on how it should be taken.

The top prescription drugs in the United States for over a decade have been cardiovascular medicines to reduce high cholesterol (statins), to treat hypertension (antihypertensives), and to thin blood (anticoagulants). These drugs reduce the risk of stroke and heart attack. The best-selling prescription drug every year since 2000 has been Lipitor, a cholesterol reducer. Other top-selling prescription drugs include antibiotics, antidepressants,

Within the context of health care, a **drug** is a substance used in the diagnosis, treatment, or prevention of an illness or disease; a drug is also known as a *medicine* or *medication*. A **prescription (Rx) drug** can be sold only by a pharmacist when authorized by a written prescription from a medical practitioner, whereas an **over-the-counter (OTC) drug** can be purchased without a doctor's prescription.

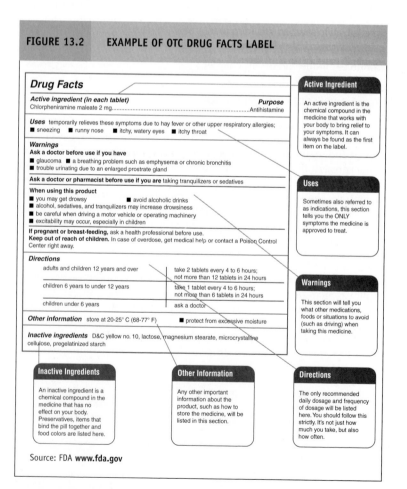

anti-ulcer drugs (for heartburn), and analgesics (for pain). In 2005, total prescription drug expenditures in the United States exceeded $250 billion, which was about $900 per American.

Finding the Right OTC Medicines

Unlike a medicine prescribed by a doctor, an OTC medicine is generally selected by the individual. The top three types of OTC medications are for colds and coughs, pain, and heartburn. The number of choices is surprisingly high and can be intimidating. Thankfully, all OTC medicines have standardized drug facts labels. This is required by the FDA so that consumers can more easily compare products. An example of a drug label with brief explanatory comments is presented in Figure 13.2.

FIGURE 13.2   EXAMPLE OF OTC DRUG FACTS LABEL

Drug Facts

Active Ingredient
An active ingredient is the chemical compound in the medicine that works with your body to bring relief to your symptoms. It can always be found as the first item on the label.

Active ingredient (in each tablet)   **Purpose**
Chlorpheniramine maleate 2 mg..Antihistamine

Uses temporarily relieves these symptoms due to hay fever or other upper respiratory allergies;
■ sneezing   ■ runny nose   ■ itchy, watery eyes   ■ itchy throat

Uses
Sometimes also referred to as indications, this section tells you the ONLY symptoms the medicine is approved to treat.

Warnings
Ask a doctor before use if you have
■ glaucoma ■ a breathing problem such as emphysema or chronic bronchitis
■ trouble urinating due to an enlarged prostrate gland

Ask a doctor or pharmacist before use if you are taking tranquilizers or sedatives

When using this product
■ you may get drowsy   ■ avoid alcoholic drinks
■ alcohol, sedatives, and tranquilizers may increase drowsiness
■ be careful when driving a motor vehicle or operating machinery
■ excitability may occur, especially in children

If pregnant or breast-feeding, ask a health professional before use.
Keep out of reach of children. In case of overdose, get medical help or contact a Poison Control Center right away.

Warnings
This section will tell you what other medications, foods or situations to avoid (such as driving) when taking this medicine.

Directions

adults and children 12 years and over	take 2 tablets every 4 to 6 hours; not more than 12 tablets in 24 hours
children 6 years to under 12 years	take 1 tablet every 4 to 6 hours; not more than 6 tablets in 24 hours
children under 6 years	ask a doctor

Other information store at 20-25° C (68-77° F)   ■ protect from excessive moisture

Inactive ingredients D&C yellow no. 10, lactose, magnesium stearate, microcrystalline cellulose, pregelatinized starch

Inactive Ingredients
An inactive ingredient is a chemical compound in the medicine that has no effect on your body. Preservatives, items that bind the pill together and food colors are listed here.

Other Information
Any other important information about the product, such as how to store the medicine, will be listed in this section.

Directions
The only recommended daily dosage and frequency of dosage will be listed here. You should follow this strictly. It's not just how much you take, but also how often.

Source: FDA **www.fda.gov**

A few precautions should be mentioned. If taking more than one OTC medicine, compare the active ingredients. You don't want to inadvertently be taking multiple doses of the same medication in different products. Also, many common brands have multiple products—often different combinations of active ingredients. The brand packaging may be similar so it's wise to double check the label each time you purchase a product. Don't misuse OTC medicines by taking them longer or in higher doses than recommended. Don't hesitate to discuss your needs with a pharmacist. Pharmacists are trained and willing to assist you in finding the right medicine for your particular condition. If symptoms persist, see your doctor.

Everyone should keep a few basic medications and medical supplies on hand to deal with minor illnesses and accidents. A basic home pharmacy should include a few common OTC drugs such as pain and fever medications, cold and allergy medications, and antacids. Each of these is briefly discussed below. In addition, your medicine kit should contain an antiseptic such as hydrogen peroxide to clean minor cuts, bandages and adhesive tape to protect such wounds, and a thermometer to check body temperature.

Pain and Fever Medications

Two main types of OTC pain and fever medications are available: nonsteroidal anti-inflammatory drugs (NSAIDs) and acetaminophen. NSAIDs include four drugs: aspirin (common brand names are Bayer and St. Joseph), ibuprofen (Advil, Motrin), naproxen (Aleve), and ketoprofen (Orudis). NSAIDs, as the name indicates, also reduce inflammation (redness and swelling) if taken in substantial dosage. The common brand name for acetaminophen is Tylenol. Some products contain both aspirin and acetaminophen (Excedrin Extra Strength, Excedrin Migraine, Vanquish).

Side effects from OTC pain relievers aren't common for healthy adults who use these medications only occasionally. However, side effects can be a concern with long-term use. For example, NSAIDs can cause gastrointestinal problems, from upset stomach to bleeding in the digestive tract. In general, acetaminophen should be the first choice for pain and fever relief in children and adults because of its greater safety. Children with fever should not be given aspirin or products containing aspirin due to the risk of developing a potentially fatal condition called Reye's syndrome. If you use pain relievers often, talk to your doctor about which drug will be most effective for you.

Cold and Allergy Medications

Common OTC cold medications such as Actifed and Contac are generally combinations of three kinds of drugs: a pain and fever reducer (acetaminophen, aspirin, ibuprofen), a decongestant such as pseudoephedrine to shrink swollen nasal passages and reduce congestion, and an antihistamine such as chlorpheniramine to dry the nasal passages and block allergies. Decongestants may cause insomnia and antihistamines drowsiness, although individual responses vary widely.

For treating colds and flu, the most important drug is the pain and fever reducer, along with standard treatment such as drinking plenty of fluids (water, fruit juices, clear soups) and getting additional rest. To treat allergy symptoms, the primary drugs are the decongestants and antihistamines. Because the cold-flu-allergy illnesses often overlap, people sometimes inadvertently overdose on these drugs by taking several products without realizing that they contain some of the same ingredients. Be sure to read the labels and know the active drugs in each medication. To be more selective in treating symptoms, you may wish to use single drugs instead of the combination medications.

Another consideration is how to treat coughs. Cough medications are often categorized into expectorants (guaifenesin), which thin mucus so that it can be coughed up more easily, and cough suppressants (dextromethorphan), which reduce coughing. Because various cough medications are available, treatment can be complicated. It's recommended that you discuss the options with your pharmacist or doctor.

Antacids and Acid Reducers
Antacids and acid reducers can help relieve an upset stomach. By neutralizing or reducing stomach acid, these medications can decrease heartburn (acid reflux disease) and gas pain. Two common antacids are calcium carbonate (such as Maalox, Tums) and sodium bicarbonate (Alka-Seltzer). The calcium carbonate antacids along with vitamin D may also be recommended for women who need additional calcium to prevent or treat osteoporosis. Bismuth subsalicylate (Pepto-Bismol, Kaopectate) is another common product that can relieve heartburn, indigestion, and nausea, as well as control diarrhea. If these common antacids aren't effective and heartburn is a recurring problem, then acid blockers (Tagamet, Pepcid) are an option. They relieve symptoms for a longer time. In any case, if you have ongoing gastrointestinal problems, you should discuss them with your doctor. Depending on the diagnosis, your doctor may prescribe a prescription medication as part of a treatment.

Tips on Reducing Medication Mistakes
Americans take more drugs per capita than people in any other nation. Based on personal experience, we know that most of us, our family members, and those we live with take one or more OTC or prescription medications on a regular or occasional basis. According to a recent estimate by the Institute of Medicine, in any given week three out of ten U.S. adults take five or more different medications. These medications can be found in many different places—a counter, a table, or a drawer in bathrooms, bedrooms, or the kitchen. With so many drugs being taken by so many people, medication errors are not uncommon. To prevent mistakes, consider applying these tips on safe storage and use of medications.

- Keep medications in their original containers.
- Store as indicated regarding temperature, light, and humidity.

- Keep your medications separate from those of others in the household as well as from pets' medications and household chemicals.
- Turn on the light when you take your medication.
- Store medicines where children can't see or reach them.
- Periodically check expiration dates and discard and replace as appropriate.
- Don't take someone else's prescription medication.

These simple steps can reduce errors, minimize confusion, and prevent anxiety and heartache.

Accessing Information on OTC and Prescription Medicines

The number of medicines available today is vast, numbering in the thousands. An Internet source that provides consumer information on both OTC and prescription medicines is the PDRhealth Web site (**www .pdrhealth.com/drug_info**) sponsored by Thomson Healthcare, the publishers of the *Physicians' Desktop Reference (PDR)* series. Updated annually, the *Physicians' Desktop Reference* is the authoritative source for prescription drug information used by physicians and other health care professionals. The 2007 edition was over 3,000 pages! A companion volume is the *PDR for Nonprescription Drugs*. The PDRhealth Web site translates information from these two PDR texts into nontechnical explanations about OTC and prescription drugs, including possible side effects and drug interactions. A second online source is the National Institute of Health's MedlinePlus Drugs, Supplements, and Herbal Information Web page, provided in cooperation with several pharmacy organizations (**www.nlm.nih.gov/ medlineplus/druginformation.html**).

COSMETIC SURGERY AND BODY ART

Although traditionally not discussed in health education, **cosmetic surgery** and body art deserve our attention because of their rapid rise in recent years. A brief overview of pertinent facts and related health issues is presented here.

Cosmetic plastic surgery is elective surgery to reshape normal facial and body structures to improve a person's appearance, often to reverse the signs of aging. By its very definition, cosmetic surgery and related procedures are not treating or curing true medical problems. Rather, these "problems" largely arise from societal attitudes that emphasize physical attractiveness and retaining a youthful look. Our aim in discussing cosmetic surgery is not to judge it but to recognize it as a growing area within medical practice and as a societal phenomenon. The demand for

---

Cosmetic surgery is elective surgery or related procedures that reshape normal facial and body structures to improve a person's appearance.

cosmetic surgery continues to rise sharply, even though these procedures are usually not covered by health insurance. Between 2000 and 2007, the total number of procedures increased by 59 percent (from 7.4 million to 11.8 million). About 90 percent of patients are women. Most patients are 40 or older, although the proportion of younger people undergoing cosmetic procedures is growing; in 2007 about 7 percent of patients were 20–29 and 19 percent were 30–39.

The most common cosmetic surgical procedures are liposuction, breast augmentation, and eyelid surgery, and the most common nonsurgical procedures are Botox injections, laser hair removal, and Hylaform injections. Liposuction is the surgical procedure in which excess fatty tissue is removed from a specific area of the body, such as the thighs or abdomen. This is done by applying suction through a narrow tube inserted through a small incision. Among nonsurgical cosmetic procedures, Botox and Hylaform injections are used to minimize wrinkles. Botox (common brand name) is derived from a botulinum toxin and works by reducing muscle contractions that form wrinkles. Hylaform (common brand name) is derived from hyaluronan, a naturally occurring substance found in skin and joint fluids; it smoothes wrinkles by adding volume under the skin. Both treatments are temporary—Botox lasts about three months and Hylaform about six months—so repeated treatments are common.

Because cosmetic surgery is lucrative and in high demand, many physicians have taken short courses to develop their skills and expanded their practice to include the most common procedures. For best results, cosmetic procedures should be performed by board-certified specialists: cosmetic surgery should be performed by plastic surgeons certified by the American Board of Plastic Surgery, and nonsurgical procedures by dermatologists certified by the American Board of Dermatology. These board-certified specialists have completed approved multi-year educational (residency) programs and have the highest level of training and experience. Plastic surgeons also perform reconstructive surgery—the reconstruction of abnormal facial and body defects due to birth disorders, trauma, burns, and disease. In reconstructive surgery, the aim is to improve function and to also approximate a normal appearance.

If you elect to undergo a cosmetic procedure, you want it done by a qualified specialist who has done the procedure hundreds, if not thousands, of times. In the hands of a qualified physician, nearly all cosmetic procedures are low risk. Most involve some discomfort and pain in the days and weeks immediately afterward. From nose reshaping, face lift, or tummy tuck to hair replacement, chemical peel, or dermabrasion, information on the entire range of cosmetic procedures can be found at the Web sites of the American Society of Plastic Surgeons (**www.plasticsurgery.org**) and the American Academy of Dermatology (**www.aad.org**).

We close this section on cosmetic surgery with a brief comment on the related topic of body art. As with cosmetic surgery, the decision to have a tattoo or body piercing is ultimately a personal one. From a health perspective, it's prudent to carefully balance the pros and cons and not rush a decision. Whereas cosmetic surgery must be performed by a licensed physician, this is clearly not the case for tattoo artwork. Laws and regulating authorities for tattooing vary widely among and within states. Consequently, additional precautions should be taken. Risks associated with tattoos and piercings include bloodborne diseases, skin infections, skin disorders such as scarring, and allergic reactions. Also, a number of the dyes used in tattooing have not been studied and little is known about their toxicity. Risks are reduced if you go to a reputable and licensed tattoo or piercing studio with trained employees who follow recommended procedures such as washing their hands, wearing gloves, using only sterile disposable needles and FDA-approved dyes, and autoclaving nondisposable instruments. Under these conditions and with proper follow-up care, medical complications appear to be low.

Dissatisfaction with tattoos over time is not uncommon. Several removal techniques are available—laser surgery, dermabrasion, surgical removal—but these require multiple visits, significant expense, and typically leave some scarring or skin imperfections. In short, investigate the risks and benefits, including advice from medical specialists in cosmetic surgery. If you proceed with some form of body art, be sure that the procedure will be done under the best of conditions and by an experienced professional.

✓ NEED TO KNOW

Medical self-care empowers people to make informed decisions and take actions to heal themselves, particularly with respect to common short-term illnesses. Knowing how to use the Internet for information on signs and symptoms, decision charts, coping with emergencies, and using medicines is key to effectively caring for yourself. A step beyond medical self-care is cosmetic surgery, which Americans are increasingly using as a means to improve appearance. Before undergoing any cosmetic procedure, carefully consider the risks and benefits including the qualifications of the doctor. Additional vigilance should be taken if considering a tattoo or body piercing because state and local oversight vary widely.

➤ Developing a Patient-Doctor Partnership

Part of medical self-care includes knowing where to draw the line between dealing with an illness on our own and needing to see a doctor. When it comes to choosing your primary care physician, just any doctor won't do. In this section, we share strategies on finding the right doctor and developing a trusting patient-doctor partnership. Over time, your end of this partnership will encompass more than just showing up at your doctor's office with a list of symptoms. As an active participant in your health care, you may need to inform yourself about various medical tests and treatments, and perhaps at some point prepare for a hospital stay. Moreover, it's certainly wise for you to maintain a complete personal medical record. We'll provide some guidelines on each of these points in the following paragraphs.

FINDING THE RIGHT DOCTOR

Regardless of how many times you may move or switch health plans, you can always use the same approach to finding a primary care doctor. Typically your insurance plan includes a directory of primary care doctors from which to choose. The size of the pool of potential physicians depends on the size of the student health center or the type of health plan, but you will generally have some latitude in selecting a doctor. As discussed in Chapter 12, selecting a board certified physician is wise. In the practice of modern medicine, having only an M.D. or D.O. degree without the additional training required for board certification is just not good enough, so it's best to check your potential doctor's credentials before you start seeing him or her. Also remember that a primary care physician is typically a family practitioner or internist, though women may have the additional option of choosing a gynecologist to be their primary care doctor.

Ask your family, friends, and coworkers for recommendations. Let them know that in addition to making sure the doctor is board certified, your aim is to find a doctor who shares your perspective about the patient-doctor relationship—that it is a partnership rather than a one-way relationship in which the doctor dispenses medical care to the patient. Another possible selection criterion is the gender of the doctor. It is natural for most people to want a doctor of the same gender. You may feel more comfortable and be better able to communicate frankly and openly with a doctor of the same gender.

In your initial office visit, you'll want to assess the manner or presence of the doctor and your comfort level with him or her. This is less tangible and involves impressions but is an important consideration. If you are not comfortable with a particular doctor, it doesn't mean he or she is not a good physician; rather the doctor may simply not be a good match for you. It may take several sessions with a doctor before you are able to decide whether he or she is the right doctor for you. To help with this process, ask yourself the following questions:

- Is this doctor a good listener?
- Does this doctor answer my questions completely and in terms I understand?

- Does this doctor ask for my input when options are available?
- Does this doctor use medicines conservatively?
- Does this doctor appear interested in me as a person and in my overall health?
- Does this doctor seem to give me quality patient time?
- Am I comfortable talking with this doctor, or am I intimidated or anxious?
- Do I have a high degree of trust and confidence in this doctor?

Answers to these questions will highlight how compatible you would be with the doctor. The more compatible you are, the more likely a meaningful patient-doctor partnership will be developed.

COMMUNICATING WITH YOUR DOCTOR

Both you and your doctor have responsibilities when it comes to making the most of an office visit and developing a solid partnership. Always remember that communicating with your doctor goes both ways. For an effective patient-doctor interaction to occur, we need to appreciate the larger health care delivery context in which doctors work. They are often overworked, behind schedule, and pressured to spend only a few minutes with each patient. Patients—in addition to being sick or having a medical concern—are often frustrated with traffic, parking, and paperwork and tired of waiting and being shuffled from one room to another. Is it so surprising that the doctor wants to immediately focus on your chief complaint, and you are less than articulate in describing the problem?

Many factors can hamper the patient-doctor visit. Intimidation, fear, and embarrassment are three common barriers to effective communication between patients and doctors. Doctors are esteemed for their intelligence and compassion. This high regard can be intimidating to some patients, particularly those with little knowledge about medical matters. Patients' fear of the unknown and the possible dire consequences of a troubling symptom or health condition can also interfere with logical thinking and clear communication. Other patients may be embarrassed to talk about highly personal or disconcerting issues that make them feel self-conscious or ill at ease. Your doctor is aware of these communication obstacles and will work to allay them. You too must be aware of them and strive to minimize such concerns and doubts by being forthright and trusting with your doctor.

As Dr. Vickery and Dr. Fries succinctly state in *Take Care of Yourself,* "You and your doctor need to be able to listen, explain, ask questions, understand each other, and choose options wisely." As a patient, you need to prepare for the office visit by being ready to describe your symptoms, their timeline, and any self-care measures you have taken, including the use of OTC medications. Ahead of time, you may want to make notes listing symptoms and key questions for reference during your visit. You

Health & the Media Communicating with Your Doctor

A humorous poster reflects the odd, uneasy feeling of sitting disrobed in an exam room waiting for the doctor. Understandably, this awkward situation puts most people at a distinct disadvantage when it comes to thinking clearly and communicating effectively during the brief few minutes they have with their doctor. Valuable tips for making the most of your medical visits are given.

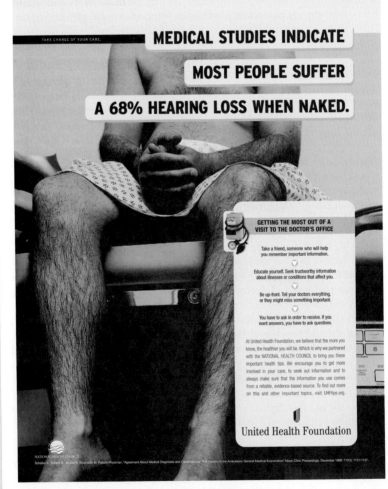

Source: United Health Foundation **www.unitedhealthfoundation.org**

should be ready to name all prescription drugs and dietary supplements that you take and all allergies and chronic medical conditions that you have. Also, it's a good idea to take a writing pad to make notes during the visit. Even a few hours later, let alone a few days later, many people have difficulty recalling the details of what their doctor said.

Depending on the severity of the illness or the complexity of the health problem, you may want to have a family member or friend take you to the doctor—not only to drive or physically assist you if needed but also to facilitate communication with the doctor. Ask someone who can ably serve as your advocate—that is, a person who can ensure that your symptoms are clearly explained and that the doctor's course of treatment is understood. Two sets of ears are always better than one.

A final point concerns advance directives. Advance directives are documents (e.g., living will, power of attorney) that specify the type of medical care you want if you are too sick to express your wishes. Although people who are terminally or seriously ill are more likely to have advance

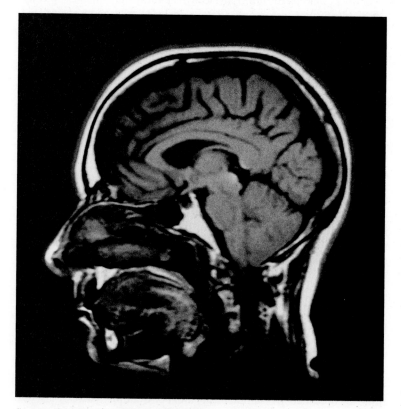

A magnetic resonance imaging (MRI) scan.

directives, those in good health may also want to consider them in case of a catastrophic accident or sudden serious illness. Advance directives deal with a variety of issues—for example, whether to resuscitate or not, use of breathing machines and feeding tubes, and organ donation. Discuss the options for medical care under these special circumstances with your doctor. Once you establish advance directives, be sure to share them with your doctor as well as your family. Knowing your wishes ahead of time will avoid confusion later.

MEDICAL TESTS AND PROCEDURES

Your physician may want to conduct tests to help make a diagnosis. Many standard tests are done on blood and urine. For example, a CBC (complete blood count) is a routine test that provides information about white blood cells, red blood cells, and platelets. Abnormal variations in the number, type, size, and shape of cells may indicate an infection, anemia, or a host of other conditions. The basic urine test, or urinalysis, screens for urinary tract infections, metabolic disease, and kidney disorders by examining the urine physically, chemically, and microscopically. The results of such tests may lead your doctor to order more specialized tests to help in making a diagnosis. Dozens of clinical lab tests are available; you can find a comprehensive resource for patient information at Lab Tests Online **(www.labtestsonline.org).**

Your doctor may order a medical imaging test, too. From routine X-rays and ultrasound imaging to more complex CT (computed tomography) and PET (positron emission tomography) scans, these tests—which fall within the specialty of radiology—can provide important clues to abnormalities that exist or may be developing within the internal tissues and organs of the body. For example, MRI (magnetic resonance imaging) uses radiofrequency waves in a strong magnetic field to generate detailed pictures of soft-tissue structures around bones. Especially useful in diagnosing sports injuries, MRI can show even small tears in ligaments and muscles around the spine and major joints (knee, shoulder, hip, elbow). RadiologyInfo **(www.radiology-info.org),** developed by the American College of Radiology, is an excellent Web site to answer consumer questions about medical imaging and radiation therapies.

The more complex your illness or disease, the more likely your doctor will refer you to a specialist for an expert opinion. This in turn may lead to further testing or medical procedures requiring specialized hospital equipment and facilities. As described in Chapter 12, this sequence reflects the widening circle of medical care from primary care to secondary and tertiary care. Ideally, your primary care physician will receive copies of the results of all tests and procedures and continue to coordinate overall medical care. For example, you can discuss a specialist's diagnosis and treatment options with your primary care doctor. If you feel uneasy or uncertain regarding a recommendation for a major surgical or medical treatment, you should not hesitate to get a second opinion. Good doctors will understand your concern and not take offense. An excellent consumer resource that provides interactive health tutorials on common diagnostic, surgical, and treatment procedures is available at MedlinePlus **(www.nlm.nih.gov/medlineplus/tutorial.html).**

There will be times when you, a family member, or a close friend must be admitted to a hospital. Many illnesses and injuries are successfully treated in hospitals. Indeed, many lives are saved. Yet, hospitals are also dangerous places; far too many errors have occurred resulting in unnecessary death and disability. Consequently, it's important to feel confident about the hospital of choice and to take reasonable precautions. Discuss this issue with your physician and ask questions about the hospital's experience in performing the particular treatment or procedure. Is it routinely done, and what is their safety record?

Once you are admitted to the hospital, consider the following tips to reduce the risk of medical errors:

- Carefully read and fully understand any consent form before signing.
- Find out why tests or treatments are being performed.
- Discuss the results of tests with your doctor.
- Know the purpose and side effects of all medications, whether given by mouth, injection, or intravenous (IV) administration.
- Be sure that all health care workers wash their hands before they have physical contact with you.
- Understand the follow-up treatment plan when you are discharged.

Remember you have the right to be fully informed of all procedures, so never hesitate to ask questions or express concerns. If necessary, be persistent: ask to speak to the supervisory nurse or discuss concerns with your doctor. If you will be incapacitated for a prolonged period, try to arrange to have a capable advocate oversee your care and ask questions on your behalf.

KEEPING MEDICAL RECORDS

Your current primary care doctor should have a complete medical file on you. However, if you are like most people, you probably have your health information scattered across multiple providers and facilities. For this reason alone, it's important to keep your own complete, updated, and easily accessible personal health record. Based on a national survey by the Harris Poll, only two in five adults keep personal or family health records, yet almost all of those who don't keep health records think it would be a good idea to do so. Simply put, it's an important task to take on and you are in the best position to do it. In fact, it's necessary if you are to be a full partner in your health care.

A personal health record is a collection of key information about your health (or the health of someone you're caring for, such as a parent or a child) that you actively maintain and update. It can contain any information that affects your health, including information that your doctor may not have, such as your exercise routines, dietary habits, and over-the-counter drugs you routinely take. Keeping a personal health record can reduce or eliminate duplicate procedures or processes, which saves health care costs, your time, and the provider's time.

A straightforward approach to a personal health record is to organize paperwork into categories such as the following:

1. *General information*: Include medical exam results, blood profiles, and other measures such as height, weight, waist circumference, and blood pressure. Organ donor authorization or living wills should also be kept here.
2. *Specific medical conditions:* Keep a separate file for these so they can be easily updated.
3. *Prescription drugs and dosages*: Keep a record of all prescription drugs, both those you take regularly and those you have taken for specific illnesses. Be sure to note any allergies or side effects.
4. *Insurance information and medical bills*: A separate file for health insurance and medical bills is necessary. Include a description of coverage, instructions and forms for filing, a ledger of payments for bills, and a log of phone calls and written communications on bills that require follow-up or resolution.

Regardless of how smart or healthy we may be, our memory alone is not adequate for keeping a personal health record! So get your records together and start filing in an organized fashion if you haven't already developed a system. Or set up your system now and start using it with your next physician visit or medical test. Like any organizational system, it takes some time at first, but it will be well worth your while.

On the horizon is the Electronic Health Record (EHR), also known as the Electronic Medical Record. An EHR is a single complete (electronic) record of a patient's profile, diagnoses, allergies, and lab results that can be continually updated by *all* clinicians involved in treating the patient. Connectivity would extend to labs, pharmacies, hospitals, and insurers as well as to the patient. EHR is a major information technology initiative within both the federal government (HHS Health Information Technology **www.hhs.gov/healthit**) and the private sector (American Health Information Management Association **www.ahima.org**). The advantages seem clear—improved efficiency and integration of medical services should result in better patient care and significant cost savings. There is little doubt that the EHR is spreading through the health care system. The question is how long it will take for widespread adoption. In the meantime, be sure to maintain your own medical records.

✓ **NEED TO KNOW**

Strategies all available to find a compatible primary care physician and to develop an effective patient-doctor partnership. Understanding how to optimize patient-doctor communication and how to access basic information about medical tests and procedures is our responsibility as active participants in our own health care. Taking precautions to minimize medical errors in hospitals and keeping an updated personal medical record are other actions that informed consumers can take to improve their health care.

➤ Understanding Health Insurance

The ideal way to have access to the services of the health care system and receive quality care at the same time is by having "good" health insurance. However, just because one has health insurance doesn't mean that worries about access to health care are over. Unfortunately, health insurance is not user-friendly. It requires knowledge to select the right plan and then to use it. A case in point—try to get a health insurance representative on the phone and you'll typically be routed through a prolonged queuing system. When you finally make contact with a live human, that person may seem disinterested and less than helpful. In this section, we'll provide practical tips on selecting and navigating the health insurance system.

HEALTH INSURANCE TERMINOLOGY

Insurance has its own language, and a common mistake consumers make is to assume they understand what a word means. Knowing the insurance language increases the likelihood of using the system more effectively and reducing health care costs. The insurance company is often called the *insurance carrier* and the insured person is the *subscriber.* Subscribers pay **premiums,** usually on a monthly basis, to hold an insurance policy. The policy is based on the (insurance) concept of indemnity, which means "assumption of risk." In the case of health insurance, the insurance company assumes the majority of medical costs within limitations defined in the policy. Many insurance plans have **deductibles,** which is the amount of money a subscriber must pay for medical services (e.g., treatments, tests, doctor's visits) before the insurance company pays.

> A **premium** is the amount of money the subscriber pays to maintain the health insurance policy. A **deductible** is the additional cost the subscriber pays per medical service before the insurance company pays.

Exclusions are those services not covered by the insurance policy. Since insurance companies are for-profit businesses, health insurance policies often control costs by excluding coverage of certain treatments, drugs, or office visits. One important type of exclusion is known as *preexisting conditions*. These are specific diseases or conditions (e.g., heart disease, cancer, diabetes) that are known to exist when you sign up for your insurance. If you have preexisting conditions, your policy may not pay for related treatments for either a specific time or ever. It is critical to carefully read and compare differences in coverage of available policies before enrolling in a specific plan.

Generally, health insurance in the United States is either private or public. Private health insurance is the most common with about 60 percent of Americans receiving coverage through employer-sponsored plans and 9 percent through individually purchased plans. Public health insurance, which includes government-supported Medicare and Medicaid, provides coverage to a smaller proportion of Americans. Both types of health insurance—private and public—will be reviewed in the following sections.

PRIVATE HEALTH INSURANCE: FEE FOR SERVICE AND MANAGED CARE

There are two basic types of plans under the private health insurance umbrella: fee for service and managed care.

Fee for Service (FFS)

A **fee-for-service plan**—also known as a *traditional indemnity plan*—was the predominant type of health insurance in the United States into the latter part of the 20th century, though it only makes up about 3 percent of policies today. There are two major components to FFS: basic and major medical. Basic health insurance is primarily hospital insurance, and major medical includes just about everything else—physicians, diagnostic testing, and medications. In both basic and major medical, a deductible must be met before the insurance begins paying for a person's medical bills. FFS plans cover a percentage of the remaining amount—typically 80 percent of the total costs. The policy holder is responsible for paying the deductible and the remaining 20 percent of the cost.

FFS has advantages. The chief advantage is the freedom to select physicians and medical care services. However, this freedom of choice comes, quite literally, at a high cost—consumers pay significantly more for medical care under the typical FFS plan than they do under a managed care plan.

Fee for service plans, or traditional indemnity plans, allow subscribers the greatest choice of doctors and hospitals but at a greater cost.

There are two primary types of **managed care plans:** Preferred Provider Organizations and Health Maintenance Organizations.

Preferred Provider Organization (PPO). Preferred Provider Organizations (PPOs) are groups of health care providers and hospitals who negotiate plans with an insurance carrier. The PPO agrees to charge the insurance company's subscribers reduced fees for their services. In exchange, the PPO-affiliated facilities and personnel get a higher volume of clients and quicker payment from the insurance company. PPO insurance policy holders can opt to go "out of network" and receive care from doctors and hospitals that are not part of their PPO. However, out-of-network services are much more expensive than in-network services.

The way most PPOs work is that a client selects a primary care physician (PCP) from a list of doctors in that particular network. The PCP will be the point of contact when medical care is being sought, providing primary care as well as coordinating any referrals to secondary care or diagnostic and treatment services. Patients can see their PCP as often as they want for a predetermined office visit co-payment. A co-payment—or simply "co-pay"—is a relatively small portion of the overall cost of the actual visit. For example, if a doctor charges $80 for an office visit, the co-pay for the patient might be only $20. The remaining $60 is paid by the insurance company.

When referred by their PCP to facilities for tests or to other in-network specialists, the patient is also charged reduced fees for those providers' services. If for some reason the patient does not get a PCP referral for secondary care or opts to go out of network, then the insurance company often still reimburses the patient for some of those costs, but not nearly as much as they do for in-network providers who were visited with a PCP referral.

A PPO is a cost-effective way to receive medical care. There are fewer out-of-pocket expenses than with a FFS plan. However, there is also less choice among doctors and treatment options. PPO administrators can be reluctant to approve payment of certain services, which means that a person with this type of insurance may need to be assertive to use the system effectively. PPOs are popular, accounting for about 50 percent of the health insurance market.

Health Maintenance Organization (HMO). Health Maintenance Organizations are plans that allow access to primary, secondary, and tertiary care within a health network. There are many slightly varying models of the HMO, and in promotional materials an insurance company may refer to a staff model, group model, independent practice association model, or point-of-service plan. But regardless of the HMO model used, the basic

Managed care plans such as PPOs and HMOs limit subscribers to specific networks of doctors and hospitals but provide medical care at lower costs.

approach is that the HMO, after premiums are paid, will provide all the medical care one "needs" for no additional charge or for a small co-pay.

For example, an HMO patient can be seen for a broad range of services from an office visit for a sore throat to tertiary care involving major surgery and only pay $10–30 per visit/service beyond the normal monthly premium. These are by far the lowest-cost plans for consumers. The downside of HMOs is that in order to receive care at rock-bottom costs, the patient abdicates most decision making and control over choice in hospitals, testing clinics, doctors, and the like. HMOs are designed to save money, and they do this by rationing services. A patient may wait for a longer period of time to receive certain diagnostic tests in an HMO than in a PPO, and treatment options may be more limited than in other types of plans.

Brief explanations of the main types of HMOs follow:

- *Staff Model HMOs* typically include a free-standing facility owned by the HMO where all the doctors and clinical professionals are salaried employees. It is a primary care version of one-stop shopping for doctor appointments, testing, and even filling of prescriptions.
- *Group Model HMO* is a group of private-practice doctors that contracts with a corporate HMO and agrees to serve HMO patients at a reduced rate. The HMO pays the group at the prenegotiated rate, and the group pays its own doctors. The Group Model HMO is a contract, not a facility. Other clinical services that an HMO patient may need are also negotiated with laboratories and pharmacies.
- *Independent Practice Association (IPA)* is another HMO structure whereby private practice physicians contract with the HMO to see HMO patients at a prenegotiated rate. Similar to the Group Model HMO, the IPA includes large numbers of private-practice physicians.
- *Point-of-Service (POS)* is a relatively new type of HMO structure. The POS allows members more choice in selecting providers and services because they have the option of going out of the network and seeing a physician of their choice, not the choice of the HMO. However, the co-pay is higher if an out of network physician is used.

Point-of-service HMOs constitute approximately 20 percent of the health insurance market, and nonpoint-of-service are 25 percent, so collectively HMOs are approximately 45 percent of the health insurance market.

Table 13.1 provides an overview of the various types of plans including what the plans offer, methods of cost control, and the advantages and disadvantages. The structures of these plans are constantly changing, and sometimes it is difficult to distinguish between an HMO and a PPO.

TABLE 13.1 PRIVATE HEALTH INSURANCE: COMPARISON OF COMMON TYPES

TYPE OF PLAN	WHAT IT OFFERS	COST CONTROL METHODS	ADVANTAGES	DISADVANTAGES
Fee for Service (Indemnity)	Services from any doctor or hospital	None except screening for fraudulent claims	Choice of any doctor or hospital	Claim forms to file; preventive services not covered
Indemnity with Utilization Review	Services from any doctor or hospital	Prior approval required for hospitalization and some outpatient procedures	Choice of any doctor and access to any hospital after prior approval	Additional paperwork to get approval for some services; preventive services not covered
Preferred Provider (PPO)	Services from any doctor or hospital, but at lower cost to those using network providers	Discounts negotiated with doctors and hospitals; prior approval required for hospitalization & some outpatient procedures	Higher rate of reimbursement when using doctors & hospitals in the network	Higher cost for services outside network; extra paperwork to get approval of some services; preventive services are not always covered
HMO—Staff/ Group Model	Services from hospitals under contract with HMO or salaried doctors at HMO medical centers	Primary care doctors at HMO medical centers manage services; hospital fees are discounted	Low co-payments; preventive care covered; no claim forms	Must use the HMO medical center doctors and hospitals
HMO—Independent Doctors (IPA)	Services from any hospital or independent doctor affiliated with HMO	Primary care doctors manage services; hospital & physician fees are discounted	Low co-payments; preventive care covered; no claim forms	Must use approved doctors and hospitals
HMO—Point of Service (POS)	Services from any doctor or hospital, but at lower cost to those using network providers	Within network, primary care doctors manage utilization of services; hospital and physician fees are discounted	Within network, lower co-payments; preventive care covered; no claim forms	Higher cost for services outside network; extra paperwork to get approval of some services

Regardless, it is imperative that consumers know what plan they have and what is covered. When you select a health insurance plan, you are entering into a business agreement.

PUBLIC HEALTH INSURANCE: MEDICARE AND MEDICAID

Since the 1960s, the federal government has provided health care to two vulnerable groups of Americans—the elderly and the poor. The program for the elderly (people age 65 and greater) is Medicare, and it is funded completely by the federal government. There are two parts to Medicare: Part A covers hospitalizations, and Part B covers medical expenses such as laboratory tests, physical therapy, and mental health services. Medical expenses are not entirely covered by either Part A or Part B. There are small premiums and deductibles and certain limitations in coverage. This can be a problem for older people of modest means. Because Medicare doesn't cover every expense, many recipients elect to purchase supplemental policies.

Medicaid, the other type of public health insurance, is for individuals whose income is below the poverty level. Medicaid is a joint federal-state program where each pays for half the program. Potential recipients must qualify for Medicaid to receive services. Like other insurance plans, both Medicare and Medicaid negotiate discounted rates of reimbursement with physicians and hospitals. With Medicaid in particular, reimbursements for providers tend to be quite low compared to what private-sector insurance companies pay for the same services—in fact they are so low that many physicians will not accept Medicaid patients.

This reduced access to health care for Medicaid patients is problematic. It results in many of the poor having to use the emergency room for their care, which can cost twenty times as much as a physician's visit. Furthermore, because of limited access, some people wait too long to be seen. When they finally are evaluated, they may be so sick that they require hospitalization or other costly medical service.

Both Medicare and Medicaid have undergone many changes over the decades and will undergo even greater changes in the years ahead. These public health programs are well intentioned but no longer cost effective. The graying of America, escalating health care costs, and the current tax system all contribute to the dilemma. The political debate will continue until a legislative solution is found. As voters we need to stay abreast of the issues and encourage legislators to explore options that are both cost effective and provide health care access to all.

CHOOSING AN APPROPRIATE PLAN

An unwise choice of a health insurance plan can have a significant negative financial impact. Simply put, choosing the wrong plan can quickly lead to excessive medical bills. This in turn can add to the emotional burden that one is already facing in dealing with a medical condition.

Having the right plan for your needs can allow you to focus on getting better without the added stress of limited access or affordability.

Health insurance plans offered as an employee benefit often have fixed benefits because the insurance was prenegotiated on the part of the organization (employer). Most often, these plans are reasonably good; however, it is still important to fully understand the choices and the specific plan and its coverage.

What Is Your Risk? Health Insurance for Young Adults?

Health insurance is about the intersection between your money and health care. People have health insurance to not only have access to medical services but also as a hedge against huge medical bills that could occur with a major injury or disease. Yet, some young adults feel that they don't need health insurance because they are young and subsequently at low risk for most diseases. But what are the facts about medical costs? Based on an annual nationwide survey, 77 percent of Americans aged 18 to 44 reported health care expenses, with the average being $2,880 (in 2005). Although health care expenses certainly rise with increasing age (90 percent of people 45–64 had health care expenses, with an average cost of $5,233, as did 97 percent of those 65 and older, with an average cost of $9,074), the statistics for the 18–44 age group remain compelling.

Listed below are national figures (2004) for diagnoses and procedures requiring hospitalization that affect young adults. The mean costs approximate what insurance companies negotiate as actual costs, and the mean charges reflect what hospitals bill patients. Not surprisingly, surgical procedures such as an appendectomy or repairing a fracture are more expensive than nonsurgical hospitalizations. It's important to point out that the mean costs do not reflect doctors' fees and may not cover costs for special lab tests. Doctors' fees may be an additional 30–50 percent of the listed mean costs.

	NO. OF CASES	MEAN CHARGES	MEAN COSTS	MEAN NO. OF DAYS	% MALE	MEAN AGE
Obstetrical procedures (childbirth)	4,177,831	$9,061	$3,297	2.6	—	28
Affective disorders such as major depression, bipolar disorder, schizophrenia	708,894	$12,301	$4,972	7.3	41%	40
Alcohol & substance-related mental disorders	450,933	$9,515	$4,151	4.7	70%	43
Asthma	418,789	$12,096	$4,611	3.4	39%	37

	NO. OF CASES	MEAN CHARGES	MEAN COSTS	MEAN NO. OF DAYS	% MALE	MEAN AGE
Appendectomy	298,420	$18,939	$7,065	2.9	54%	32
Poisoning	254,725	$13,054	$4,909	2.7	44%	39
Fracture or dislocation of lower extremity (other than hip or femur)	192,845	$24,756	$9,487	4.0	50%	47
Fracture of skull and face	54,900	$25,509	$9,638	3.6	72%	35
Headache including migraine	81,717	$10,759	$4,048	2.8	26%	42
Burns	32,470	$40,729	$17,323	8.9	70%	35

Clearly, a hospitalization of only a few days could easily range from $5,000–6,000 on the low end (hospital cost plus doctors' fees) to $10,000–20,000. If you have health insurance, most of these costs would be covered. If you don't, then you would be responsible for all costs and legally bound to honor your debt. From these examples, you can see that just a few days in the hospital can result in a huge cost. Consider finding a health care plan that protects you against large medical bills and pay the couple hundred dollars a month in insurance premiums for peace of mind. Being uninsured is a calculated risk; but if you lose, you may lose big.

Sources: Medical Expenditure Panel Survey (MEPS) and Healthcare Cost and Utilization Project (HCUP) at Agency for Healthcare Research and Quality (**www.ahrq.gov**)

There is no one-size-fits-all "best" insurance plan. What is best for an individual depends on a variety of factors including age, gender, personal health history, current health status, family situation, and financial means. These factors must be considered along with whether you are willing to pay more to have more control over your treatment or prefer to pay less and are willing to relinquish control. Here are some key issues to consider as you formulate questions to ask about health insurance plans.

Choice of Doctors
Does a particular doctor you already see accept the insurance you are considering? Or are there a large number of doctors in the network?

Facilities—Proximity and Quality
Is the insurance plan–sponsored hospital too far from your home to be convenient? The hospital or clinic might be nearby, but does it have a reputation for quality care? What are the out-patient and in-patient facilities like? Will you have access to diagnostic tools like MRIs and CT scans?

Waiting Periods
Is there a waiting period if you have a preexisting condition such as asthma, diabetes, heart disease, or cancer? If there is a waiting period, can you afford to pay for treatment out of pocket in the interim? Make sure your treatments won't be excluded indefinitely before you sign up for a plan.

Health Screenings

How easy is it to get routine health screenings like cholesterol profiles, Pap smears, and mammograms? Does the plan let women go to a gynecologist for an annual exam without going through their primary care physician?

Other Features/Options

If you (or your spouse) is or may become pregnant, what type of prenatal coverage is available? If a family member needs long-term care, is convalescent care provided in the plan? Are dental and vision care covered?

Once a decision has been made regarding appropriate services, then cost becomes a major factor. Be sure you understand how much the premiums, deductibles, and co-pays are. For employer-sponsored plans, talk to a benefits officer and ask a lot of what-if questions. Create possible scenarios for yourself (and family), and see if the answers are acceptable. If they are acceptable, then most likely you have appropriate coverage. If not, you may want to add additional services to your coverage or purchase a different policy.

Prices of policies purchased on the open market as an individual or family are determined by age, previous medical conditions, family history, and results of a comprehensive physical exam. It is not inexpensive, but it is necessary. Remember that not knowing what is covered or how a policy works is not an acceptable excuse for avoiding a health care bill. It is only through appropriate health care coverage that heath care needs can be realized.

✓ NEED TO KNOW

Private health insurance plans can be broadly categorized as fee-for-service or managed care. Fee-for-service plans provide maximum choice but can require significant out-of-pocket expenses. Managed care is generally offered as either a Preferred Provider Organization (PPO) or a Health Maintenance Organization (HMO). PPOs provide some choice in providers and facilities, yet keep out-of-pocket costs fairly low. HMOs provide comprehensive care within a specific network of doctors and facilities while minimizing out-of-pocket expenses. Medicare and Medicaid are government-funded programs that provide health care for the elderly and the indigent, respectively. When choosing a health care plan, take the time to carefully study the available options and select the plan that best meets your needs.

➤ Striving for Optimal Health

In Chapter 1, we set up a personal health roadmap directing you to selected destinations on fundamental health behaviors, medical conditions, and health care topics. Our aim has been to provide you with the knowledge, confidence, and motivation to explore a variety of paths in pursuit of a healthier life. As we come to the end of the last chapter, we're completing our trip on the personal health circuit by returning to the start-

FIGURE 13.3   DETERMINANTS OF HEALTH

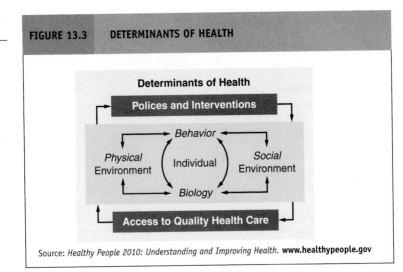

Source: *Healthy People 2010: Understanding and Improving Health.* **www.healthypeople.gov**

ing point. As seen in Figure 13.3, let's remember that our health is determined by a combination of interacting factors including genetics, behaviors, environments, policies and interventions, and access to health care. All factors can contribute to varying degrees based on an individual's circumstances and surroundings. However, for most Americans, health is largely determined by lifestyle choices and behaviors. The fact that each of us has the potential to significantly affect our own health may seem obvious to us today. In actuality, the necessary knowledge and resources to support this statement have only been realized within the last few generations.

We trust that you view the concept of health much differently now. At this point, defining health as simply the absence of disease and illness seems short-sighted and self-limiting. We hope you have gained an appreciation for health as a multidimensional concept directly related to your quality of life. And this includes your quality of life *right now and in the weeks and months ahead.* Striving for optimal health is just not about reducing chronic disease and disability in middle age and beyond; it's also about feeling good and functioning at a high level today. To this end, staying informed and practicing prevention go hand in hand with living a healthy lifestyle.

STAYING INFORMED

Staying informed is all about health literacy. As discussed in Chapter 1, *health literacy* means having the knowledge and skills to successfully access, analyze, and interpret relevant information to answer personal health questions. Common questions relate to seeking guidance on dealing with a health condition or changing a health behavior. Health literacy also encompasses a working knowledge of the health care system, which has been the focus of this and the previous chapter.

Self-directed learning, effective communication, and critical thinking—three threads of health literacy—have been emphasized throughout the book. It's important to continue to develop your skills in these areas beyond this course. Health literacy also assumes a mindfulness and a curiosity that motivates continual learning. Hopefully, this mindset is present or will develop with time. Recommended Internet sites on general health information for the consumer are listed at the end of the chapter.

PRACTICING PREVENTION

As shown in Figure 13.4, health care encompasses four areas: acute care, chronic care, palliative care, and preventive care. The majority of all health care involves treatment of acute illnesses and injuries and control of chronic diseases. Acute care is predominant among younger adults, while chronic care is more common among middle-aged and older adults. Palliative care is an emerging area of care that focuses on improving the quality of life of people who have a serious or life-threatening disease by controlling pain and providing comfort.

Preventive care, the fourth area of care, has historically received little emphasis because most medical systems are designed to treat and cure illness, not prevent it. The tide is turning though. The value of keeping people healthy upfront—rather than treating them *after* they develop disease—has become clear. Preventive medicine makes sense in several ways—it's less costly, it contributes to a more productive workforce, it

FIGURE 13.4   HEALTH CARE EMPHASIS AREAS

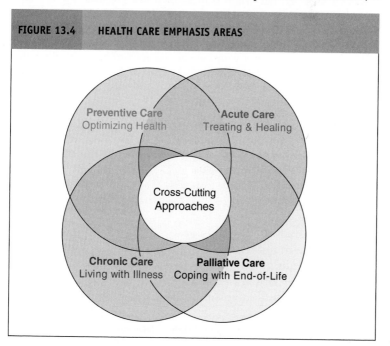

Preventive Care
Optimizing Health

Acute Care
Treating & Healing

Cross-Cutting
Approaches

Chronic Care
Living with Illness

Palliative Care
Coping with End-of-Life

reduces human suffering, and it generally improves overall quality of life. Preventive care comprises healthy behaviors, regular wellness exams, and consulting a doctor about relevant medical and lifestyle strategies for your individual situation.

Responsibility for preventive health care ultimately rests with each individual. Selecting a prevention-minded doctor and a health insurance plan that encompasses prevention are important choices. Following through by undergoing age- and gender-appropriate screening tests according to evidence-based guidelines is an important habit to establish. These tests are listed under "Adult Health Resources" on the Web site of the Agency for Healthcare Research and Quality **(www.ahrq.gov/ppip/ adguide).** Yet, as discussed throughout this book, perhaps the most important steps are those we take everyday—our personal actions, especially those related to eating, exercising, sexual behavior, drug use, and managing stress.

Many of you now have a better appreciation for the challenges involved with changing a health behavior. It's generally much more complex than initially thought, particularly today when social conditioning and environmental design often favor health-compromising behaviors. Developing healthy behaviors requires planning and strategies. Conceptual frameworks and examples have been provided to help you implement positive lifestyle changes.

Always remember that health is more than just physical health—it's a multidimensional concept encompassing physical, emotional, intellectual, social, and spiritual elements. Striving for optimal health is an active, ongoing process. Fundamental health-promoting actions are listed in Table 13.2. As you chart your own course toward better health, tailor

TABLE 13.2	**TEN ACTION STEPS TO BEING HEALTHY**

1. Focus your efforts on things that matter; inform yourself about risks and benefits.
2. Don't smoke or use tobacco products.
3. Eat a balanced diet and handle foods safely.
4. If you drink alcoholic beverages, keep your intake moderate.
5. Exercise regularly.
6. Achieve and maintain a healthy weight.
7. Protect yourself against AIDS and other sexually transmitted infections.
8. See your doctors for scheduled screening and preventive maintenance.
9. Always separate drinking and driving.
10. Use safety devices—such as seat belts, helmets, safety glasses—every time.

Source: Adapted from Make 2008 the Healthiest Year Yet, American Council on Science and Health. **www.acsh.org/publications/pubID.1648/pub_detail.asp**

your own list and map out a plan. Maintain your positive actions, work to strengthen other healthy behaviors, and resolve to stay on track. Good health habits provide a strong foundation for a full life. Making informed decisions about health care and practicing prevention further strengthen this foundation.

✓ **NEED TO KNOW**

Our health is determined by a combination of factors from the realms of heredity, lifestyle, environment, and health care policy and access. All factors can contribute to varying degrees based on a person's circumstances and surroundings. However, for most Americans, our health is largely determined by our own lifestyle choices and behaviors. We each chart a course that either strengthens or weakens our health. Staying informed and practicing prevention are two key elements in striving for optimal health.

Web Site Resources

General

Agency for Healthcare Research and Quality
www.ahrq.gov
Food and Drug Administration
www.fda.gov
Joint Commission on Accreditation of Healthcare Organizations
www.jointcommission.org/GeneralPublic
Kaiser Family Foundation
www.kff.org

Common Medical Problems

American Academy of Family Physicians (Search by Symptom)
http://familydoctor.org/online/famdocen/home/tools/symptom.html
Merck Manual of Medical Information, Home Edition
www.mercksource.com/pp/us/cns/cns_merckmanualhome.jsp

Handling Medical Emergencies

CPR and First Aid courses: Contact your local chapter
- American Heart Association
  www.americanheart.org
- American Red Cross
  www.redcross.org
- National Safety Council
  www.nsc.org

Mayo Clinic First Aid Guide
www.mayoclinic.com/health/FirstAidIndex/FirstAidIndex

OTC and Prescription Medicines

MedlinePlus Drug Information
www.nlm.nih.gov/medlineplus/druginformation.html
National Council on Patient Information and Education
www.talkaboutrx.org
PDRhealth (Physicians' Desktop Reference)
www.pdrhealth.com/drugs/drugs-index.aspx

Cosmetic Surgery

American Academy of Dermatology
www.aad.org
American Society of Plastic Surgeons
www.plasticsurgery.org

Finding the Right Doctor

American Board of Medical Specialties
www.abms.org/Who_We_Help/Consumers/
Specialty Boards, American Osteopathic Association
www.do-online.osteotech.org/index.cfm?PageID=crt_memboards

Medical Tests and Procedures
Lab Tests Online
www.labtestsonline.org
MedlinePlus Health Tutorials
www.nlm.nih.gov/medlineplus/tutorial.html
RadiologyInfo
www.radiologyinfo.org

Understanding Health Insurance
Agency for Healthcare Research and Quality (Choosing a Health Plan)
www.ahrq.gov/consumer/qnt/qnthplan.htm
America's Health Insurance Plans (AHIP)
www.ahip.org/content/default.aspx?bc=41

Staying Informed
Centers for Disease Control and Prevention (CDC)
www.cdc.gov
Columbia University's Health Q & A
www.goaskalice.columbia.edu
healthfinder®
www.healthfinder.gov
Healthline
www.healthline.com
Mayo Clinic
www.mayoclinic.com
MedlinePlus
http://medlineplus.gov

Practicing Prevention
Adult Health Resources
www.ahrq.gov/ppip/adguide

Knowing the Language

cosmetic surgery
deductible
fee-for-service plans
managed care plans
medical self-care

over-the-counter (OTC) drug
premium
prescription drug (Rx)
sign
symptom

Understanding the Content

1. What are signs, symptoms, and decision charts?
2. What are three common types of OTC medications that should be available in every home?

3. What characteristics would you like to see in a primary care physician?
4. What is a personal health record? What information should it include?
5. What are the two main types of private health insurance? Contrast and compare.

Exploring Ideas

1. A key to effective medical self-care is knowing how much to do on your own and knowing when to contact your doctor. Think of two instances in which you were sick and sought medical care. Apply the signs and symptoms in each instance to the self-care resources (familydoctor.org, mercksource.com) and see what steps are recommended. Are the steps similar to or different from how you proceeded when you were sick?
2. Our current health care system offers several levels of care to diagnose and treat a vast array of illnesses and injuries from the simplest to the most complex. As a patient, how can one efficiently access and utilize medical care? What health care suggestions about finding a doctor or using a hospital would you give to a friend who is moving to the United States from another country?
3. Typically, young adults can choose from many different health plans. Assume a 25-year-old had two major medical costs in a year: $1,700 for an emergency room visit to check on a possible concussion and $450 incurred from a visit to his primary care physician to treat an infection (including blood tests and Rx drug). To what degree would these charges be covered by your health plan versus different plans of two friends? Compare bottom line costs by incorporating insurance premiums and deductibles.

Selected References

Agency for Healthcare Research and Quality. Choosing a Health Plan (AHRQ). **www.ahrq.gov/consumer/qnt/qnthplan.htm**

AHRQ. Healthcare Cost and Utilization Project. **www.ahrq.gov/data/hcup**

AHRQ. Medical Expenditure Panel Survey. **www.ahrq.gov/data/mepsix.htm**

AHRQ. 20 Tips to Help Prevent Medical Errors. **www.ahrq.gov/consumer/20tips.htm**

America's Health Insurance Plans (AHIP). Questions and Answers about Health Insurance: A Consumer Guide. August 2007. **www.ahip.org/content/default.aspx?bc=41|329|20888**

American Society of Plastic Surgeons. Cosmetic Surgery Statistics, 2007. **www.plasticsurgery.org/media/statistics/index.cfm**

Aspden P, Wolcott J, Bootman J, Cronenwett L (eds). *Preventing Medication Errors.* Washington, DC: Institute of Medicine, National Academies Press, 2007.
http://books.nap.edu/catalog.php?record_id=11623

Center on Budget and Policy Priorities. More Americans, including more children, now lack health insurance. August 31, 2007.
www.cbpp.org/8-28-07health.htm

Consumer Healthcare Products Association. OTC Facts and Figures. February 2006.
**www.chpa-info.org/ChpaPortal/PressRoom/Statistics/
OTCFactsandFigures.htm**

Drug Topics. Pharmacy Facts And Figures.
www.drugtopics.com/Pharmacy+Facts+And+Figures

Harris Interactive. Two in Five Adults Keep Personal or Family Health Records and Almost Everybody Thinks This Is a Good Idea. August 10, 2004.
www.harrisinteractive.com/news/allnewsbydate.asp?NewsID=832

Kaiser Family Foundation. *Trends and Indicators in the Changing Health Care Marketplace 2005.* February 2, 2005.
www.kff.org/insurance/7031/index.cfm

Johns Hopkins Pathology. Personal Stories: Carolyn Benivegna
www.ovariancancer.jhmi.edu/stories2.cfm?personID=15

MayoClinic.com. Tattoos: Risks and precautions to know first. February 16, 2008.
www.mayoclinic.com/health/tattoos-and-piercings/MC00020

National Coalition on Health Care. Health Insurance Cost.
www.nchc.org/facts/cost.shtml

Ornish D. *The Spectrum: A Scientifically Proven Program to Feel Better, Live Longer, Lose Weight, and Gain Health.* New York: Ballantine, 2007.

Ornish D. Yes, prevention is cheaper than treatment. *Newsweek* April 24, 2008.
www.newsweek.com/id/133751/

Pantell RH, Fries JF, Vickery DM. *Taking Care of Your Child: A Parent's Illustrated Guide to Complete Medical Care* (7th ed.). Cambridge, MA: Da Capo Press, 2006.

United Health Foundation. Communicate with Your Health Care Team.
www.unitedhealthfoundation.org/comm.html

U.S. Department of Health and Human Services. Medicare.
www.medicare.gov

U.S. News and World Report. America's best health plans 2007. October 25, 2007.
http://health.usnews.com/sections/health/health-plans/index.html

Vickery DM, Fries JF. *Taking Care of Yourself: The Complete Illustrated Guide to Medical Self-Care* (8th ed.). Cambridge, MA: Da Capo Press, 2005.